PRIMARY PULMONARY HYPERTENSION

LUNG BIOLOGY IN HEALTH AND DISEASE

Executive Editor

Claude Lenfant
Director, National Heart, Lung and Blood Institute
National Institutes of Health
Bethesda, Maryland

1. Immunologic and Infectious Reactions in the Lung, *edited by Charles H. Kirkpatrick and Herbert Y. Reynolds*
2. The Biochemical Basis of Pulmonary Function, *edited by Ronald G. Crystal*
3. Bioengineering Aspects of the Lung, *edited by John B. West*
4. Metabolic Functions of the Lung, *edited by Y. S. Bakhle and John R. Vane*
5. Respiratory Defense Mechanisms (in two parts), *edited by Joseph D. Brain, Donald F. Proctor, and Lynne M. Reid*
6. Development of the Lung, *edited by W. Alan Hodson*
7. Lung Water and Solute Exchange, *edited by Norman C. Staub*
8. Extrapulmonary Manifestations of Respiratory Disease, *edited by Eugene Debs Robin*
9. Chronic Obstructive Pulmonary Disease, *edited by Thomas L. Petty*
10. Pathogenesis and Therapy of Lung Cancer, *edited by Curtis C. Harris*
11. Genetic Determinants of Pulmonary Disease, *edited by Stephen D. Litwin*
12. The Lung in the Transition Between Health and Disease, *edited by Peter T. Macklem and Solbert Permutt*
13. Evolution of Respiratory Processes: A Comparative Approach, *edited by Stephen C. Wood and Claude Lenfant*
14. Pulmonary Vascular Diseases, *edited by Kenneth M. Moser*
15. Physiology and Pharmacology of the Airways, *edited by Jay A. Nadel*
16. Diagnostic Techniques in Pulmonary Disease (in two parts), *edited by Marvin A. Sackner*
17. Regulation of Breathing (in two parts), *edited by Thomas F. Hornbein*
18. Occupational Lung Diseases: Research Approaches and Methods, *edited by Hans Weill and Margaret Turner-Warwick*
19. Immunopharmacology of the Lung, *edited by Harold H. Newball*
20. Sarcoidosis and Other Granulomatous Diseases of the Lung, *edited by Barry L. Fanburg*

21. Sleep and Breathing, *edited by Nicholas A. Saunders and Colin E. Sullivan*
22. *Pneumocystis carinii* Pneumonia: Pathogenesis, Diagnosis, and Treatment, *edited by Lowell S. Young*
23. Pulmonary Nuclear Medicine: Techniques in Diagnosis of Lung Disease, *edited by Harold L. Atkins*
24. Acute Respiratory Failure, *edited by Warren M. Zapol and Konrad J. Falke*
25. Gas Mixing and Distribution in the Lung, *edited by Ludwig A. Engel and Manuel Paiva*
26. High-Frequency Ventilation in Intensive Care and During Surgery, *edited by Graziano Carlon and William S. Howland*
27. Pulmonary Development: Transition from Intrauterine to Extrauterine Life, *edited by George H. Nelson*
28. Chronic Obstructive Pulmonary Disease: Second Edition, Revised and Expanded, *edited by Thomas L. Petty*
29. The Thorax (in two parts), *edited by Charis Roussos and Peter T. Macklem*
30. The Pleura in Health and Disease, *edited by Jacques Chrétien, Jean Bignon, and Albert Hirsch*
31. Drug Therapy for Asthma: Research and Clinical Practice, *edited by John W. Jenne and Shirley Murphy*
32. Pulmonary Endothelium in Health and Disease, *edited by Una S. Ryan*
33. The Airways: Neural Control in Health and Disease, *edited by Michael A. Kaliner and Peter J. Barnes*
34. Pathophysiology and Treatment of Inhalation Injuries, *edited by Jacob Loke*
35. Respiratory Function of the Upper Airway, *edited by Oommen P. Mathew and Giuseppe Sant'Ambrogio*
36. Chronic Obstructive Pulmonary Disease: A Behavioral Perspective, *edited by A. John McSweeny and Igor Grant*
37. Biology of Lung Cancer: Diagnosis and Treatment, *edited by Steven T. Rosen, James L. Mulshine, Frank Cuttitta, and Paul G. Abrams*
38. Pulmonary Vascular Physiology and Pathophysiology, *edited by E. Kenneth Weir and John T. Reeves*
39. Comparative Pulmonary Physiology: Current Concepts, *edited by Stephen C. Wood*
40. Respiratory Physiology: An Analytical Approach, *edited by H. K. Chang and Manuel Paiva*
41. Lung Cell Biology, *edited by Donald Massaro*
42. Heart–Lung Interactions in Health and Disease, *edited by Steven M. Scharf and Sharon S. Cassidy*
43. Clinical Epidemiology of Chronic Obstructive Pulmonary Disease, *edited by Michael J. Hensley and Nicholas A. Saunders*
44. Surgical Pathology of Lung Neoplasms, *edited by Alberto M. Marchevsky*

45. The Lung in Rheumatic Diseases, *edited by Grant W. Cannon and Guy A. Zimmerman*
46. Diagnostic Imaging of the Lung, *edited by Charles E. Putman*
47. Models of Lung Disease: Microscopy and Structural Methods, *edited by Joan Gil*
48. Electron Microscopy of the Lung, *edited by Dean E. Schraufnagel*
49. Asthma: Its Pathology and Treatment, *edited by Michael A. Kaliner, Peter J. Barnes, and Carl G. A. Persson*
50. Acute Respiratory Failure: Second Edition, *edited by Warren M. Zapol and Francois Lemaire*
51. Lung Disease in the Tropics, *edited by Om P. Sharma*
52. Exercise: Pulmonary Physiology and Pathophysiology, *edited by Brian J. Whipp and Karlman Wasserman*
53. Developmental Neurobiology of Breathing, *edited by Gabriel G. Haddad and Jay P. Farber*
54. Mediators of Pulmonary Inflammation, *edited by Michael A. Bray and Wayne H. Anderson*
55. The Airway Epithelium, *edited by Stephen G. Farmer and Douglas Hay*
56. Physiological Adaptations in Vertebrates: Respiration, Circulation, and Metabolism, *edited by Stephen C. Wood, Roy E. Weber, Alan R. Hargens, and Ronald W. Millard*
57. The Bronchial Circulation, *edited by John Butler*
58. Lung Cancer Differentiation: Implications for Diagnosis and Treatment, *edited by Samuel D. Bernal and Paul J. Hesketh*
59. Pulmonary Complications of Systemic Disease, *edited by John F. Murray*
60. Lung Vascular Injury: Molecular and Cellular Response, *edited by Arnold Johnson and Thomas J. Ferro*
61. Cytokines of the Lung, *edited by Jason Kelley*
62. The Mast Cell in Health and Disease, *edited by Michael A. Kaliner and Dean D. Metcalfe*
63. Pulmonary Disease in the Elderly Patient, *edited by Donald A. Mahler*
64. Cystic Fibrosis, *edited by Pamela B. Davis*
65. Signal Transduction in Lung Cells, *edited by Jerome S. Brody, David M. Center, and Vsevolod A. Tkachuk*
66. Tuberculosis: A Comprehensive International Approach, *edited by Lee B. Reichman and Earl S. Hershfield*
67. Pharmacology of the Respiratory Tract: Experimental and Clinical Research, *edited by K. Fan Chung and Peter J. Barnes*
68. Prevention of Respiratory Diseases, *edited by Albert Hirsch, Marcel Goldberg, Jean-Pierre Martin, and Roland Masse*
69. *Pneumocystis carinii* Pneumonia: Second Edition, Revised and Expanded, *edited by Peter D. Walzer*
70. Fluid and Solute Transport in the Airspaces of the Lungs, *edited by Richard M. Effros and H. K. Chang*

71. Sleep and Breathing: Second Edition, Revised and Expanded, *edited by Nicholas A. Saunders and Colin E. Sullivan*
72. Airway Secretion: Physiological Bases for the Control of Mucous Hypersecretion, *edited by Tamotsu Takishima and Sanae Shimura*
73. Sarcoidosis and Other Granulomatous Disorders, *edited by D. Geraint James*
74. Epidemiology of Lung Cancer, *edited by Jonathan M. Samet*
75. Pulmonary Embolism, *edited by Mario Morpurgo*
76. Sports and Exercise Medicine, *edited by Stephen C. Wood and Robert C. Roach*
77. Endotoxin and the Lungs, *edited by Kenneth L. Brigham*
78. The Mesothelial Cell and Mesothelioma, *edited by Marie-Claude Jaurand and Jean Bignon*
79. Regulation of Breathing: Second Edition, Revised and Expanded, *edited by Jerome A. Dempsey and Allan I. Pack*
80. Pulmonary Fibrosis, *edited by Sem Hin Phan and Roger S. Thrall*
81. Long-Term Oxygen Therapy: Scientific Basis and Clinical Application, *edited by Walter J. O'Donohue, Jr.*
82. Ventral Brainstem Mechanisms and Control of Respiration and Blood Pressure, *edited by C. Ovid Trouth, Richard M. Millis, Heidrun F. Kiwull-Schöne, and Marianne E. Schläfke*
83. A History of Breathing Physiology, *edited by Donald F. Proctor*
84. Surfactant Therapy for Lung Disease, *edited by Bengt Robertson and H. William Taeusch*
85. The Thorax: Second Edition, Revised and Expanded (in three parts), *edited by Charis Roussos*
86. Severe Asthma: Pathogenesis and Clinical Management, *edited by Stanley J. Szefler and Donald Y. M. Leung*
87. *Mycobacterium avium*–Complex Infection: Progress in Research and Treatment, *edited by Joyce A. Korvick and Constance A. Benson*
88. Alpha 1–Antitrypsin Deficiency: Biology • Pathogenesis • Clinical Manifestations • Therapy, *edited by Ronald G. Crystal*
89. Adhesion Molecules and the Lung, *edited by Peter A. Ward and Joseph C. Fantone*
90. Respiratory Sensation, *edited by Lewis Adams and Abraham Guz*
91. Pulmonary Rehabilitation, *edited by Alfred P. Fishman*
92. Acute Respiratory Failure in Chronic Obstructive Pulmonary Disease, *edited by Jean-Philippe Derenne, William A. Whitelaw, and Thomas Similowski*
93. Environmental Impact on the Airways: From Injury to Repair, *edited by Jacques Chrétien and Daniel Dusser*
94. Inhalation Aerosols: Physical and Biological Basis for Therapy, *edited by Anthony J. Hickey*
95. Tissue Oxygen Deprivation: From Molecular to Integrated Function, *edited by Gabriel G. Haddad and George Lister*
96. The Genetics of Asthma, *edited by Stephen B. Liggett and Deborah A. Meyers*

97. Inhaled Glucocorticoids in Asthma: Mechanisms and Clinical Actions, *edited by Robert P. Schleimer, William W. Busse, and Paul M. O'Byrne*
98. Nitric Oxide and the Lung, *edited by Warren M. Zapol and Kenneth D. Bloch*
99. Primary Pulmonary Hypertension, *edited by Lewis J. Rubin and Stuart Rich*
100. Lung Growth and Development, *edited by John A. McDonald*

ADDITIONAL VOLUMES IN PREPARATION

Parasitic Lung Diseases, *edited by Adel A. F. Mahmoud*

Pulmonary and Cardiac Imaging, *edited by Caroline Chiles and Charles E. Putman*

Inhalation Delivery of Therapeutic Peptides and Proteins, *edited by Lex A. Adjei and P. K. Gupta*

Treatment of the Hospitalized Cystic Fibrosis Patient, *edited by David M. Orenstein and Robert C. Stern*

Dyspnea, *edited by Donald A. Mahler*

Lung Macrophages and Dendritic Cells, *edited by Mary F. Lipscomb and Stephen W. Russell*

$Beta_2$-Agonists in Asthma Treatment, *edited by Romain Pauwels and Paul M. O'Byrne*

Gene Therapy for Diseases of the Lung, *edited by Kenneth L. Brigham*

Oxygen, Gene Expression, and Cellular Interaction, *edited by Donald J. Massaro and Linda Clerch*

PRIMARY PULMONARY HYPERTENSION

Edited by

Lewis J. Rubin

University of Maryland
School of Medicine
Baltimore, Maryland

Stuart Rich

University of Illinois
at Chicago
Chicago, Illinois

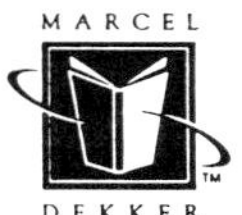

MARCEL DEKKER, INC. NEW YORK • BASEL

ISBN: 0-8247-9505-9

The publisher offers discounts on this book when ordered in bulk quantities. For more information, write to Special Sales/Professional Marketing at the address below.

This book is printed on acid-free paper.

Marcel Dekker, Inc.
270 Madison Avenue, New York, New York 10016

Current printing (last digit):
10 9 8 7 6 5 4 3 2

PRINTED IN THE UNITED STATES OF AMERICA

INTRODUCTION

The history of the pulmonary circulation in health and disease is a fascinating subject. For most of modern times, at least since the seventeenth century, William Harvey has been unquestionably recognized and acclaimed as the discoverer of the pulmonary circulation. Indeed, one must acknowledge the monumental treatise of William Harvey, *Exercitatio Anatomica De Motus Cordis et Sanguinis in Animali* (1628), which includes a chapter titled "The blood permeates from the right ventricle of the heart through the parenchyma of the lungs into the vein-like artery and the left ventricle." It is said that this description put to rest Galen's misconception that the blood moved from one ventricle to the other because of the existence of invisible pores in the septum.

Yet students of history know that long before Harvey, Abu al Hassan al Kurashic Ibn al Nafis—the head of a Cairo hospital in the thirteenth century—had established that Galen's concepts and statements were incorrect. He demonstrated that the blood flowed from one side of the heart to the other through the lungs. His error, however, was to hypothesize that in the lungs the blood "mix with what there is of air there and be cooked in it until it is tempered and become fit for the nourishment of the spirit, and afterward pass to the spirit that is in the heart...."

One may wonder why it took another 400 years to recognize the existence of the pulmonary circulation. In his splendid book *Discoverers of Blood Circulation*, T. Doby (1963) provides a fascinating explanation, particularly when considered with the perception of modern times. He wrote:

> Another thing which might have increased [Ibn al Nafis'] unpopularity was the fact that he was a bachelor. In the Caliph's city, the more wives he possessed, the greater his prestige would have been, yet he had none at all. A man about whose love life nothing is known, what sort of man could that be?

Well! So much for the history of pulmonary circulation in health! What about pulmonary circulation in disease?

The reactivity of pulmonary circulation to respiratory gases and to their abnormalities has been known for many years, especially since the advent of catheterization. In contrast, as stated by Drs. Rubin and Rich in their Preface to this volume, "until recently [primary pulmonary hypertension] has been poorly characterized throughout the medical literature."

Today, primary pulmonary hypertension has become the focus of great investigative interest that has led to significant advances in our understanding of and our ability to treat it. Unquestionably, a momentum has gathered and further progress is at our doorstep.

Drs. Rubin and Rich have inspired and pioneered some of the most valuable research into primary pulmonary hypertension during the last two decades. Their acceptance of the invitation to edit this volume represented an extraordinary opportunity because we knew then, and still believe, that this is the first book on the subject. They enlisted the contributions of experts from many countries to ensure that this monograph will be not only a landmark, but also a stepping-stone for more novel investigations and discoveries. Will we ever be able to control this disease? It seems that the odds are now on the side of optimism.

The patients who suffer from primary pulmonary hypertension live in the hope that someday survival will improve because a treatment, or even a cure, will be available. To achieve these goals, research is needed, and I believe that this volume will stimulate such effort. Undoubtedly, its editors and authors will consider this the best reward for their work.

As the Executive Editor of the series of monographs Lung Biology in Health in Disease, I am grateful for this contribution, which adds so much to this series.

Claude Lenfant, M.D.
Bethesda, Maryland

PREFACE

The story of primary pulmonary hypertension (PPH) is a fascinating account of how physicians have studied a difficult-to-characterize disease at the bedside, tested hypotheses in the laboratory, and returned to the bedside with effective diagnostic and treatment strategies. Although PPH is not a new illness, until recently it has been poorly characterized throughout the medical literature. Descriptions of young people dying of right heart failure for unexplained reasons existed in the older medical literature, but it was not until 1951 that Robert Dresdale published findings on a small series of patients and used the appellation "primary pulmonary hypertension." This fostered clinical interest in PPH, although the rareness of the disease clearly stifled progress. In 1967 an "epidemic" of PPH occurred in Europe following the introduction of aminorex fumarate, an appetite-suppressant medication, into the community. The newly heightened interest in PPH led to a World Health Organization Symposium in 1973, which brought together world leaders in pulmonary vascular disease to produce a monograph that provided a clinical description of the pathology, presumed pathogenesis, diagnosis, and treatment. However, little progress was made in our understanding of the biological basis for PPH or in effective clinical treatments for the next decade. In 1981 the National Institutes of Health sponsored the Patient Registry for the Characterization of Primary Pulmonary Hypertension, which provided the prospective collection of 194 patients with PPH to allow a better understanding of the clinical features, current treatments, pathology, and survival rates of PPH.

Simultaneous with this has been a rapid advancement in our understanding of vascular biology at the basic science level. The role of the endothelium in regulating vascular smooth muscle cell tone and proliferation, in generating local mediators to regulate vascular contraction and coagulation, and in the vascular response to injury has provided a basis to explore the mechanisms by which pulmonary hypertension can occur in humans. Studies on patients with various secondary forms of pulmonary hypertension have given insight into how various stimuli can trigger the vascular changes typical of PPH. Our understanding of cellular mechanisms has provided answers regarding the control of the pulmonary vascular bed in general, as well as insights into the clinical features of the disease. In 1995 the Food and Drug Administration approved epoprostenol as the first indicated treatment of PPH. The development of prostacyclin, which is protective and therapeutic when administered, demonstrates the marriage of progress in cellular science and clinical medicine to produce a peptide that is believed to be deficient in these patients.

This book reviews the current knowledge and optimism in the field of PPH to date. The pathology of PPH has now been very well characterized in several large series and is consistent with cellular mechanisms and the clinical expression of the disease. The actual pathogenesis of the disease has yet to be fully elucidated. However, the uncovering of endothelial mediators of vascular tone and growth, and the potential role of cytokines and other mediators of vascular injury, lead us to believe that the elucidation of the pathobiological pathway in PPH will be coming shortly. The epidemiology of PPH is equally fascinating. Although it is a rare disease, it does appear that in the majority of cases some type of risk factor or trigger can be identified that may explain the clinical expression of the disease in a given patient at a given time. That some underlying genetic predisposition exists in these patients is further underscored by the development of our understanding of the familial patterns of inheritance of patients with familial PPH. The identification of a gene, or genes, responsible for developing PPH is also on our doorstep.

Advances in our understanding of ventricular function and its characterization have provided better insights into the hemodynamics of PPH and the clinical manifestation of systolic and diastolic left and right heart failure in association. The interplay between pulmonary pressure and pulmonary blood flow, as a feature of pulmonary vascular resistance, is also better understood. We now have a clear definition of the natural history of PPH and the impact of new therapies. The effectiveness of anticoagulants, oral calcium channel blockers, intravenous prostacyclin, and lung transplantation indicates that there is a treatment for patients with PPH at virtually every stage of the disease. If the progress of therapy follows the traditional course of medical advancement, these "first generation" treatments are likely to be improved upon in the years to come.

We sincerely hope that this book provides an informative and authoritative update on PPH for the generalist and specialist alike. Having managed patients in an era when there was no effective therapy, into the current period of great hope and optimism, we feel a particular sense of personal pride and gratification with this book.

Lewis J. Rubin
Stuart Rich

CONTRIBUTORS

Lucien Abenhaim, M.D., M.Sc., Sc.D. Associate Professor, Department of Biostatistics, McGill University, and Director, Center for Clinical Epidemiology and Community Studies, Sir Mortimer B. Davis Jewish General Hospital, Montreal, Quebec, Canada

Robyn J. Barst, M.D. Associate Professor of Pediatrics, Department of Pediatrics, Columbia University College of Physicians and Surgeons, New York, New York

François Brenot, M.D.† Assistant, Department of Pulmonary and Critical Care Medicine, University of Paris XI School of Medicine, and Antoine Béclère Hospital, Clamart, France

Bruce H. Brundage, M.D. Professor of Medicine and Radiological Sciences, Department of Medicine, UCLA School of Medicine, and Chief, Division of Cardiology, Harbor–UCLA Medical Center, Torrance, California

Tiesheng Cao, M.D. Professor of Medicine and Chief-Physician, Fourth Military Medical University, Xian, People's Republic of China, and Research Associate, Department of Medicine, Harbor–UCLA Medical Center, Torrance, California

†Deceased.

George Cremona, M.D., Ph.D. Senior Transplant Fellow, Department of Respiratory Physiology, Papworth Hospital NHS Trust, Cambridge, England

Gilbert E. D'Alonzo, D.O. Professor of Medicine, Division of Pulmonary and Critical Care, Temple University Health Science Center, Philadelphia, Pennsylvania

David R. Dantzker, M.D. President, Long Island Jewish Medical Center, New Hyde Park, and Professor, Department of Medicine, Albert Einstein College of Medicine, Bronx, New York

Alfred P. Fishman, M.D., M.S. William Maul Measey Professor of Medicine, Department of Medicine, University of Pennsylvania School of Medicine, Philadelphia, Pennsylvania

Demetrios Georgiou, M.D. Assistant Professor of Medicine, UCLA School of Medicine, and Director, Cardiology Clinic/Ultrafast CT Scanner, Division of Cardiology, Saint John's Cardiovascular Research Center and Harbor–UCLA Medical Center, Torrance, California

Leonard E. Ginzton, M.D. Associate Professor of Medicine, UCLA School of Medicine, and Director of Echocardiography, Division of Cardiology, Harbor–UCLA Medical Center, Torrance, California

Timothy Higenbottam, M.D. Department of Respiratory Physiology, Papworth Hospital NHS Trust, Cambridge, England

Yoshihiko Katayama, M.D. Department of Respiratory Physiology, Papworth Hospital NHS Trust, Cambridge, England

James E. Loyd, M.D. Associate Professor of Medicine, Department of Medicine, Vanderbilt University School of Medicine, Nashville, Tennessee

Michael D. McGoon, M.D. Associate Professor of Medicine, Division of Cardiovascular Diseases, Mayo Clinic, Rochester, Minnesota

Yola Moride, Ph.D. Assistant Professor, Department of Epidemiology and Biostatistics, McGill University, and Project Director, Center for Clinical Epidemiology and Community Studies, Sir Mortimer B. Davis Jewish General Hospital, Montreal, Quebec, Canada

John H. Newman, M.D. Professor of Medicine, Department of Medicine, Vanderbilt University School of Medicine, Nashville, Tennessee

Giuseppe G. Pietra, M.D. Professor of Pathology, Department of Pathology and Laboratory Medicine, University of Pennsylvania School of Medicine, Philadelphia, Pennsylvania

Marlene Rabinovitch, M.D. Professor of Pediatrics, Pathology, and Medicine, University of Toronto, and Director, Cardiovascular Research, The Hospital for Sick Children, Toronto, Ontario, Canada

Stuart Rich, M.D. Professor of Medicine, Department of Medicine, University of Illinois at Chicago, Chicago, Illinois

Lewis J. Rubin, M.D. Professor of Medicine and Physiology and Head, Division of Pulmonary and Critical Care Medicine, University of Maryland School of Medicine, Baltimore, Maryland

Charles L. Selby, M.D.† Chief, Department of Rheumatology, Germantown Hospital and Medical Center, Philadelphia, Pennsylvania

Shelley M. Shapiro, M.D., Ph.D. Associate Professor of Medicine, Department of Medicine, UCLA School of Medicine, and Cardiology Division, Harbor–UCLA Medical Center, Torrance, California

Gérald Simonneau, M.D. Department of Pulmonary and Critical Care Medicine, University of Paris XI School of Medicine, and Antoine Béclère Hospital, Clamart, France

Rubin M. Tuder, M.D. Assistant Professor of Pathology and Medicine, Department of Pathology, University of Colorado Health Sciences Center, Denver, Colorado

Norbert F. Voelkel, M.D. Professor of Medicine, Department of Medicine, and Director, Pulmonary Hypertension Center, University of Colorado Health Sciences Center, Denver, Colorado

John Wallwork, B.Sc., M.B.Ch.B., F.R.C.S.(E), F.R.C.S., M.A. Consultant Cardiothoracic Surgeon and Director of Transplant Service, Surgical Unit, Papworth Hospital NHS Trust, Cambridge, England

E. Kenneth Weir, M.D., F.R.C.P. Professor of Medicine, Department of Medicine, University of Minnesota, and Department of Veterans Affairs Medical Center, Minneapolis, Minnesota

Jiwei Xu Department of Epidemiology and Biostatistics, McGill University, Montreal, Quebec, Canada

---

†Deceased.

CONTENTS

1

A Century of Primary Pulmonary Hypertension

ALFRED P. FISHMAN

University of Pennsylvania School of Medicine
Philadelphia, Pennsylvania

I. Introduction

Primary pulmonary hypertension simply means unexplained pulmonary hypertension. Since the first descriptions of this entity a century ago (1), it has been a diagnosis of exclusion, reached by weighing and then discounting all recognizable cause of pulmonary hypertension. Since diagnostic capabilities have increased greatly over the years, it is not surprising that many instances of pulmonary hypertension originally designated as "primary" would now be considered to be "secondary," or at least unproved.

II. The First Fifty Years

Before the turn of this century, pulmonary arteriosclerosis ("pulmonary vascular sclerosis") was a familiar finding at autopsy in patients with diseases of the heart, lungs, or pleura. However, in 1891, Romberg reported a case of pulmonary vascular sclerosis in which extensive search at autopsy failed to disclose any conceivable cause (1). During life, his patient manifested severe right ventricular failure and cyanosis; at autopsy, the findings were those of "pulmonary vascular sclerosis," which he found impossible to explain. Neither the clinical nor pathological findings were pathognomonic of the disease: the clinical evidences of severe heart failure were nonspecific (i.e., they could have been due to right ventricular failure of any cause); nor were the pathological findings particularly distinctive (i.e., the label of pulmonary vascular sclerosis did not even distinguish between arteriosclerosis of large vessels and obliterative disease of the small vessels). Moreover, although the arteriosclerosis did suggest that the patient had had pulmonary hypertension, it could not settle whether the pulmonary hypertension was the cause or a consequence of the pulmonary arteriosclerosis.

Romberg's original report did not even hint at an etiology for the mysterious malady, "primary pulmonary vascular sclerosis." However, 10 years later a series of reports, predominantly from Argentina, began to popularize the idea that syphilitic pulmonary arteritis was the root cause of primary pulmonary hypertension.

This detour in the search for etiology began in 1901, with an unpublished lecture by Abel Ayerza, Professor of Clinical Medicine at the National University of Buenos Aires, in which he described a group of patients with cyanosis, dyspnea, and precordial pain, who died in right ventricular failure. Because of the intensity of the cyanosis, Ayerza designated these patients as "cardiacos negros." His description was entirely clinical (2,3). In 1905, his pupil Escudero, associated the clinical syndrome with severe atherosclerosis of the major pulmonary arteries. In 1909, Marty, also of the Buenos Aires school, became the first to use the term "Ayerza's disease" in his doctoral thesis, *La Tension Arterial En La Tuberculosis Pulmonar* (4).

In 1913, in a doctoral thesis that dealt with 11 cases of cardiacos negros (cardiaques noirs), Arrillaga invoked syphilitic pulmonary endarteritis as the cause of Ayerza's disease (2). Not all endorsed this view. Barbaro of the same school doubted that Ayerza's disease was a clinical entity and that syphilis was its cause. Conversely, Warthin, an American, lent great support to Arrillaga's belief by a case report of a patient who had widespread syphilis and a positive Wasserman test, even though spirochetes were not found in the pulmonary artery at autopsy (4). The lines were drawn. In 1924, Arrillaga published seven more cases in support of his theory (3); the idea was challenged the next year by Brachetto-Brian, also of Argentina, who shared Barbaro's misgivings (5).

The final nail in the coffin of Ayerza's disease was driven home by Brenner 10 years later in a landmark series of papers on the pathology of the pulmonary circulation (6). Oscar Brenner, an Assistant Physician at the Queens Hospital in Birmingham, England, came to the Massachusetts General Hospital in 1931 on the last leg of a Rockefeller Foundation Traveling Fellowship (8). During his 7 months as a member of the cardiology section under Paul D. White, he devoted himself to the review of the autopsy material on pulmonary hypertension in the pathology department of the Massachusetts General Hospital. He wrote up his research after returning to England, supplementing his personal observations with a review of published reports (6).

Brenner's review of 20 presumed cases of Ayerza's disease in the literature led him to conclude that there is no "universally acceptable definition of Ayerza's disease ...; the lesions ... were merely those of chronic pulmonary disease with moderate atherosclerosis of the pulmonary vessels and hypertrophy of the right ventricle; and the symptoms were those of heart failure associated with chronic disease of the lung.... There seems to be no good reason for retaining the term 'Ayerza's disease.' " This judgment is in keeping with the current view that considers many of Ayerza's cases as instances of secondary pulmonary hypertension caused by either congenital and acquired heart disease, or by chronic obstructive lung disease.

Brenner also noted that there is an "undue tendency, especially on the part of French and South American authors, to exaggerate the frequency of syphilis of the pulmonary vessels and the importance of syphilis in the pathology of the vessels of the pulmonary circulation." In his own series of 100 cases of pulmonary hypertension, he could identify only one instance of syphilis of the pulmonary artery.

Before Brenner, with the major exception of Posselt, who reported many cases of pulmonary atherosclerosis without shedding light on pathogenesis (7), most reports were descriptions of individual cases, some of which may have been instances of primary pulmonary hypertension. In most of these reports, the coexistence of acquired or congenital cardiac or of chronic pulmonary disease was considered to be a contributing factor, rather than the cause of the right heart enlargement and failure. Only a few authors envisaged a connection between the pulmonary vascular sclerosis and the cardiac disease; others attributed both to a common cause, rather than to a cause–effect relationship.

Brenner's major contribution was painstaking descriptions of the pathological changes in the pulmonary vessels, consisting of proliferation of the intima, hypertrophy of the media, and fibrosis of the media. From his observations, he was able to conclude that, "It is, therefore, obvious that primary sclerosis is not a pathologic entity, but several different conditions are included under the same name." Turning to the literature, his review of 66 published cases left him with only 16 who satisfied the necessary criteria for primary pulmonary hypertension, which he identified as follows:

1. "All factors commonly ... sought to cause secondary pulmonary vascular sclerosis must be absent."
2. "There must be marked hypertrophy of the right ventricle."

Brenner's papers also reflected the state of knowledge about pulmonary vasomotricity in the 1930s. He knew that both constrictor and dilator fibers run to the pulmonary vessels (9,10). However, he was uncertain about the function of these fibers; that is, the "extent [to which] independent contraction of the pulmonary vessels in response to nervous or chemical stimuli influences the pulmonary circulation is still disputed." He discounted the prevalent idea that "primary sclerosis [of the pulmonary vessels] ... is due either to spasm of the pulmonary arterioles ... or to a congenital narrowness of the main pulmonary veins ...," and judged "that the pulmonary circulation is largely regulated by the output of the right ventricle and the resistance in the left auricle and that the effects of these are greatly modified by the ready mechanical distensibility of the small pulmonary vessels...."

Unfortunately, he found it difficult to imagine a relationship between the obliterative pulmonary vascular disease and the right ventricular hypertrophy. He states, "On the whole, therefore, it seems unlikely that the hypertrophy of the right ventricle and the heart failure are directly due to the lesions in the pulmonary vessels...." He was not the last to hold this view (11,12). He suggested instead "that the pulmonary vascular lesions and the ventricular hypertrophy and failure are due to some unknown common cause rather than they are related as cause and effect." Relative to the effects of acetylcholine, he found that the literature to date "produced varied results." He certainly did not picture this pharmacological agent as a pulmonary vasodilator of therapeutic importance.

III. The Second Fifty Years

During the second 50 years (i.e., since the 1950s), insights into primary pulmonary hypertension were gained principally along two separate fronts: physiological and pathological. Although clinical insights were also gained, they did more to underscore the multiplicity of the causes of primary pulmonary hypertension and to elaborate the manifestations of the late stages of primary pulmonary hypertension, than to shed light on the pathogenesis of the disease.

A. The Physiological Revolution

Until the 1950s, those interested in the etiology of primary pulmonary hypertension generally focused their attention on structural changes in the pulmonary vessels, generally underestimating or discounting the possibility that heightened pulmonary vascular tone might play a role in its pathogenesis. This was true, even though it was known since Romberg's time that the pulmonary vessels were innervated, that they could respond to direct stimulation of nerves to the lungs, and that the pulmonary circulation could respond to vasoactive drugs (13). However, these observations were based almost exclusively on animal experiments and abnormal preparations (14,15). Not until pulmonary arterial pressures could be recorded directly and safely in humans would it become possible to test the significance of these observations for the normal and abnormal human pulmonary circulations (16–18).

One of the first reports of pulmonary vasomotricity in humans was by Motley et al., in 1947, from the laboratory of Cournand and Richards at Bellevue Hospital in New York City (19). In five human subjects, they found that breathing 10% O_2 for 10 min elicited an increase in pulmonary arterial pressure accompanied by a decrease in cardiac output that they calculated by applying the Fick principle. The direct determination of mean pulmonary arterial pressure, the calculated cardiac output, and the assumption of an unchanged left atrial pressure, enabled them to calculate the pulmonary vascular resistance before and after exposure to acute hypoxia. They concluded that acute hypoxia elicited pulmonary vasoconstriction. Although their application of the Fick principle subsequently proved to be in error, because the duration of the exposure to acute hypoxia was too brief for a steady state to be achieved, the direction of change in calculated resistance proved to be correct (20). Their observations immediately attracted worldwide attention for two reasons: (1) the results in humans studied under near-natural conditions reinforced those of Euler and Liljestrand made in open-chest cats; and (2) the results also reinforced the Euler–Liljestrand hypothesis that local concentrations of the respiratory gases adjusted ventilation–perfusion relationships (21). From then on, interest has continued unabated in the mechanisms responsible for the hypoxic pressor response (22–24) and in the possibility that pulmonary vasomotor activity might play an important role in the pathogenesis of different types of pulmonary hypertension (25–27).

In 1951, David Dresdale (Fig. 1) sparked new interest in pulmonary vasomotricity by demonstrating the effectiveness of tolazoline (Priscoline) in lowering pulmonary arterial pressure in a young woman with primary pulmonary hypertension (17). Dresdale, a former resident of D. W. Richards, had been motivated by him to engage in human research first at the Bellevue Hospital Laboratory (19) and, subsequently, at the Presbyterian Hospital, where Eleanor Baldwin, Richards and he set up a cardiac catheterization unit modeled after the Bellevue Hospital Laboratory. In 1948, after setting up his own laboratory at the Maimonides Hospital in Brooklyn, he was faced with the management of a young woman with primary pulmonary hypertension. Based on previous reports (28) and his own experience with tolazoline as a systemic vasodilator, he administered the drug in the attempt to relieve the pulmonary hypertension by causing pulmonary vasodilation. The result was an impressive decrease in pulmonary arterial pressure and in calculated pulmonary vascular resistance, with virtually no effect on the systemic circulation. Unfortunately, he was unable to turn the favorable acute vasodilator response to the patients' lasting benefit, since there was no drug available to sustain this effect on an ambulatory basis.

The next major step in the study of pulmonary vasomotor activity was

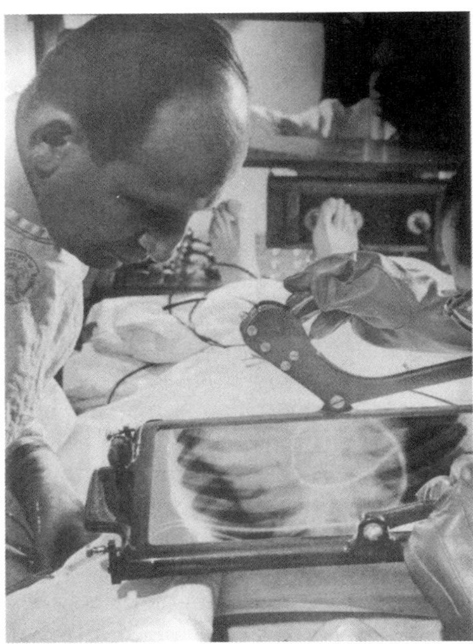

Figure 1 Dr. David Dresdale, left, performing right-heart catheterization at the Maimonides Hospital in 1953.

initiated by Peter Harris, who was appointed Senior Registrar at King's College Hospital in 1952 under the mentorship of the distinguished cardiologist, Terence East (29; Fig. 2). At that time, cardiac catheterization was being done only at the Hammersmith Hospital (MacMichael) and the National Heart Hospital (Wood). East asked Harris to set up cardiac catheterization at King's College Hospital. Harris, excited by the large number of uninvestigated patients with all sorts of cardiac and pulmonary diseases to study, made the human pulmonary circulation the subject of his Ph.D. thesis.

Harris was aware of the work of Dresdale using tolazoline. However, he could not imagine how to distinguish secondary effects of this agent on the pulmonary circulation (i.e., passive effects owing to systemic vascular dilation) from direct effects on the pulmonary vasculature. This distinction was a problem for other agents that affected both the systemic and pulmonary circulations (30,31). To circumvent this problem, Harris resorted to the intracardiac administration of acetylcholine, anticipating that its vasodilator would be confined to the pulmonary circulation if it were destroyed in the blood before reaching the systemic circulation (32).

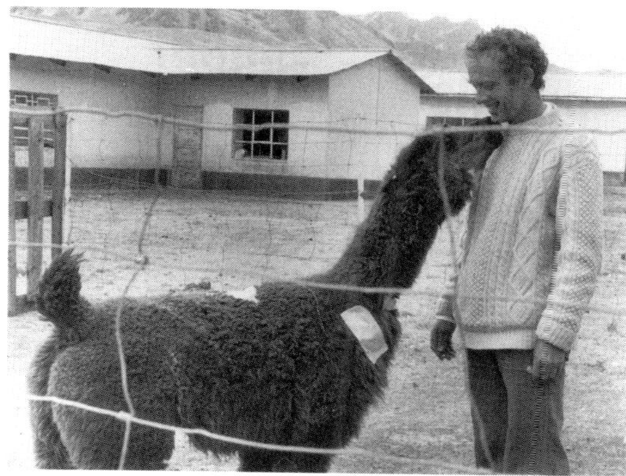

Figure 2 Professor Peter Harris with an alpaca that he had subjected to cardiac catheterization at LaRaya (4200 m) in August 1979. (Courtesy Dr. David R. Williams, also appears as the frontispiece to Heath D, Williams DR, eds. Man at High Altitude, 2nd ed, Edinburgh: Churchill Livingstone, 1981.)

The effects of acetylcholine on the lungs had been tested for many years before then (33,34); however, as Brenner indicated, the results were difficult to interpret. Harris administered acetylcholine to patients with various types of pulmonary hypertension (32,35), injecting the drug as a single bolus into the pulmonary artery through a cardiac catheter. He recorded only changes in pulmonary and systemic arterial pressures. He found that pulmonary arterial pressures fell in some, but not all patients. In his 1955 Ph.D. thesis, *Influence Of Acetylcholine On The Pulmonary Artery Pressure*, Harris concluded that acetylcholine caused vasodilation in patients with moderate, but not in severe, pulmonary hypertension. He attributed this difference in response to pathological changes in the pulmonary arterial wall (i.e., muscular hypertrophy vs. medial fibrosis). This interpretation was subsequently supported by Donald Heath on histological grounds (36). In 1955, at a meeting of the Junior Cardiac Club, Harris told of his results with acetylcholine in patients with pulmonary hypertension. In the same year he submitted his paper to the *British Heart Journal*, in which it was published in 1957 (32).

Wood (Fig. 3) and his associates had accumulated a large experience with congenital and acquired heart disease, particularly Eisenmenger's complex and mitral stenosis (37–40). In Eisenmenger's complex, Wood had become convinced that it was the pulmonary vascular disease, rather than the anatomical level of systemic–pulmonary communication, that determined the natural history of the disorders (41). He perceived similarities in the pathology of severe pulmonary hypertension in Eisenmenger's complex, mitral stenosis, and primary pulmonary hypertension (42). He and his colleagues were receptive to the idea of inducing

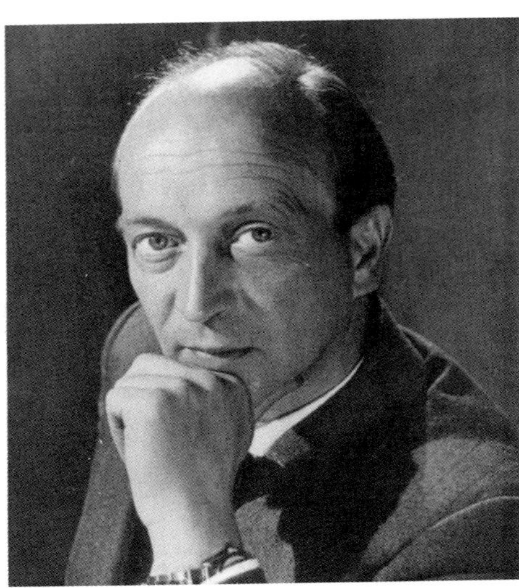

Figure 3 Dr. Paul Hamilton Wood (1907–1962). (Courtesy of Dr. E. Grey Dimond.)

pulmonary vasodilation in these disorders. Wood's acceptance of a vasoconstrictive element in the pathogenesis of pulmonary hypertension differed strongly from that of Evans, who believed that, irrespective of cause, patients with pulmonary hypertension suffered from a congenital weakness of the media, and that familial pulmonary hypertension illustrated the idea of congenital weakness of the media (43,44).

In 1957, two articles on the use of acetylcholine as a pulmonary vasodilator appeared, back-to-back, in the same issue of the *British Heart Journal*. One was by Harris, the paper originally submitted in 1955 (32); the other, by Wood and associates (45), does not mention the prior work by Harris; nor is Harris' use of acetylcholine acknowledged in a subsequent paper by Wood on pulmonary hypertension (46). As McIlroy, a senior registrar of Wood's in the mid-1950s points out, "Harris' work clearly antedated Wood's" (29).

In the paper by Wood et al. in 1957 (45), the idea is advanced that "functional pulmonary vasoconstriction plays an important part in initiating and maintaining the high [pulmonary] resistance." Wood believed that precapillary vasoconstriction was "protective" against pulmonary edema and dyspnea. Harking back to Brenner, Wood et al. recognized similarities in the histological appearance of the pulmonary arteries and arterioles in severe pulmonary hypertension of different etiologies, including Eisenmenger's complex, mitral stenosis, and primary pulmonary hypertension. Wood et al. appreciated that the histology of the lung in primary pulmonary hypertension resembles that of the Eisenmenger's syndrome, "medial hypertrophy and intimal proliferation, thrombosis and recanalization of medium lung arteries, together with angiomatoid and glomera-like vascular formation adjacent to obstructive vessels—the hallmarks of pulmonary hypertension in its severest form" (40).

In 1957, Harris left England for 1 year of research in the Cournand–Richards laboratory. During that year he and his new co-workers extended his earlier observations by showing that acetylcholine was virtually without effect on the normal pulmonary circulation, whereas it produced vasodilation when normal tone was increased by exposure to acute hypoxia (47).

In the 1968 edition of his book, Paul Wood, drawing on his large experience "of approximately 10,000 cases of cardiovascular disease of all types personally examined by the author," summarized what he had learned from 17 instances of primary pulmonary hypertension (48). He invoked "reactive pulmonary hypertension" in the pathogenesis of primary pulmonary hypertension. Twelve of his 17 patients underwent right heart catheterization, and the pulmonary vascular resistance averaged about eight times normal "the same as is commonly found in fully developed reactive pulmonary hypertension in mitrostenosis and the Eisenmenger group." He found the cardiac output in these patients to be low and, on effort, the right ventricle was readily overloaded "so that the output may fall and result in syncope, whilst the reduced coronary flow may cause angina pectoris." The response to acetylcholine (1 mg) injected "quickly into the pulmonary artery ... proves conclusively that some degree of vasoconstriction, whether physiological or pathological, is present in these cases." He discounts as therapeutic agents pulmonary vasodilators such as tolazoline (Priscol) and aminophylline, ganglion blocking agents, and cortisone; he also dismisses the Blalock operation and anticoagulation therapy.

In contrast to Brenner (6), Wood implicated "the high pulmonary vascular resistance" afforded by the small arteries and arterioles in the pathogenesis of the right ventricular hypertrophy. He underscored the great variability of the pulmonary vascular lesions and recognized that atherosclerosis is common in the major arteries, especially in older patients, that it is a secondary change, and that secondary thrombosis may occur. But, "it is in the small arteries and arterioles that the most significant lesions are found." Wood recognized that the "degree and extent of proliferative changes in the small arteries and arterioles was usually quite outside the range of what may be seen in controls." Interest in the contribution of pulmonary vasoconstriction to the pathogenesis of primary pulmonary hypertension, and the effectiveness of acetylcholine as a pulmonary vasodilator, continues unabated to the present (49).

B. Clinical Insights

By the time of Wood's 1968 edition, a great deal had been learned about the clinical manifestation of primary pulmonary hypertension, particularly about the later stages of the disease. In addition, syndromes that featured primary pulmonary hypertension as a component excited new ways of thinking about possible etiologies. The association of liver cirrhosis and primary pulmonary hypertension prompted speculation about the "liver–lung axis" (50–52). Familial primary pulmonary hypertension, first described by Clarke in 1927 (53), was redescribed by Lange in 1948 (54) by Dresdale et al. in 1954 (55), and subsequently, by others (56). The syndrome of persistent fetal circulation also began to be reported in the 1950s (57).

However, the next major surge of interest in primary pulmonary hypertension came from another direction (i.e., epidemiology). In the late 1960s, an epidemic of pulmonary hypertension occurred in three European countries, Switzerland, Austria, and the Federal Republic of Germany. It was attributed to the ingestion of aminorex, an oral anorexigenic agent that was sold over-the-counter (58). At autopsy, the histological appearance was identified by pathologists with primary pulmonary hypertension: it afforded a population of cases for study, suggested that an agent taken by mouth could cause so-called primary pulmonary hypertension, and pinpointed aminorex as the cause, since the epidemic ceased once the aminorex was discontinued. It also brightened prospects for patients with primary pulmonary hypertension, since, contrary to expectations, many affected individuals recovered.

Attempts to reproduce the human disease in animals by administering aminorex were unsuccessful. However, seeds of *Crotalaria spectabilis* given to rats did cause pulmonary hypertension by way of hepatotoxic injury followed by pulmonary arteritis (59,60). Although the pulmonary vascular lesions produced by *Crotalaria* spp. and related substances differed from those usually identified with primary pulmonary hypertension, they did reaffirm the point that toxic materials taken by mouth could cause pulmonary hypertension (i.e., they supported the idea of a "dietary" type of primary pulmonary hypertension (61). This conclusion was further reinforced subsequently by an epidemic caused by the ingestion of toxic, denatured, and refined rapeseed oil (62).

C. Reorientation in Pathology

Before the advent of cardiac catheterization, primary pulmonary hypertension, or its pathological congenor "primary pulmonary vascular sclerosis," was sufficiently rare to be reported case-by-case (26,63–73). Three reasons can be identified for the sustained interest that prompted these individual case reports: (1) part of the mystery about the etiology and pathogenesis of the disease was attributed to its rarity, which precluded the accumulation by large clinics of large series for systematic study; (2) the disease was recognizable only late in its course, so that extrapolations to etiology and pathogenesis were debatable; and (3) pathologists, who had the last word in making the diagnosis, strove to identify distinctive lesions (e.g., plexiform and angiomatoid lesions) and debated with each other and with clinicians about the causes and nature of these lesions (69,74–78).

In the few sizable series that were gathered, misgivings were voiced about the authenticity of many of the case reports in the literature. In 1935, Brenner could find only 16 cases of primary pulmonary vascular sclerosis (6). By 1950, Brill and Kryger accepted only 31 cases as authentic, more than half of which had previously been endorsed by Brenner (79). In contrast, by 1958, less than a decade after the use of cardiac catheterization had become widespread, Yu could add 50 additional cases (73).

Before cardiac catheterization, there were three main reasons why the case reports were suspect: (1) failure to distinguish between arteriosclerosis of major pulmonary arteries and obliterative disease of small muscular arteries and arterioles; (2) failure to relate obliterative disease of the small muscular pulmonary arteries and arterioles to the right ventricular enlargement, leading to the notion that the pulmonary vascular disease and the disease of the heart were coincident, rather than cause and effect (11,12); and (3) underestimation of the etiological importance of concomitant intrathoracic disease, so that instead of recognizing pulmonary vascular sclerosis as secondary, pathologists often invoked underlying congenital infirmities or mysterious infections of the pulmonary vessels.

Pathologists drew on a large experience with pulmonary vascular disease in patients who underwent cardiac catheterization for acquired, and congenital heart disease to sort out the diagnostic features of primary pulmonary hypertension and to identify successive stages in the evolution of the disease (72,80–86).

In 1973, prompted in large part by the aminorex epidemic, the World Health Organization convened a working group to assess the scientific understanding of primary pulmonary hypertension (87). The major outcome of this meeting, in which the pathologists were on the firmest footing, was a histopathological classification of the disease, in which plexiform and angiomatoid lesions featured prominently. Subsequently, this classification was revamped, based on the experience of a nationwide registry that collected and analyzed data from 35 medical centers on unexplained (primary) pulmonary hypertension (88). The registry strengthened the view that the clinical syndrome of primary pulmonary hypertension could result from diverse etiologies and different types of vascular lesions. Meanwhile, independent observations on familial primary pulmonary hypertension showed conclusively that a wide variety of histological lesions and constellations, other than plexiform and dilatation lesions, could be involved in the pathogenesis of the clinical syndrome (89). Among these are isolated medial hypertrophy, intimal and medial hypertrophy, thrombotic lesions, and necrotizing arteritis. Moreover, it has turned out that the clinical syndrome of primary pulmonary hypertension can be produced not only by different types and constellations of histological lesions, but also by lesions affecting vascular segments other than the small pulmonary arteries and arterioles (e.g., pulmonary veno-occlusive disease and pulmonary capillary hemangiomatosis (90,91).

IV. Treatment of Primary Pulmonary Hypertension

Once it was shown that pulmonary vasoconstriction contributed to the high pulmonary arterial pressure in some patients with primary pulmonary hypertension, the race was on to develop pulmonary vasodilators that could be used to treat the disease. From the beginning, the search for pulmonary vasodilators has drawn heavily on agents developed as systemic vasodilators for the management of chronic congestive heart failure. As appreciated by Dresdale (17), Harris (32), and Wood (45), the sine qua non is that the action of the vasodilator be confined entirely, or almost entirely, to the pulmonary circulation (49). For a long time, this criterion could be satisfied only by agents that had to be administered intravenously. This limitation severely limited opportunities for maintenance therapy. More recently, agents that can be administered orally have been used to great advantage in the third of the population of patients with primary pulmonary hypertension in whom pulmonary vasoconstriction is an important pathogenetic factor. When this form of medical treatment is either impractical or inapplicable, a new horizon has been opened by the advent of lung or heart–lung transplantation. These therapeutic modalities are considered in detail elsewhere in this volume.

V. Concluding Comment

The history of primary pulmonary hypertension consists fundamentally of two eras: pre- and postcardiac catheterization in humans. For the first 50 years, clinicians and pathologists groped for etiology, relying primarily on autopsy findings to prove that the cause of the pulmonary vascular sclerosis (primary hypertension) was a mystery. However, extrapolating from autopsy findings of an unexplainable disease to its origins was virtually impossible.

In the 1950s, the widespread adoption of right heart catheterization for the study of heart and lung disease in humans, revolutionized the understanding of the disease. Many more instances of primary pulmonary hypertension were identified, the functional (vasoconstrictive) component was appreciated, and fresh therapeutic interventions could be applied. A wide variety of clues and associations suggested that the clinical syndrome could originate from diverse causes, heterogeneous pulmonary vascular lesions, and different vascular sites.

Despite this remarkable growth of understanding, a unifying concept of etiology and pathogenesis is difficult to construct, primarily because the disease becomes clinically manifest only in its late stages. The occurrence of epidemics of primary pulmonary hypertension and the increased awareness of familial pulmonary hypertension has greatly increased the prospects for further insights into etiologies and pathogenesis. The search for etiology and pathogenesis now awaits new tools that will enable early clinical diagnosis and experimental models that will enable induction of the disease at consecutive stages in its evolution.

Acknowledgment

This manuscript was reviewed for accuracy by Drs. David Dresdale, Peter Harris, and Donald Heath. I am grateful to them for their advice and help.

References

1. Romberg E. Ueber Sklerose der Lungen arterie. Dsch Archiv Klin Med 1891; 48: 197–206.
2. Arrillaga FC. Sclérose de l'artére pulmonaire secondaire à certains états pulmonaries chroniques. Arch Mal Coeur 1913; 6:518–529.
3. Arrillaga FC. Sclérose de l'artére pulmonaire (cardiaques noirs). Bull Mem Soc Méd Hop Paris 1924; 48:292–303.
4. Warthin AS. A case of Ayerza's disease: chronic cyanosis, dyspnea and erythremia, associated with syphilitic arteriosclerosis of the pulmonary arteries. Trans Assoc Am Physicians 1919; 34:219–239.
5. Brachetto-Brian D. Concepto anatomo-pathologico de los cardiacos negros de Ayerza. Rev Soc Med Int Soc Tisiol 1925; 1:821–931.
6. Brenner O. Pathology of the vessels of the pulmonary circulation. Arch Intern Med 1935; 56:211–237,457–497,724–752,976–1014,1190–1241.
7. Posselt A. Die Erkrankungen der Lungenschlagader. Ergeb Alleg Pathol Pathol Anat 1909; 13:298–526.
8. Rosenbaum T. Personal communication re Dr. Oscar Brenner. Rockefeller Foundation Archives, RG10, Medical and Natural Sciences, Great Britain, Brenner, Jan 13, 1931.
9. Daly I deB, Hebb CO. Pulmonary and Bronchial Vascular Systems. London: Edward Arnold, 1966.
10. Daly I deB, von Euler V. The functional anatomy of the vasomotor nerves to the lungs in the dog. Proc R Soc Lond B 1932; 110:92–111.
11. De Navasquez S, Forbes JR, Holling HE. Right ventricular hypertrophy of unknown origin; so-called pulmonary hypertension. Br Heart J 1940, 2:177–188.
12. East T. Pulmonary hypertension. Br Heart J 1940; 2:189–200.
13. Bradford JR, Dean HP. The Pulmonary Circulation. 1894; 16:34–96.
14. Duke HN. The effect of adrenergic alpha-blocking agents on the pulmonary vasoconstrictor response to hypoxia in isolated cat lungs. J Physiol (Lond) 1968; 196:59–61P.
15. Szidon JP, Fishman AP. Autonomic control of the pulmonary circulation. In: Fishman AP, Hecht H, eds. Pulmonary Circulation and Interstitial Space. Chicago: University of Chicago Press, 1969:239–264.

16. Cournand A, Ranges HA. Catheterization of right auricle in man. Proc Soc Exp Biol Med 1941; 46:462.
17. Dresdale DT, Schultz M, Michtom RJ. Primary pulmonary hypertension. I. Clinical and haemodynamic study. Am J Med 1951; 11:686–705.
18. Fowler NO, Westcott RN, Hauenstein VD, Scott RC, McGuire J. Observations on autonomic participation in pulmonary arteriolar resistance in man. J Clin Invest 1950; 29:1387.
19. Motley HL, Cournand A, Werko L, Himmelstein A, Dresdale DT. The influence of short periods of induced anoxia upon pulmonary artery pressure in man. Am J Physiol 1947; 150:315–320.
20. Fishman AP, McClement J, Himmelstein A, Cournand A. Effects of acute anoxia on the circulation and respiration in patients with chronic pulmonary disease studied during the "steady state." J Clin Invest 1952; 31:770–781.
21. von Euler US, Liljestrand G. Observations on the pulmonary arterial blood pressure in the cat. Acta Physiol Scand 1946; 12:301–320.
22. Fishman AP. Hypoxia on the pulmonary circulation. How and where it acts. Circ Res 1976; 38:221–231.
23. Fishman AP. Respiratory gases in the regulation of the pulmonary circulation. Physiol Rev 1961; 41:214–280.
24. Fishman AP, ed. The Pulmonary Circulation: Normal and Abnormal. Mechanisms, Management and the National Registry. Philadelphia: University of Pennsylvania Press, 1990.
25. Daley R, Wade JD, Maraist F, Bing RJ. Pulmonary hypertension in dogs induced by injection of lycopodium spores into the pulmonary artery, with special reference to the absence of vasomotor reflexes. Am J Physiol 1951; 164:380–390.
26. Hart C. Ueber die isolierte Sklerose der Pulmonalarterie. Berl Klin Wochenschr 1916; 53:304–306.
27. Kuida H, Dammin G, Haynes F, Rapaport E, Dexter L. Primary pulmonary hypertension. Am J Med 1957; 23:166–182.
28. Chess D. Yonkman FF. Adrenolytic and sympatholytic actions of Priscol (benzylimidazoline). Proc Soc Exp Biol Med 1946; 61:127.
29. McIlroy MB. Commentary. Paul Wood Revisited. Am J Cardiology 1972; 30:170–171.
30. Greene DG, Bunnell IL. Vasomotor tone in the lesser circulation, and its inhibition by tetraethylammonium chloride. J Clin Invest 1950; 29:818.
31. Lyons RH, Moe GK, Neligh RB, Hoobler SW, Campbell KN, Berry RL, Rennick BR. The effects of blockade of the autonomic ganglia in man with tetraethylammonium. Am J Med Sci 1947; 213:315–323.
32. Harris P. Influence of acetylcholine on the pulmonary arterial pressure: Br Heart J 1957; 19:272–286.
33. Carmichael EA, Fraser FR. The effects of acetylcholine in man. Heart 1933; 16: 262–274.
34. Hunt R. Vasodilator reactions. Am J Physiol 1917; 45:197–230.
35. Harris P. Patent ductus arteriosus with pulmonary hypertension. Br Heart J 1955; 17:85–92.

36. Heath D. Structural alterations of pulmonary vessels in response to pulmonary hypertension. In: Adams WR, Veith I, eds. Pulmonary Circulation. An International Symposium, Sponsored by the Chicago Heart Association, New York: Grune & Stratton, 1959:122–125.
37. Wood P. An appreciation of mitral stenosis. Br Med J 1954; 1:1051–1063, 1113–1124.
38. Wood P. Diseases of the Heart and Circulation. Philadelphia: JB Lippincott, 1950: 461–464.
39. Wood P. Pulmonary hypertension. Br Med Bull 1952; 8:348–353.
40. Wood P. The Eisenmenger syndrome. Br Med J 1958; 2:701–709, 755–762.
41. Hudson REB. Commentary. The Eisenmenger syndrome. Am J Cardiol 1972; 30: 172–174.
42. Eisenmenger V. Die angeborenen Defecte der Kammerscheidewand des Herzen. Z Klin Med 1897; 32:1–28.
43. Evans W, Short DS. Pulmonary hypertension in congenital heart disease. Br Med J 1958; 20:529–551.
44. Gilmour JR, Evans W. Primary pulmonary hypertension. J Pathol Bacteriol 1946; 58: 687–697.
45. Wood P, Besterman EM, Towers MK, McIlroy MB. The effect of acetylcholine on pulmonary vascular resistance and left atrial pressure in mitral stenosis. Br Heart J 1957; 19:279–286.
46. Wood P. Pulmonary hypertension with special reference to the vasoconstrictive factor. Br Heart J 1958; 21:557–570.
47. Fritts HW, Harris P Jr, Clauss RH, Odell JE, Cournand A. The effect of acetylcholine on the human pulmonary circulation under normal and hypoxic conditions. J Clin Invest 1958; 37:99–108.
48. Wood P. Diseases of the Heart and Circulation. Philadelphia: JB Lippincott, 1968: 976–983.
49. Palevsky HI, Long W, Crow J, Fishman AP. Prostacyclin and acetylcholine as screening agents for acute pulmonary vasodilator responsiveness in primary pulmonary hypertension. Circulation 1990; 82:2018–2026.
50. Rutishauser E, Blanc W. Anastomoses artério-veineuses glomiques du poumon avec syndrome d'insuffisance droite et cyanose. Schweiz Z Allg Pathol Bacteriol 1950; 13:61–65.
51. Groves BM, Brundage BH, Elliott CG, Koerner SK, et al. Pulmonary hypertension associated with hepatic cirrhosis. In: Fishman AP, ed. The Pulmonary Circulation: Normal and Abnormal. Mechanisms, Management and the National Registry. Philadelphia: University of Pennsylvania Press, 1990; 359–369.
52. Levine OR, Harris RC, Blanc WA, Mellins RB. Progressive pulmonary hypertension in children with portal hypertension. J Pediatr 1973; 83:964–972.
53. Clarke RC, Coombs CF, Hadfield G, Todd AT. On certain abnormalities, congenital and acquired of the pulmonary artery. Q J Med 1927; 21:51–70.
54. Lange F. Die Essentielle Hypertonie der Lungenstrombahn und ihr familiares Vorkommen. Dtsch Med Wochenschr 1948; 73:322–326.
55. Dresdale DT, Michtom RF, Schultz M. Recent studies in primary pulmonary hyper-

tension including pharmacodynamic observations on pulmonary vascular resistance. Bull NY Acad Med 1954; 30:195–207.
56. Newman JH, Loyd JE. Genetic basis of pulmonary hypertension. Semin Respir Med 1986; 7:343–352.
57. Berthong M, Cochran TH. Pathological findings in nine children with "primary" pulmonary hypertension. Bull Johns Hopkins Hosp 1955; 97:69–111.
58. Gurtner HP. Aminorex pulmonary hypertension. In: Fishman AP, ed. The Pulmonary Circulation: Normal and Abnormal. Mechanisms, Management and the National Registry. Philadelphia: University of Pennsylvania Press, 1990:397–411.
59. Kay JM, Harris P, Heath D. Pulmonary hypertension produced in rats by ingestion of *Crotalaria spectabilis* seeds. Thorax 1967; 22:176–179.
60. Lalich JJ, Merkow L. Pulmonary arteritis produced in rats by feeding *Crotalaria spectabilis*. Lab Invest 1961; 10:744–750.
61. Fishman AP. Dietary pulmonary hypertension. Circ Res 1974; 35:657–660.
62. Lopez-Sendon J, Gomez-Sanchez M, Mestre deJuan M, Coma-Canella I. Pulmonary hypertension in the toxic oil syndrome. In: Fishman AP, ed. The Pulmonary Circulation: Normal and Abnormal. Mechanisms, Management and the National Registry. Philadelphia: University of Pennsylvania Press, 1990; 385–395.
63. Krutsch G. Über rechtsseitige Herzhypertrophie durch Einengung des Gesamtquerschnittes der kleineren und kleinsten Lungenarterien. Frankfurt Z Pathol 1920; 23: 247–271.
64. Kucsko L. Über arteriovenöse Verbindungen in der menschlichen Lunge und ihre funktionelle Bedeutung. Frankfurt Z Pathol 1953; 64:54–83.
65. Ljungdahl M. Unterschungen über die Arteriosklerose des kleinen Kreislaufs. Weisbaden: JF Bergmann, 1915:147–155.
66. MacCallum WG. Obliterative pulmonary arteriosclerosis. Bull Johns Hopkins Hosp 1931; 49:37–48.
67. McQuire J, Scott RC, Helm RA, et al. Is there an entity primary pulmonary hypertension? Arch Intern Med 1957; 99:917–931.
68. Mönckeberg JG. Ueber die genuine Arteriosklerose der Lungenarterie. D Med Wchnschr 1907; 33:1243–1246.
69. Moschcowitz E, Rubin E, Strauss L. Hypertension of pulmonary circulation due to congenital glomoid obstruction of pulmonary arteries. Am J Pathol 1961; 39:75–93.
70. Rich AR. A hitherto unrecognized tendency to the development of widespread pulmonary vascular obstruction in patients with congenital pulmonary stenosis (tetralogy of Fallot). Bull Johns Hopkins Hosp 1948; 82:389–401.
71. Rogers L. Extensive atheroma and dilatation of the pulmonary arteries, without marked valvular lesions, as a not very rare cause of fatal cardiac disease in Bengal. Q J Med 1908; 2:1–18.
72. Spencer H. Primary pulmonary hypertension and related vascular changes in lungs. J Pathol Bacteriol 1950; 62:75–84.
73. Yu PN. Primary pulmonary hypertension: report of 6 cases and review of literature. Ann Intern Med 1958; 49:1138.
74. Naeye RL, Vennart GP. Structure and significance of pulmonary plexiform structures. Am J Pathol 1960; 36:593–606.

75. Fishman AP. Plexiform lesions. Pathol Microbiol 1975; 43:242–245.
76. McCormack LJ. Glomoid hyperplasia of the pulmonary vasculature; a phenomenon in severe pulmonary hypertension (abstr). Am J Pathol 1959; 35:668.
77. Naeye RL. "Primary" pulmonary hypertension with coexisting portal hypertension. A retrospective study of 6 cases. Circulation 1960; 22:376.
78. Senior RM, Britton RC, Turino GM, Wood JA, Langer GA, Fishman AP. Pulmonary hypertension associated with cirrhosis of the liver and with portacaval shunts. Circulation 1968; 37:88–96.
79. Brill IC, Krygier CK. Primary pulmonary vascular sclerosis. Arch Intern Med 1941; 68:560–577.
80. Civin WH, Edwards JE. Pathology of the pulmonary vascular tree. I. A comparison of the intrapulmonary arteries in the Eisenmenger complex and in stenosis of ostium infundibuli associated with biventricular origin of the aorta. Circulation 1950; 2: 545–552.
81. Edwards JF. Functional pathology of the pulmonary vascular tree in congenital cardiac disease. Circulation 1957; 15:164–196.
82. Heath D, Edwards JE. Pathology of hypertensive pulmonary vascular disease: description of six grades of structural changes in pulmonary arteries with special reference in congenital cardiac septal defects. Circulation 1958; 18:533–547.
83. Larrabee WF, Parker RL, Edwards JE. Pathology of intrapulmonary arteries and arterioles in mitral stenosis. Proc Mayo Clin 1949; 24:316–326.
84. Wagenvoort CA. Morphology of certain vascular lesions in pulmonary hypertension. J Pathol Bacteriol 1959; 78:503–511.
85. Wagenvoort CA, Wagenvoort H. Primary pulmonary hypertension: a pathologic study of the lung vessels in 156 classically diagnosed cases. Circulation 1970; 42:1163–1184.
86. Wagenvoort CA. Vasoconstriction and medial hypertrophy in pulmonary hypertension. Circulation 1960; 22:535.
87. Hatano S, Strasser T, eds. Primary pulmonary hypertension. World Health Organization, Geneva, 1975.
88. Pietra GG. The histopathology of primary pulmonary hypertension. In: Fishman AP, ed. The Pulmonary Circulation: Normal and Abnormal. Mechanisms, Management and the National Registry. Philadelphia: University of Pennsylvania Press, 1990: 459–472.
89. Loyd JE, Atkinson JB, Pietra GG, Virmani R, Newman JH. Heterogeneity of pathological lesions in familial primary pulmonary hypertension. Am Rev Respir Dis 1988; 138:952–957.
90. Wagenvoort CA, Wagenvoort N, Takahashi T. Pulmonary veno-occlusive disease: involvement of pulmonary arteries and review of the literature. Hum Pathol 1985; 16:1033–1041.
91. Wagenvoort CA. Capillary haemangiomatosis of the lung. Histopathology 1978; 2: 401–406.

2

The Pathology of Primary Pulmonary Hypertension

GIUSEPPE G. PIETRA

University of Pennsylvania School of Medicine
Philadelphia, Pennsylvania

I. Introduction

Primary pulmonary hypertension (PPH) is defined as a clinical condition characterized by persistent elevation of the pulmonary artery pressure without any demonstrable cause. Thus, PPH is not a disease process with a well-defined pathogenesis and unique pathology, but a clinical syndrome with a variety of underlying vascular pathological changes. In the past, it was recognized that three types of pathological vascular lesions—plexogenic arteriopathy, thromboembolic arteriopathy, and pulmonary venoocclusive disease—could be found in patients with a clinical diagnosis of PPH (1). Because only plexogenic arteriopathy was considered as being the morphological hallmark of primary chronic vasoconstriction (1,2), only those patients with that type of vascular pathology were recognized as having genuine PPH. Therefore, the task of the pathologist was to distinguish between the "primary lesions" of plexogenic arteriopathy and thromboembolic arteriopathy. The latter was considered "secondary" to unrecognized chronic pulmonary embolism (2,3). More recent studies have shown that both plexogenic and thromboembolic arteriopathy may be present in patients with unequivocal PPH and that "thromboembolic" pulmonary vascular disease (or arteriopathy) is often present in the absence of clinical or pathological evidence of chronic pulmonary embolism (4,5). Accordingly, the notion of primary in situ thrombosis as an important pathogenetic mechanism for the development of PPH has gained wider recognition and acceptance (4–6).

The purpose of this chapter is to review, first, the general histological features of the normal and hypertensive pulmonary vasculature and, then, the pathology of PPH.

II. The Normal Pulmonary Vasculature

The lung is unique in having a double arterial blood supply, from the pulmonary and the bronchial arteries, as well as a double venous drainage into the pulmonary and azygos veins.

The right and left pulmonary arteries, which carry the entire output of the right ventricle, enter the respective lung at the hilum in a loose connective tissue sheath adjacent to the main bronchus. Inside the lung, each pulmonary artery invariably accompanies the appropriate generation bronchus and divides with it, down to the level of the respiratory bronchioles. However, besides the "conventional" branches that accompany the bronchi, additional "supernumerary" branches originate without relation to bronchial divisions and directly penetrate into the lung parenchyma. The diameter of the arteries decreases more rapidly than that of the airways they accompany, so that in the lung periphery the diameters of the arteries are smaller than those of the adjacent airways. Within the respiratory units (the acini), the pulmonary arteries and arterioles (intracinar arteries) are centrally located and give rise to precapillary arterioles, from which a network of capillaries radiate into the alveolar walls (Fig. 1). Blood carried in the alveolar capillaries collects at the periphery of the acini into venules (Fig. 2), which then drain into larger veins located within the interlobular and interlobar septa. Owing to histological similarities, arterioles and veins can be correctly identified only by their location in relation to the airways. The arteries are closely associated with the airways, whereas the veins are at a distance from them.

Histologically, the pulmonary arteries are classified as elastic or muscular on the basis of the structure of their tunica media. The elastic arteries include the pulmonary trunk and its intrapulmonary branches, down to vessels of about 0.5 mm in diameter. Elastic arteries are conducting vessels, highly distensible at low transmural pressures. In normal adults, the extrapulmonary portions of the elastic arteries contain a multilayer lattice of coarse elastic fibers of different size and orientation; however, within the lung, the elastic laminae become more regular (Fig. 3). The space between the fibers is filled with connective tissue and smooth-muscle cells. As the arteries decrease in size, the number of elastic laminae decreases and the smooth muscle increases. Eventually, in vessels with a diameter between 1000 and 500 μm, the elastic tissue is lost altogether from the media, and the arteries become muscular (discussed later).

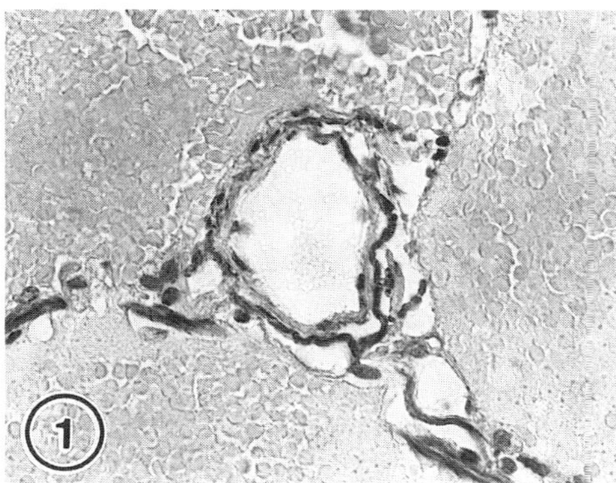

Figure 1 Transverse section of a nonmuscular pulmonary arteriole from an 18-year-old man who died of traumatic hemorrhagic pulmonary edema. The vessel wall consists of only a thin intima and a single elastic lamina (Verhoeff-van-Gieson's [VvG], × 300).

The intima of the pulmonary arteries is thin, consisting of a single layer of endothelial cells and their basement membrane. However, with increasing age, intimal fibrous or atheromatous patches develop, particularly in relation to branching points. These age-related changes should not be considered diagnostic for pulmonary hypertension. The adventitia is composed of dense connective tissue in direct continuity with the peribronchial connective tissue sheath.

The muscular arteries are vessels of about 500 μm in diameter or less, characterized by a muscular media bounded by internal and external elastic laminae (Fig. 4). In normal adults, in comparison with systemic arteries, the lumen

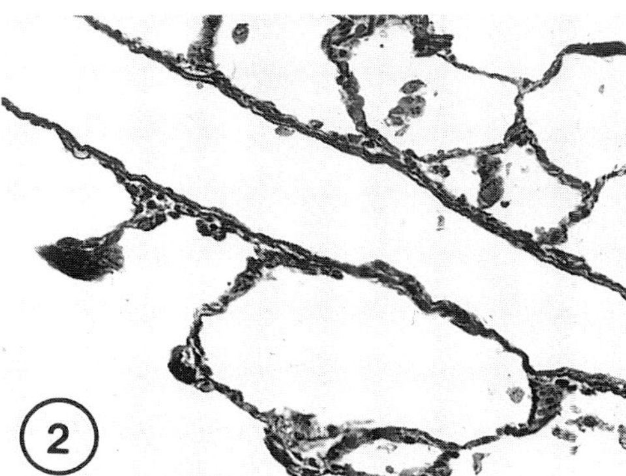

Figure 2 Pulmonary venule coursing within an interlobular septum (Hematoxylin–eosin [HE], × 160).

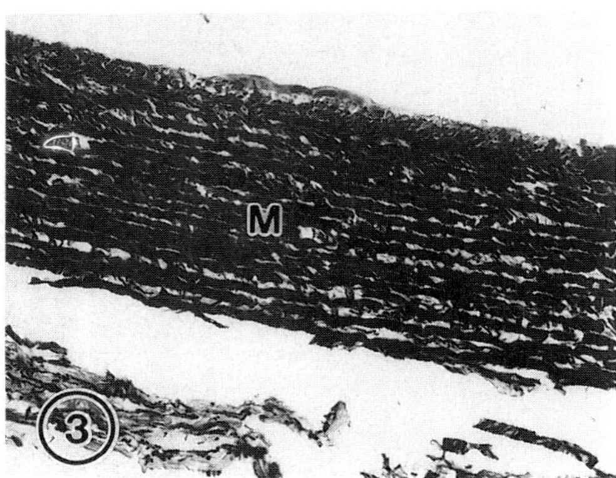

Figure 3 Lobar pulmonary artery with a media (M) composed of regular, parallel elastic laminae. The separation of the media from the underlying adventitia is due to sectioning artifact (VvG, × 150).

is wide and the media is thin representing less than 10% of the arterial cross-sectional area (see Fig. 4). Although the intima is normally composed of a single layer of endothelial cells, with aging, patchy eccentric fibrosis or bundles of longitudinal muscle develop (Fig. 5). Longitudinal muscle bundles are normally present in fetal life, but disappear in postnatal life; they reappear in hypoxic

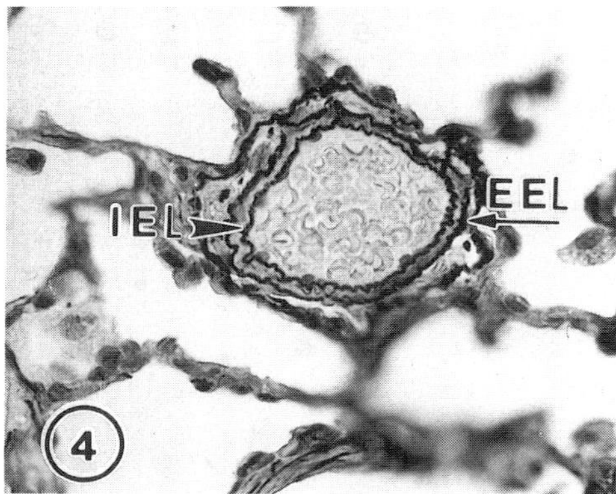

Figure 4 Transverse section of a normal muscular pulmonary artery. Note the relatively wide lumen and thin media bounded by internal (IEL) and external elastic laminae (EEL) (VvG, × 300).

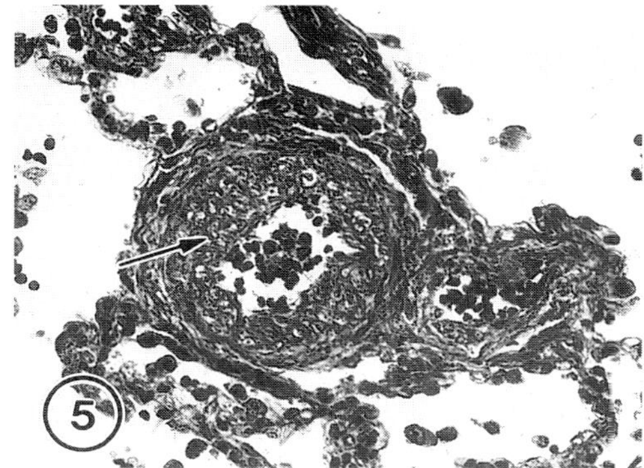

Figure 5 Transverse section of a muscular pulmonary artery with luminal narrowing caused by subintimal longitudinal bundles of smooth muscle (arrow) (HE, × 200).

pulmonary hypertension, in patients with chronic bronchitis, and in older individuals in whom they may be related to smoking habits (7,8).

Arterioles have been defined as precapillary arteries, smaller than 100 μm in outer diameter composed solely of a thin intima and a single elastic lamina (see Figs. 1 and 6). This definition, based on size only, has been criticized because the transition from muscular arteries to arterioles is not uniform for vessels of the same size in all segments of the pulmonary vasculature and at all ages. Thus,

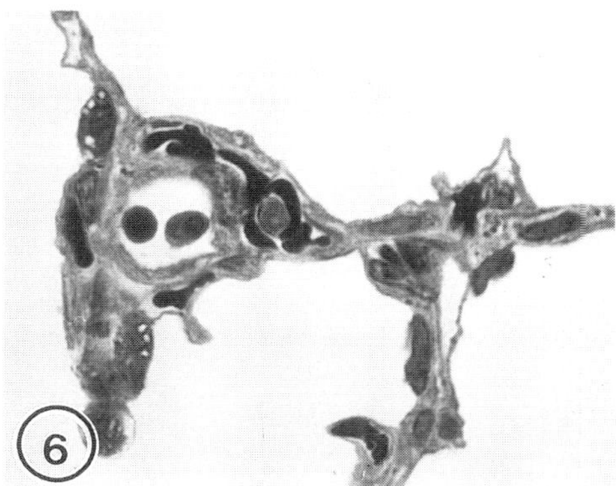

Figure 6 Transverse section of a nonmuscular pulmonary arteriole in the wall of a respiratory bronchiole. The vessel is lined by the endothelium, its basement membrane, and a single poorly developed elastic lamina (resin-embedded tissue, toluidine-blue stain, × 350).

arteries smaller than 100 μm can possess a complete or partial muscular medial coat. To characterize these vessels, the terms muscular, partially muscular, and nonmuscular arteries have been proposed (9). This terminology is cumbersome, and the term arteriole is well entrenched in the medical literature; hence, it will be retained in this chapter, in spite of its limitations. Nonmuscular arterioles are histologically indistinguishable from postcapillary venules unless either special injection techniques are used to identify them, or their origin from parent arteries is traced in serial sections.

The alveolar capillaries are lined by a continuous layer of endothelium resting on a continuous basement membrane and focally connected to scattered pericytes located beneath the basement membrane.

As described earlier, postcapillary venules, up to 70–80 μm in diameter, have a structure similar to that of the precapillary nonmuscular arterioles. These venules feed into interlobular veins, larger than 100 μm in diameter, that possess a tunica media composed of scattered smooth-muscle fibers and irregular elastic fibers (Fig. 7). Larger veins within the interlobar septa have a well-developed media composed of connective tissue, smooth muscle, and a distinct internal elastic lamina. Since there is no external elastic lamina, the media is poorly demarcated from the adventitia, which is composed of several layers of irregular

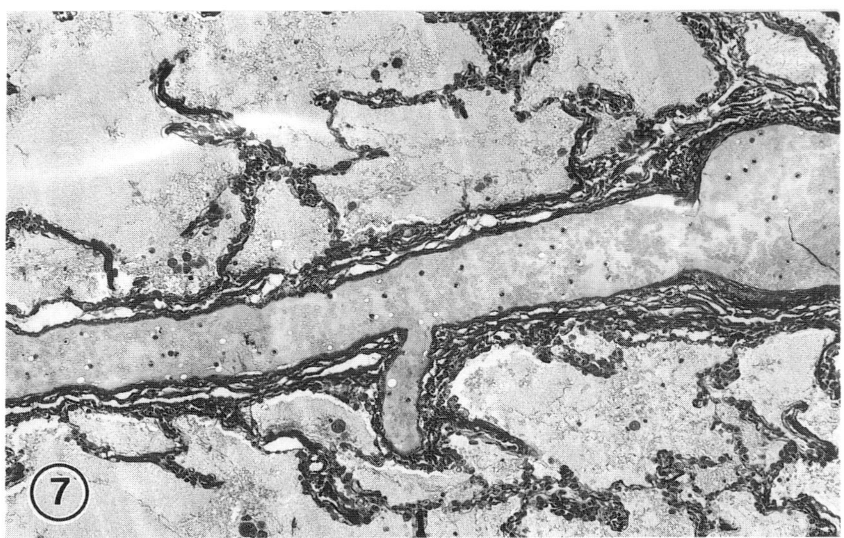

Figure 7 Pulmonary vein with the media composed of irregular layers of elastic fibers (VvG, × 100).

elastic fibers, connective tissue, and smooth muscle. With advancing age, fragmentation of the elastic laminae and sclerosis of the intima and media are commonly found (Fig. 8).

The bronchial arteries arise directly or indirectly from the aorta and provide metabolic substrates, primarily to the airways, the pulmonary arteries, and the lymph nodes, down to the level of the terminal bronchioles. In physiological conditions, the bronchial arterial flow is 0.5–1.5% of the cardiac output (10), but may greatly increase in pathological conditions. The bronchial arteries are systemic arteries, with a thick media composed of circularly oriented smooth muscle. They can be distinguished from the pulmonary arteries by the thick internal elastic lamina and absent, or indistinct, external elastic lamina. Perhaps in response to repeated longitudinal stresses in relation to their location within the walls of the bronchi, bronchial arteries develop layers of longitudinally oriented bundles of smooth muscle often separated by elastic fibers (Fig. 9).

The bronchial veins drain the proximal bronchovascular bundles into the azygos and hemiazygos veins; in the lung periphery, the bronchial veins empty into the pulmonary veins. Thus, the potential for extensive pathological shunting of the bronchopulmonary venous flow to the alveolar capillaries does exist.

Pulmonary artery–pulmonary vein shunts and bronchial artery–pulmonary artery shunts have been shown to be present in the normal adult lung. Their extent

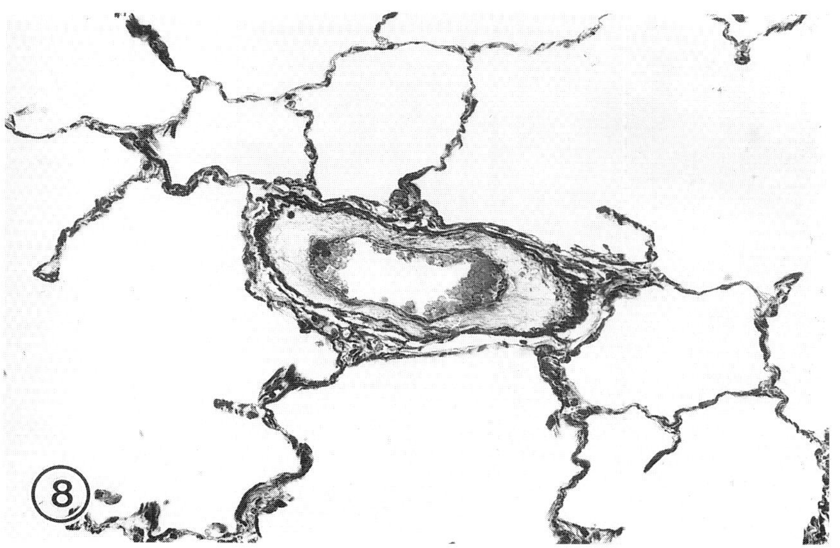

Figure 8 Pulmonary vein showing intimal fibrosis as an age-related change (VvG, × 200).

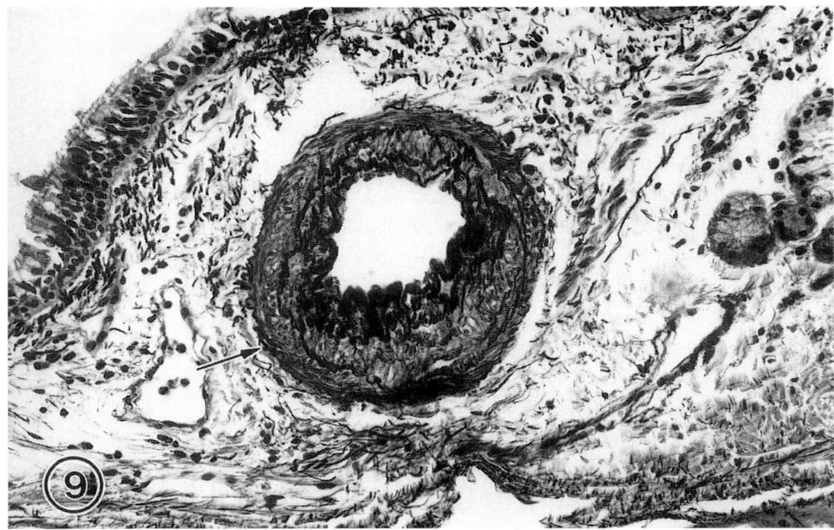

Figure 9 Transverse section of a bronchial artery showing wall thickening by subintimal longitudinal bundles of smooth muscle and elastic fibers. The vessel can be distinguished from a muscular pulmonary artery with medial hypertrophy by the poorly developed external elastic lamina (arrow) (VvG, × 200).

and significance is not well known, but their number and size can increase in primary and secondary pulmonary hypertension (11,12).

III. General Histopathological Features of Hypertensive Angiopathy

A. Arteriopathy

The structure of pulmonary arteries reflects the postnatal low-pressure and low-resistance environment of the normal pulmonary circulation. In comparison with systemic arteries, the pulmonary arteries are very compliant and can readily accommodate large increments in blood volume in response to orthostatic changes or exercise. This property has been attributed to the relatively small number of muscle fibers in the media of the muscular pulmonary arteries and arterioles. In pulmonary hypertension, widespread vascular changes are found in these vessels. Typically, they consist of thickening of the media and intima and of complex lesions involving the lumen and the arterial wall.

Medial Hypertrophy

Medial hypertrophy is characterized by an increase in the medial smooth muscle of muscular arteries (Figs. 10 and 11) and the development of a well-defined muscle layer in nonmuscularized arterioles (Figs. 12 and 13). In muscular arteries it is also associated with the development (reduplication) of several layers of elastic tissue and a variable amount of connective tissue matrix (see Fig. 10). Medial hypertrophy is a general response of the arterial wall to increased pressure, therefore, it is present in all forms of chronic pulmonary hypertension, regardless of its etiology. However, its severity varies from vessel to vessel within the same lung and with the pathogenesis of the hypertensive disease. Medial hypertrophy is not an isolated lesion, but most often, it is associated with other vascular lesions involving the intima or adventitia, as will be described later.

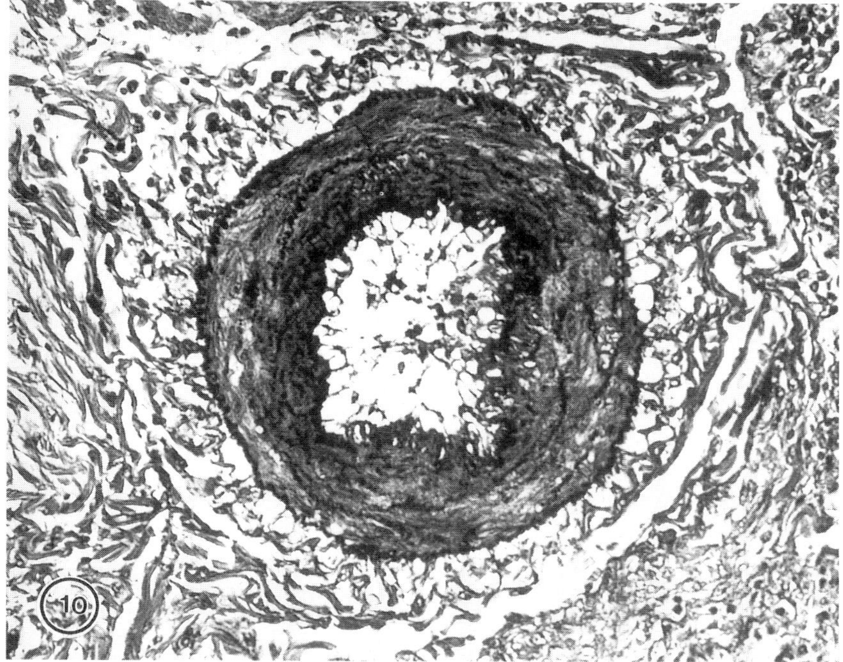

Figure 10 Transverse section of a muscular pulmonary artery with medial hypertrophy. The media occupies 30% of the cross-sectional area (VvG, × 100).

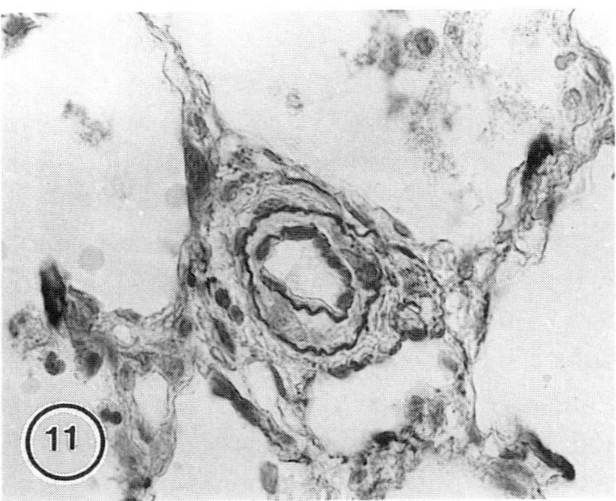

Figure 11 Medial hypertrophy of an intra-acinar muscular pulmonary artery (VvG, × 400).

Medial hypertrophy and muscularization of arterioles are the morphological hallmarks of chronic vasoconstriction. Elegant ultrastructural studies of experimental pulmonary hypertension have shown that medial hypertrophy and muscularization of arterioles result from the recruitment of fibroblasts and myofibroblasts that develop into smooth-muscle cells (9,13). Since the increase in medial muscle mass in hypertensive vessels is due to both proliferation of precursor smooth muscle cells and to hypertrophy of preexisting muscle fibers, the designation of medial thickening, rather than medial hypertrophy, has been recommended (14).

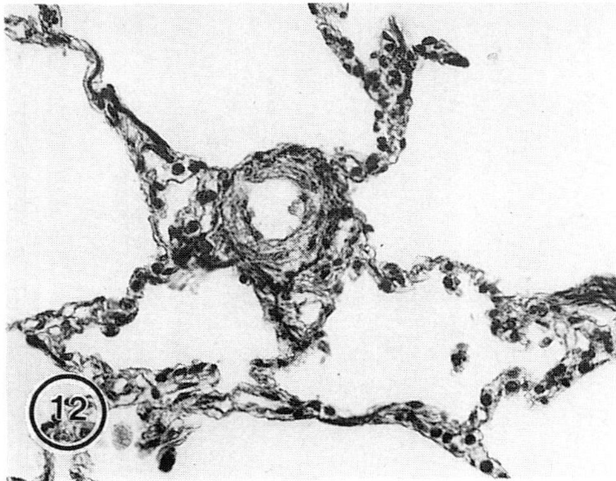

Figure 12 Muscularized pulmonary arteriole. Concentric layers of smooth muscle fibers have developed between the intima and the external elastic lamina (HE, × 160).

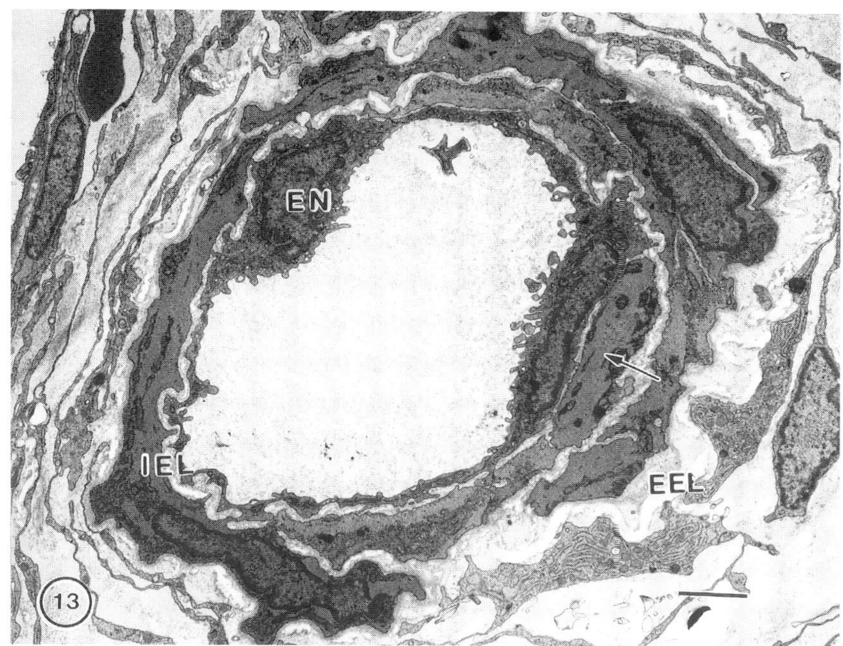

Figure 13 Electron microphotograph of a muscularized pulmonary arteriole from a case of PPH. The external elastic lamina (EEL) represents the original elastic lamina; a discontinuous internal elastic lamina (IEL) has been formed below the endothelium (EN). Between the two elastic laminae are circularly oriented smooth-muscle cells (arrow) (uranyl acetate–lead citrate, × 4000, bar = 5 μm).

Experimental data have shown that the vascular endothelium plays a role in the modulation of medial smooth-muscle contractility (15–18) and smooth-muscle proliferation (19,20). Thus, it appears likely that endothelial dysfunction might play a critical role in the pathogenesis of chronic vasoconstriction, which has been postulated to be the initiating event in PPH (21).

Medial smooth muscle may become atrophic or undergo degeneration and replacement by fibrous tissue (Fig. 14). Atrophy and fibrosis of the medial muscle results in dilatation of the lumen and thinning of the media. Medial atrophy is often a complication of severe intimal fibrosis, but it is not known whether the atrophy is the cause or the consequence of the intimal thickening. Whether these morphological alterations influence the response of the arterial wall to vasodilators is unknown.

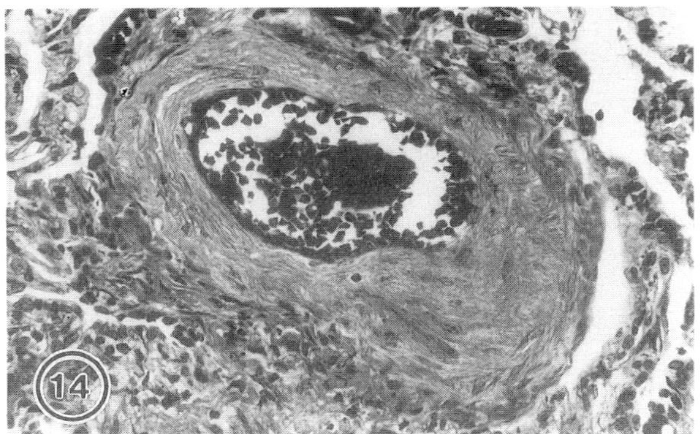

Figure 14 Transverse section of a muscular pulmonary artery with medial fibrosis. The thickened media consists predominantly of cellular connective tissue that has replaced the atrophic smooth muscle (Mallory's trichrome, × 200).

In certain forms of pulmonary hypertensions, such as in hypoxia and in pulmonary venous hypertension, medial thickening may also be associated with thickening of the adventitia.

Intimal Thickening

Intimal thickening is found in arteries with normal, hyperplastic, or atrophic media; it may involve only a segment of the intima (eccentric fibrosis), or its entire circumference (concentric laminar or concentric nonlaminar fibrosis). Intimal thickening is due to the proliferation of smooth-muscle cells, myofibroblasts, or fibroblasts, and the deposition of a variable amount of elastic fibers, collagen fibers, and matrix. Depending on the predominant component, intimal thickening may be cellular or acellular. In the absence of medial hypertrophy, acellular intimal thickening by itself is not pathognomonic of hypertensive arteriopathy. Both types may occur as age-related changes in individuals with normal pulmonary artery pressures, particularly in the lung's upper lobes.

Eccentric Intimal Fibrosis and Concentric Nonlaminar Intimal Fibrosis

Eccentric intimal and concentric nonlaminar intimal fibrosis (EIF; CnLIF) are part of a spectrum of lesions characterized by cushion-like or concentric patches of proliferated myofibroblasts, fibroblasts, and connective tissue (Figs. 15 and 16). These lesions may result from mural organization of thrombi or emboli, or from the stimulation of mesenchymal intimal cells by poorly defined growth factors and cytokines.

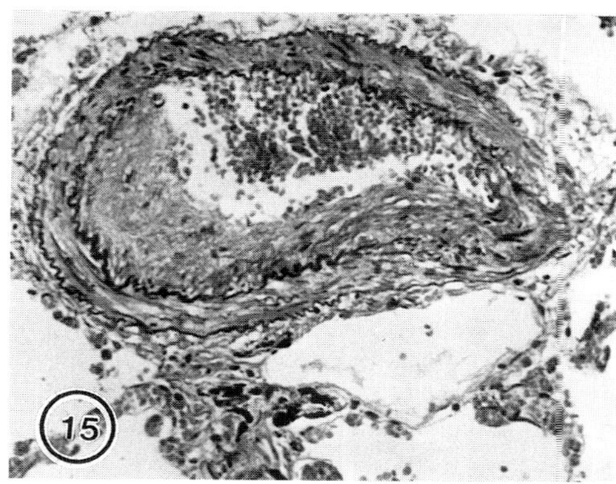

Figure 15 Muscular pulmonary artery with eccentric intimal fibrosis (EIF). A crescent-shaped layer of cellular fibrous tissue is present between the lumen and the internal elastic lamina (VvG, × 100).

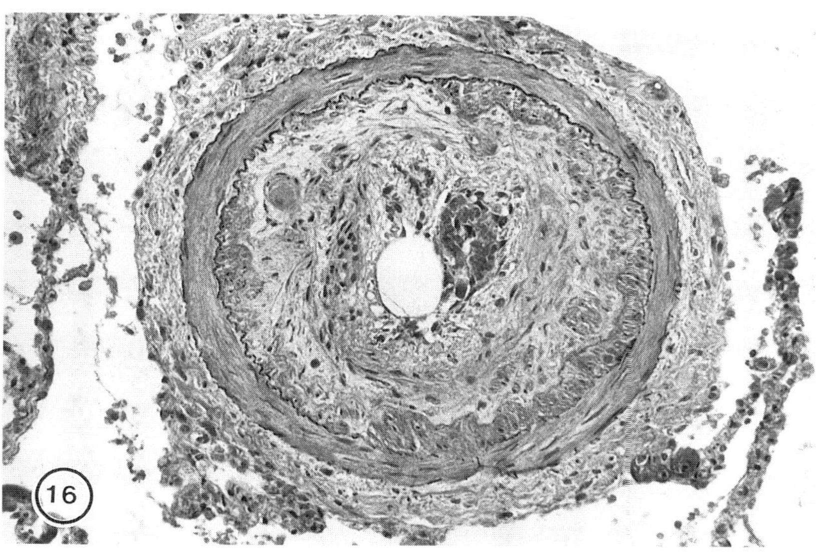

Figure 16 Concentric but nonlaminar fibrosis (CnLF) resulting from organization of thrombus in a muscular pulmonary artery (VvG, × 120).

Concentric Laminar Fibroelastosis

Concentric laminar fibroelastosis (CLIF) is a highly characteristic lesion composed of concentric, onion skin-like layers of myofibroblasts that are often separated by newly formed elastic fibers and abundant connective tissue matrix (22; Figs. 17 and 18). This lesion is not unique to hypertensive arteriopathy, but it occurs in pulmonary or systemic muscular arteries in progressive systemic sclerosis and in chronic allograft rejection, suggesting a stereotyped response of the arterial endothelium to a variety of injuries.

Complex Arterial Wall Lesions

The term *complex arterial wall lesions* includes arteritis, plexiform (or glomoid) lesions, and dilatation (or angiomatoid) lesions. These are destructive and reparative processes affecting several layers of the arterial wall and often the lumen.

The Arteritis

Arteritis is an inflammatory process involving primarily an artery or arteriole. The inflammatory infiltrate can be composed of polymorphonuclear leukocytes or mononuclear cells (Fig. 19). Fibrinoid necrosis is a necrotizing arteritis characterized by wall necrosis and infiltration of the arterial wall with fibrin and plasma proteins (Fig. 20). Healing of the arteritis can result in occlusive intimal fibrosis or deposition of iron–calcium salts on damaged elastic laminae, a process designated as ferruginization.

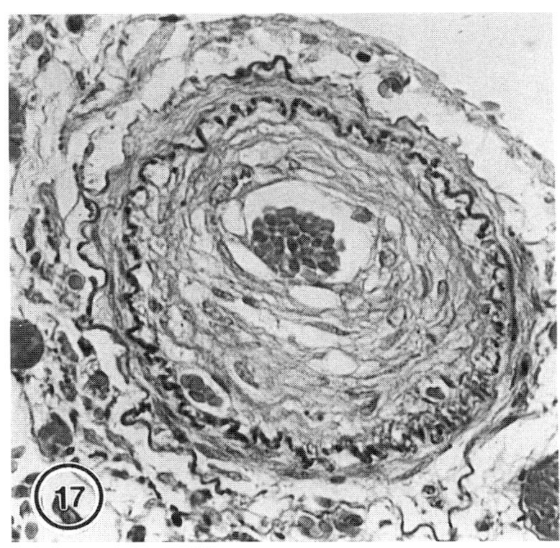

Figure 17 Muscular pulmonary artery with marked luminal narrowing by concentric–laminar intimal fibrosis (CLIF) (VvG, × 340).

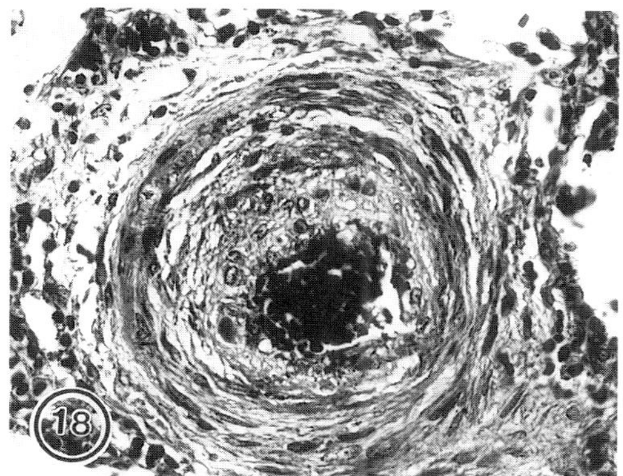

Figure 18 Another example of muscular pulmonary artery with medial hypertrophy and concentric laminar fibrosis (HE, × 400).

The Plexiform Lesion

The plexiform lesion is an aneurysmatic dilation of a muscular artery distal to its origin from a larger parent vessel that is obstructed by intimal fibroelastosis (Figs. 21–23). It is associated with an exuberant proliferation of thin-walled microvessels filling the lumen of the aneurysm and extending into the periarterial connective tissue sheath (see Figs. 21–23). These vessels can be partially thrombosed. Distally, the plexiform lesion feeds into a network of dilated thin-walled sinusoidal channels (see Fig. 22).

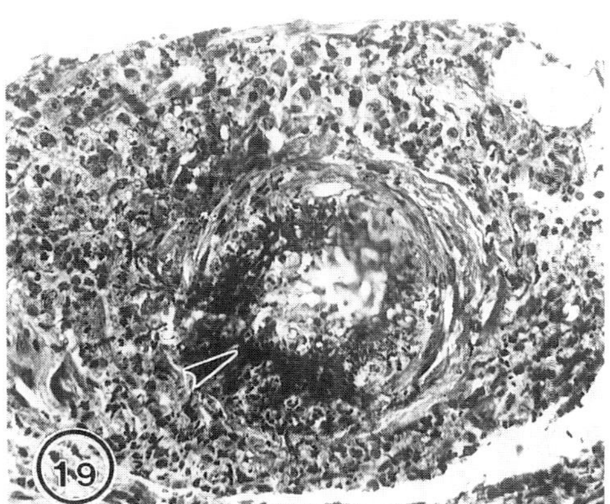

Figure 19 Necrotizing arteritis—the wall is infiltrated by mononuclear inflammatory cells and fibrin (arrowhead) (HE, × 100).

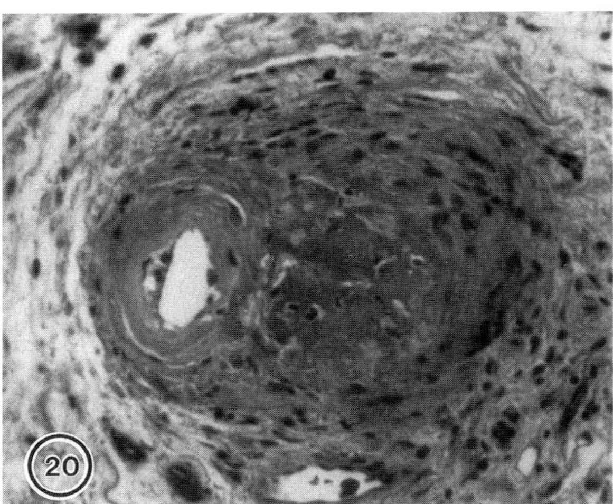

Figure 20 Muscular pulmonary artery with fibrinoid necrosis (HE, × 200).

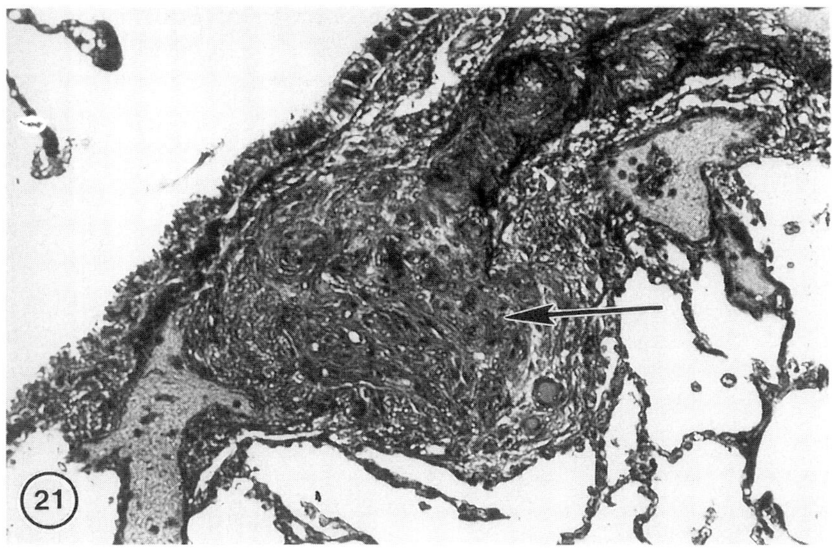

Figure 21 Plexiform lesions (arrow) arising from a stenotic muscular pulmonary artery and feeding into dilated thin-walled arteries (VvG, × 100).

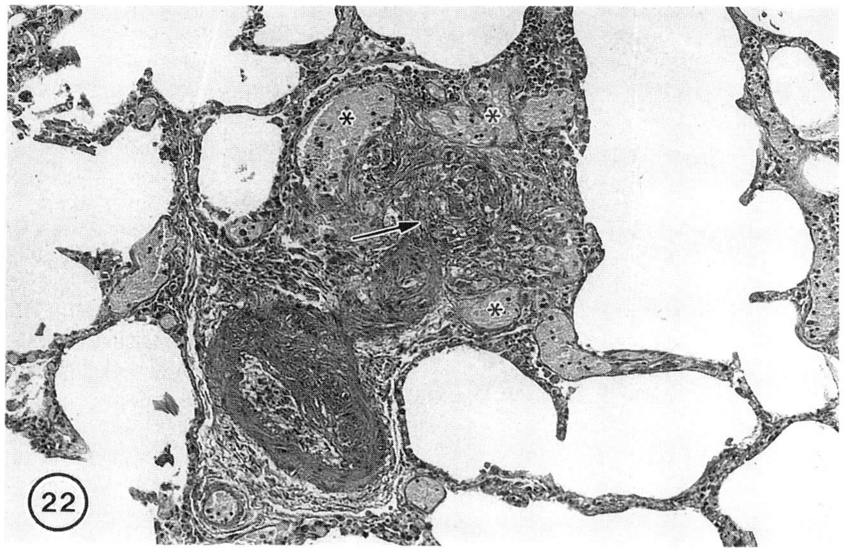

Figure 22 Another example of plexiform lesion (arrow), arising from a stenotic muscular pulmonary artery. Distally, the plexiform lesion communicates with a network of dilated thin-walled vessels, the dilatation lesions (*) (HE, × 100).

The pathogenesis of the plexiform lesion is controversial. Originally it was considered a congenital malformation (23). Others have suggested that it is an aneurysm formed at sites of congenitally weak media (24), or at branching sites of supernumerary arteries (25). Alternatively, it may result from weakening of the arterial wall at branching points by mechanical injury, or by necrotizing arteritis (Figs. 24 and 25) (2,5). By creating surgical shunts between pulmonary and systemic circulation in dogs, it has been possible to demonstrate experimentally that exposure of the pulmonary vessels to high systemic pressures causes necrotizing arteritis of small, muscular arteries, followed by the development of plexiform lesions. The experimental evidence suggests that the plexiform lesions represent a process of repair, recanalization, and formation of collateral small channels that are believed to arise largely from the bronchial circulation (26).

The Dilatation Lesion

The dilatation lesion consists of clusters of dilated thin-walled vessels (Fig. 26) not associated with the plexiform lesion. It may be associated with necrotizing arteritis, or it may be located distal to obstructive luminal lesions.

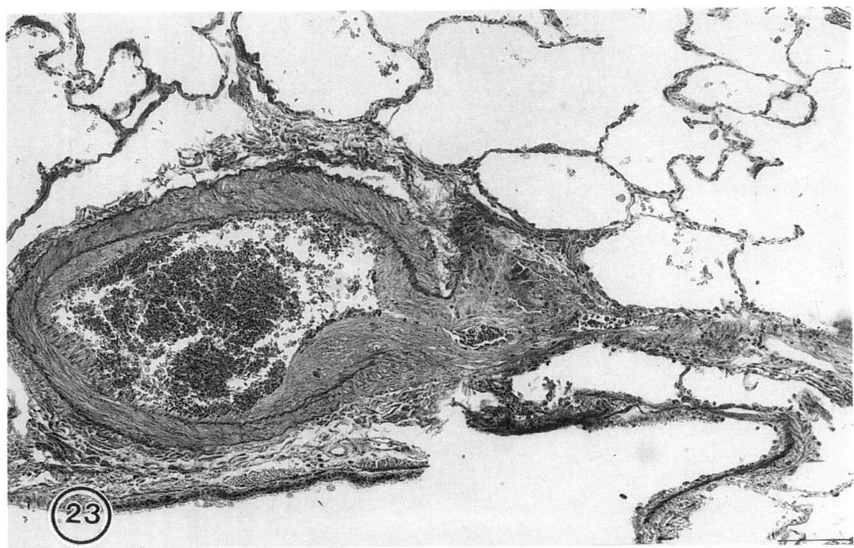

Figure 23 Muscular pulmonary artery with medial hypertrophy and occlusive intimal fibrosis giving rise to a plexiform lesion at the site of origin of a smaller branch (VvG, × 80).

B. Venopathy

Intimal fibrosis may be present in pulmonary veins located downstream from obstructed pulmonary arteries, most likely secondary to low blood flow and thrombosis. In cases of postcapillary obstruction to pulmonary blood flow, there is dilatation and arterialization of the pulmonary veins. Arterialized veins are characterized by the development of a muscular tunica media bounded by distinct internal and external elastic laminae (Fig. 27). The arterialized veins can be distinguished from arteries by their location at the periphery of the lobules, rather than within the peribronchial interstitial space, and by the incomplete development of the muscular layers in the media (see Fig. 27).

Obstructive intimal fibrous cushions and tortuous sinusoidal channels, filling the lumens of lobular and lobar veins (Fig. 28), are pathognomonic features of pulmonary veno-occlusive disease (PVOD), which is thought to be caused by venous thrombosis (see later).

As a consequence of increased venous pressure, the alveolar capillaries are dilated and congested, the pleural and pulmonary lymphatics are dilated, and the interstitial space edematous. Eventually, capillary engorgement results in diapedesis of red blood cells into the alveolar interstitium and into the air spaces.

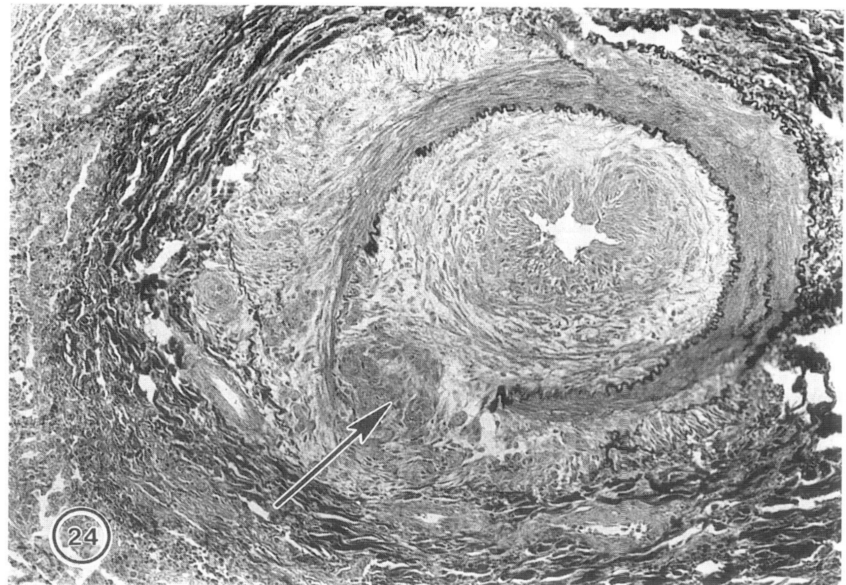

Figure 24 Muscular pulmonary artery in a 14-year-old boy with PPH with segmental necrosis of the wall and early development of a plexiform lesion (arrow) (VvG, × 250).

IV. Pathology of Primary Pulmonary Hypertension

The pathological changes of PPH may be limited to the pulmonary arterial circulation (hypertensive pulmonary arteriopathy), or may involve veins, capillaries, and arteries (pulmonary veno-occlusive disease and capillary hemangiomatosis; Table 1).

A. Hypertensive Pulmonary Arteriopathy

Several studies on the pulmonary vascular pathology of patients diagnosed clinically as having PPH have shown that hypertensive pulmonary arteriopathy is the most common underlying vascular pathology (Table 2). In the prospective study of the National Institutes of Health Registry on PPH, in which the diagnosis of PPH was established by well-standardized clinical and laboratory criteria, hypertensive pulmonary arteriopathy was present in 85% of the cases in which lung tissue was available for independent review by a panel of three pathologists (5).

Hypertensive pulmonary arteriopathy in PPH is a disease of the muscular arteries and arterioles. Changes in the elastic arteries are secondary and non-

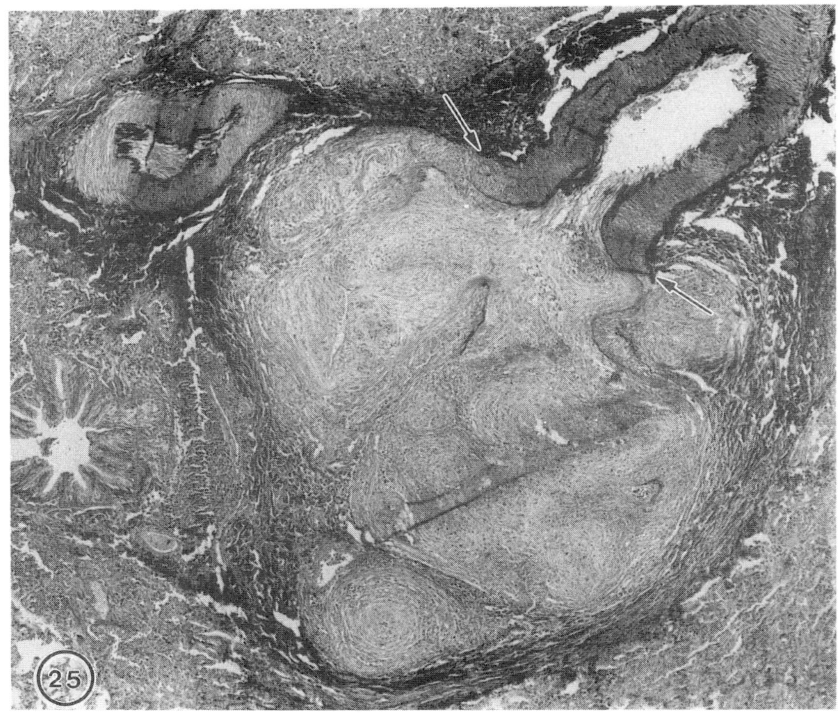

Figure 25 Same patient. Aneurysmatic dilatation of a pulmonary muscular artery with proliferating small blood vessels. This represents an early stage in the development of a plexiform lesion. Arrows indicate the destroyed arterial wall (VvG, × 40).

specific, consisting of dilatation, medial degeneration, and intimal atheromas (Figs. 29 and 30) and, rarely, aneurysms (28).

In the microcirculation there is widening of the pericapillary interstitium and duplication of the capillary basal lamina (Fig. 31). These lesions are probably secondary to ischemic injury and repair. As in all forms of pulmonary hypertension, marked right ventricular hypertrophy is commonly found at autopsy (Fig. 32).

On the basis of histological features, four subsets of hypertensive pulmonary arteriopathy can be identified: isolated medial hypertrophy (IMH), plexogenic pulmonary arteriopathy (PPA), thrombotic pulmonary arteriopathy (TPA), and isolated pulmonary arteritis (4,5). The characteristic histopathological features are summarized in Table 1. Although it is uncertain whether these subsets represent different pathogenetic mechanisms or different manifestations of the same disease

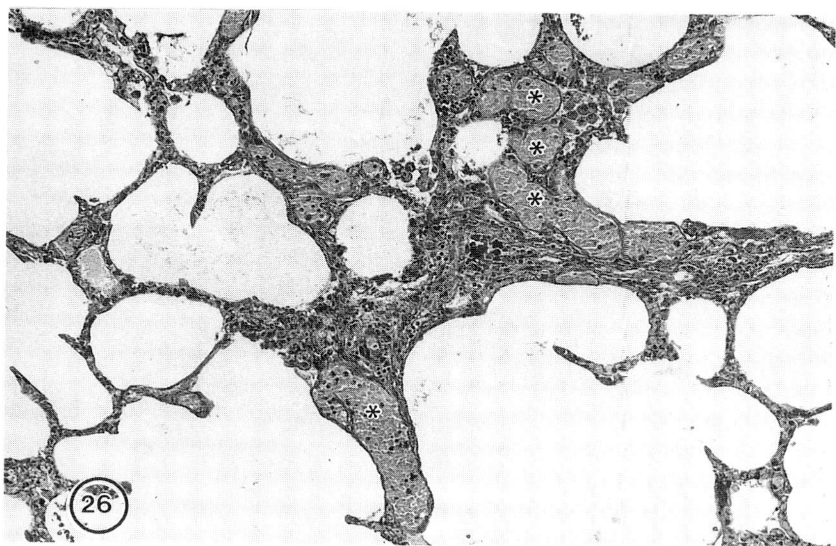

Figure 26 Dilatation lesion consisting of several dilated thin-walled vascular channels (*) (HE, × 80).

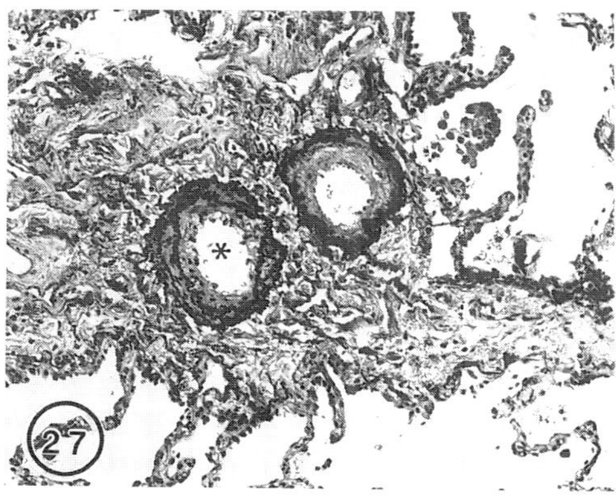

Figure 27 Arterialized interlobular vein. The vessel in the middle of the field (*) shows a distinct media sandwiched between two distinct elastic laminae. The confusion with a muscular artery can be avoided by noting the location of this vessel at a distance from an airway and the incomplete muscularized media (VvG, × 60).

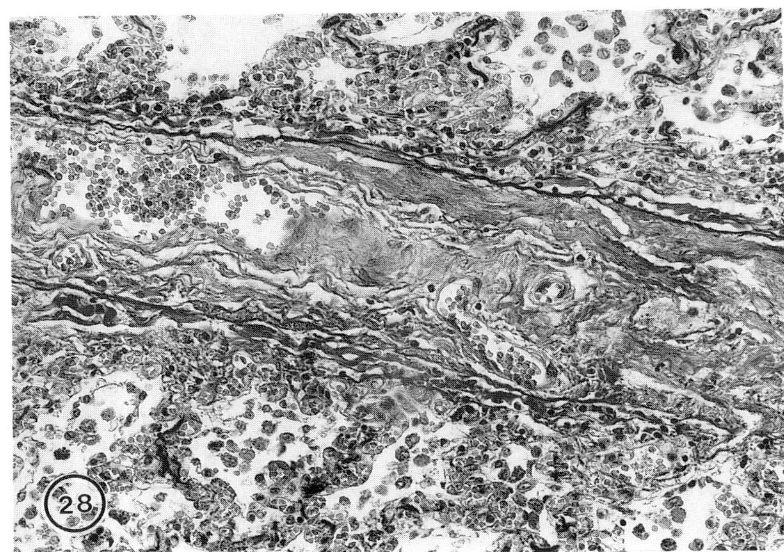

Figure 28 Pulmonary veins from a patient with veno-occlusive disease. The lumen of the vessel is obliterated by fibrous tissue in which there are several small blood channels. The alveolar space contains numerous hemosiderin-laden macrophages, and the alveolar capillaries are congested (VvG, × 120).

(4,5,29), the histopathological distinction is important, since it provides a morphological basis for classification and for evaluating the effects of various therapeutic protocols in PPH. The relative distribution of the different subsets in different pathology series is shown in Table 2.

Pulmonary Artery Medial Hypertrophy

Medial hypertrophy is present in all forms of pulmonary hypertension, either as an isolated lesion (IMH; see Figs. 10–13, 33, 34), or associated with intimal or luminal lesions. Some authors (2,3,28,30) consider IMH an early stage of development of plexogenic pulmonary arteriopathy (PPA). Since the pathogenesis of PPA is unknown, and quantitative studies of vascular lesions in patients with PPH have failed to demonstrate a correlation between age of the patients and frequency of IMH (29), it is preferable to separate the pure form of IMH from the classic PPA, because the former is a potentially reversible type of arteriopathy, which may be amenable to medical treatment with vasodilators. When strict criteria for diagnosis of IMH are applied (4,5), its incidence among adolescents and adults with PPH is between 2 and 4% (see Table 2).

Table 1 Histopathological Classification of Primary Pulmonary Hypertensive Angiopathy

Classification	Characteristic histopathological features
A. Arteriopathy	
Isolated medial hypertrophy (IMH)	Medial hypertrophy: increase of medial muscle in muscular arteries, muscularization of nonmuscularized arterioles; no appreciable intimal or luminal obstructive lesions. No plexiform lesions.
Plexogenic pulmonary arteriopathy (PPA)	Plexiform and dilatation lesions. Medial hypertrophy;[a] eccentric or concentric-laminar and nonlaminar intimal thickening; fibrinoid necrosis, arteritis, and thrombotic lesions.
Thrombotic pulmonary arteriopathy (TPA)	Thrombi (fresh, organizing, or organized, and colander lesions). Eccentric and concentric nonlaminar intimal thickening, varying degrees of medial hypertrophy. No plexiform lesions.
Isolated pulmonary arteritis	Active or healed arteritis. Limited to pulmonary arteries; varying degrees of medial hypertrophy, intimal fibrosis, and thrombotic lesions. No plexiform lesions. No systemic arteritis.
B. Venopathy	
Pulmonary veno-occlusive disease (PVOD)	Eccentric intimal fibrosis and recanalized thrombi within pulmonary veins and venules; arterialized veins, capillary congestion, alveolar edema and siderophages, dilated lymphatics, pleural and septal edema and arterial medial hypertrophy,[a] intimal thickening and thrombotic lesions.
C. Microangiopathy	
Pulmonary capillary hemangiomatosis (PCH)	Infiltrating thin-walled blood vessels throughout pulmonary parenchyma, pleura, bronchi, and walls of pulmonary veins and arteries. Medial hypertrophy and intimal thickening of muscular pulmonary arteries and arterioles.

[a]Medial hypertrophy includes muscularization of arterioles.

In children, IMH may be associated with a variable degree of adventitial fibrosis (see Fig. 33).

Plexogenic Pulmonary Arteriopathy

In the absence of congenital heart disease with left-to-right shunts, plexogenic pulmonary arteriopathy was considered the hallmark of PPH (2,3,28). This view is no longer valid because PPA can occur in pulmonary hypertension associated with a variety of noncardiac conditions, such as liver diseases and portal hypertension (31–33), the use of certain appetite suppressants (34,35), consumption of de-

Table 2 Histopathological Types of Pulmonary Angiopathy in Seven Series of PPH

Type	1970 (2) $n = 156$	1980 (46) $n = 40$	1985 (4) $n = 80$	1987 (44) $n = 26$	1989 (5)[a] $n = 58$	1989 (70)[a] $n = 19$	1991 (30) $n = 86$	Total $n = 465$
Arteriopathy	n (%)	n (%)	n (%)	n (%)	n (%)	n (%)	n (%)	n (%)
IMH[b]	—	—	3 (4)	—	1 (2)	3 (16)	—	} 48 (10)
MH+IF	30 (21)	—	—	—	4 (7)	—	7 (7)	
PPA[b]	80 (51)	14[c] (35)	22 (28)	23[d] (88)	25 (43)	6 (32)	41 (41)	211 (46)
TPA[b]	31 (20)	12 (30)	45 (56)	2 (8)	19 (33)	10 (53)	13 (13)	132 (28)
Isolated arteritis	—	—	3 (4)	—	—	—	—	3 (0.6)
PVOD[b]	5 (3)	2 (5)	5 (6)	1 (4)	7 (12)	—	25 (29)[e]	45 (10)
PCH[b]	—	—	—	—	—	—	—	— (0)
Others[f]	10 (6)	12 (30)	2 (3)	—	2 (3)	—	—	26 (6)

[a]Prospective series with standardized clinical and laboratory criteria for diagnosis of PPH.

[b]IMH, isolated medial hypertrophy; PPA, plexogenic pulmonary arteriopathy; TPA, thrombotic pulmonary arteriopathy; PVOD, pulmonary veno-occlusive disease; PCH, pulmonary capillary hemangiomatosis.

[c]Includes four cases without plexogenic lesions.

[d]Includes two cases with arteritis as the predominant lesion.

[e]Includes cases of PCH.

[f]Includes pulmonary venous hypertension, sarcoidosis, hypoxic arteriopathy, schistosomiasis, and normal vessels.

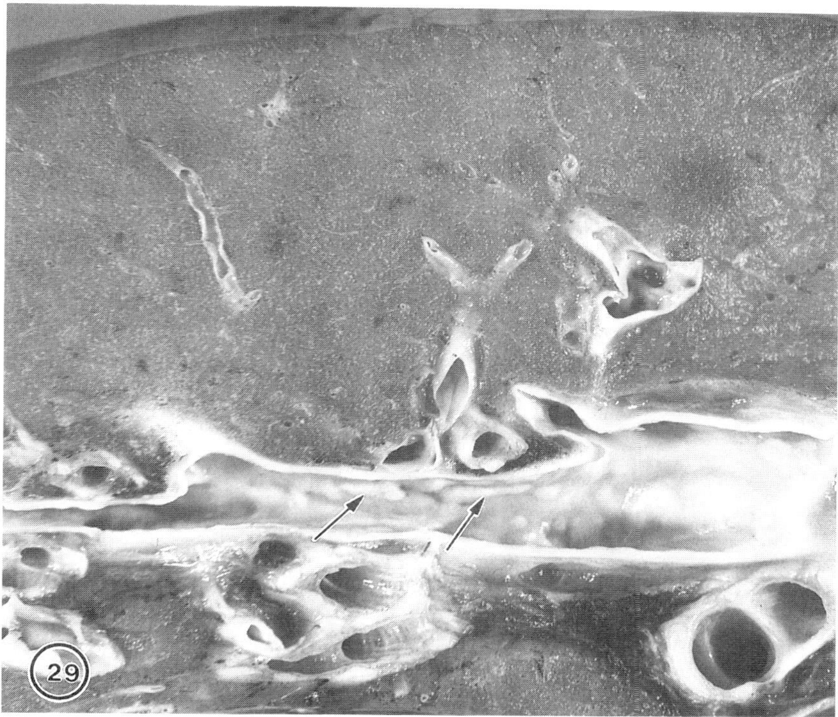

Figure 29 Atherosclerotic plaques (arrows) and dilatation of lobar pulmonary artery and its branches from a patient with PPH.

natured rapeseed oil (36,37), human immunodeficiency virus (HIV) infection (38–42), or intravenous chemotherapy (43).

Nevertheless, plexogenic pulmonary arteriopathy (PPA) is the most common type of pulmonary hypertensive arteriopathy in PPH patients, accounting for about 45% of the cases (see Table 2). In the National Institutes of Health Registry on PPH, the male/female ratio for PPA was 1:2. Patients with this type of arteriopathy were on average 10 years younger and appeared to have a worse prognosis than those with thrombotic arteriopathy (5). It is unclear whether the greater incidence of PPA in young women indicates different pathogenetic mechanisms, or a greater reactivity to nonspecific hypertensive stimuli (29).

Plexogenic pulmonary arteriopathy is characterized by a constellation of lesions that include medial hypertrophy, muscularization of arterioles, intimal proliferation, and complex lesions (2–5,28,30,44). The intimal lesions are of three types: concentric laminar intimal fibroelastosis (CLIF; see Figs. 17 and 18),

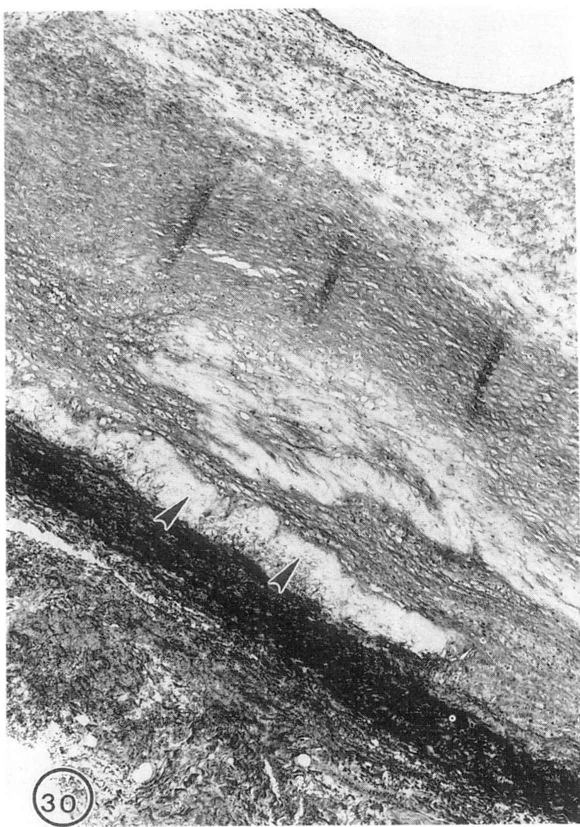

Figure 30 Main pulmonary artery from a patient with PPH. There is marked intimal thickening with fibrosis and atheromatous material and patchy degeneration of elastic laminae in the media (arrowheads) (VvG, × 80).

eccentric intimal fibrosis (EIF; see Fig. 15), and concentric nonlaminar fibrosis (CnLIF; see Fig. 16) (4,5,28,30,44). The relative proportion of CLIF, EIF, and CnLIF varies from case to case and in different regions of the same lung. Since EIF and CnLIF are generally considered markers of thrombotic arteriopathy, it has been proposed that their presence in PPA is a secondary complication of the hypertension, rather than a primary lesion (45). The main argument for the secondary nature of thrombotic lesions is their absence or paucity in children. On the other hand, quantitative analysis of vascular lesions has shown lack of correlation between the frequency of thrombotic lesions, age of patients, or length of

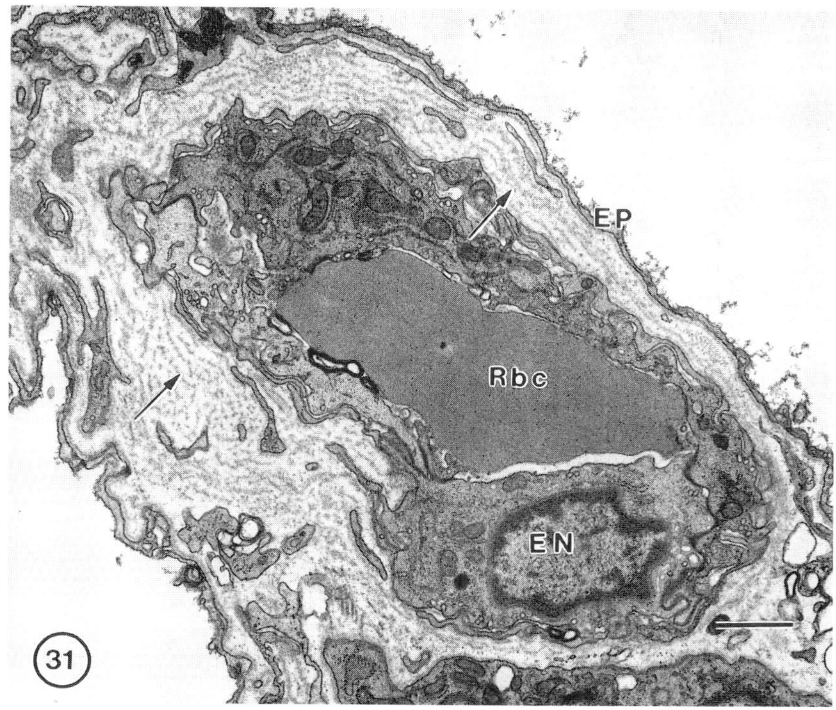

Figure 31 Representative electron microphotograph of alveolar capillaries from a 36-year-old woman with PPH who underwent a lung transplant. The capillary basal lamina is composed of multiple layers (arrows). (EN, endothelium; EP, alveolar epithelium; Rbc, red blood cell) (uranyl acetate, lead citrate, × 10,000; bar = 1 μm).

survival after diagnosis (29). Moreover, in a high proportion of well-documented cases of PPH, thrombotic arteriopathy is the only pulmonary vascular pathology (4,5). It is always difficult to extrapolate pathogenetic mechanisms from morphological observations on end-stage diseases in which secondary events and reparative processes are superimposed on primary lesions. Nevertheless, the experimental evidence that the pulmonary endothelium plays a critical role in modulating medial muscle tone and proliferation (15–20) suggests that thromboembolic lesions could be the morphological markers of a primary endothelial injury, rather than secondary changes related to long-standing hemodynamic injury.

Typically, in addition to medial and intimal changes, a variable number of complex lesions involving all the components of the arterial wall are present in

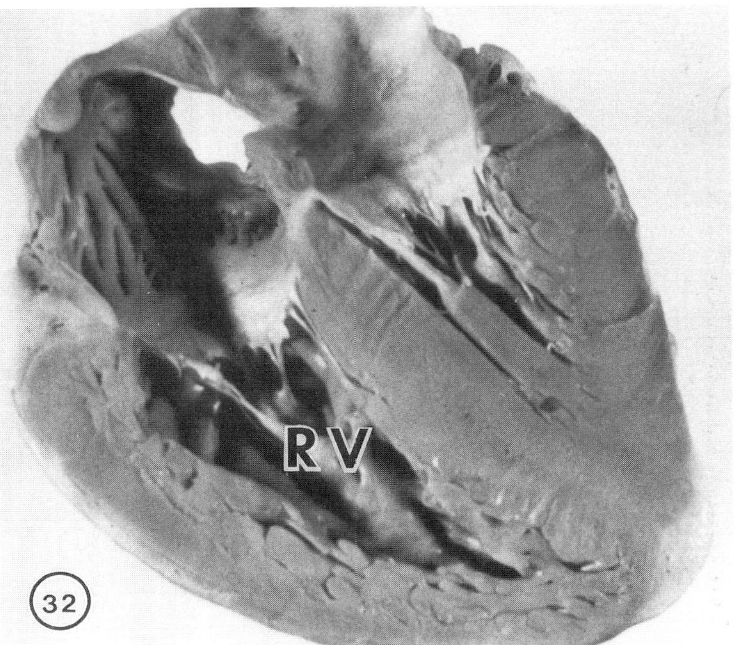

Figure 32 Bisected heart from a patient with PPH showing the marked hypertrophy of the right ventricle (RV) and dilatation of the right atrium.

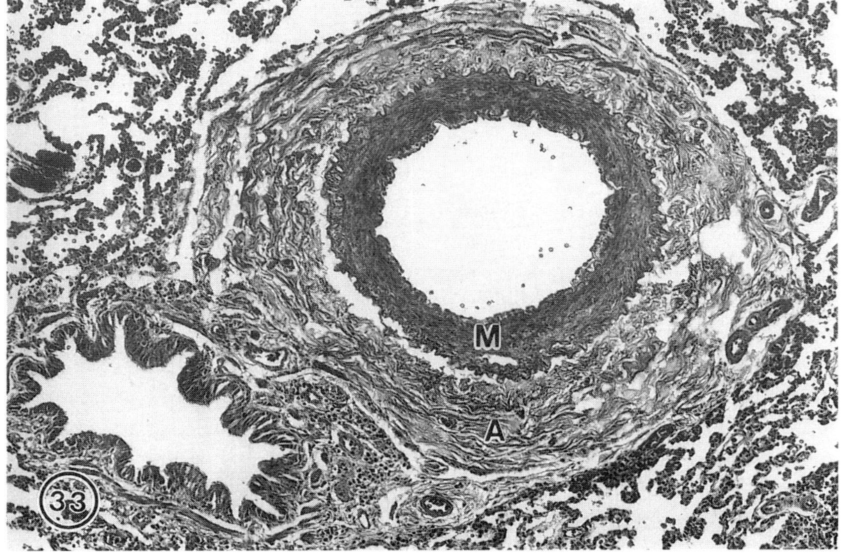

Figure 33 Isolated medial hypertrophy from an 11-year-old boy with PPH. There is thickening of both media (M) and adventitia (A).

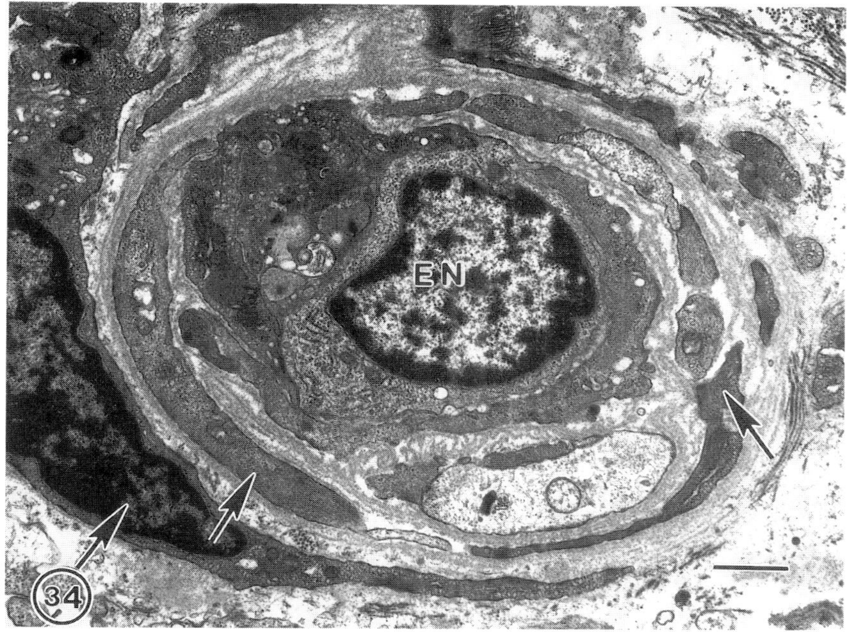

Figure 34 Electron micrograph of a muscularized precapillary arteriole from a 33-year-old woman with PPH. The lumen is nearly obliterated by a plump endothelial cell (EN). Smooth-muscle cells (arrows) form several concentric layers within the multilayered basal lamina (uranyl acetate, lead citrate, × 4000; bar = 5μm).

PPA. These lesions include the plexiform lesions (see Figs. 21–23), the dilatation lesions (see Fig. 26), and necrotizing arteritis (see Figs. 19,20,24). Although plexiform lesions are interesting pathological processes associated with severe pulmonary hypertension, their diagnostic and prognostic significance has been greatly overemphasized. The frequency of plexiform lesions varies greatly (Fig. 35); plexiform lesions may involve less than 10% of muscular arteries (5,35) and, therefore, can be absent in a lung biopsy sample if only a limited number of muscular arteries are present. Plexiform lesions are not specific for PPH, since they have been found in a variety of secondary forms of pulmonary hypertension (36–42).

Pathologists unfamiliar with pulmonary vascular diseases may have difficulties in distinguishing between plexiform lesions and recanalized thrombi, also called "colander-like lesions" (Figs. 36 and 37; 3). Although at times difficult (27), the distinction between plexiform lesions and recanalized thromboemboli can be made by noting that recanalized thromboemboli are randomly distributed

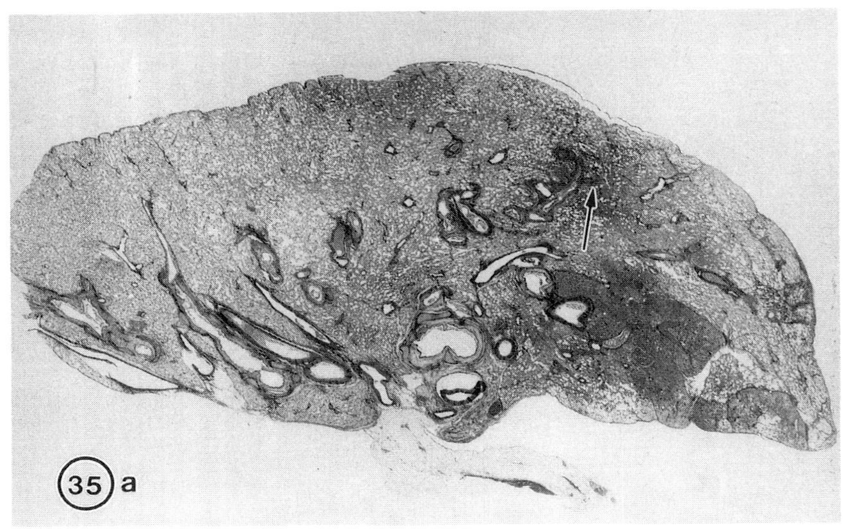

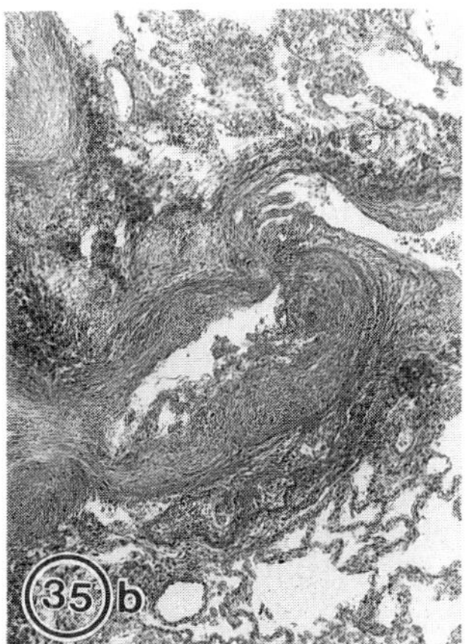

Figure 35 (a) Coronal section of an entire lung lobe from a patient with PPA. Only one single plexiform lesion was found in the entire section (arrow) (VvG, reduced 20% from natural size). (b) Magnified area from (a) to show the plexiform lesion (VvG, × 20).

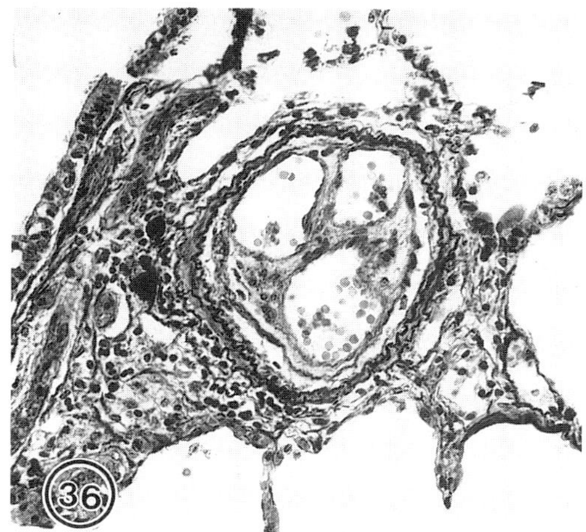

Figure 36 "Classic" colander-like lesion in a muscular pulmonary artery. There is no medial hypertrophy and the recanalization of a thromboembolus has created large channels lined by endothelium (VvG, × 150).

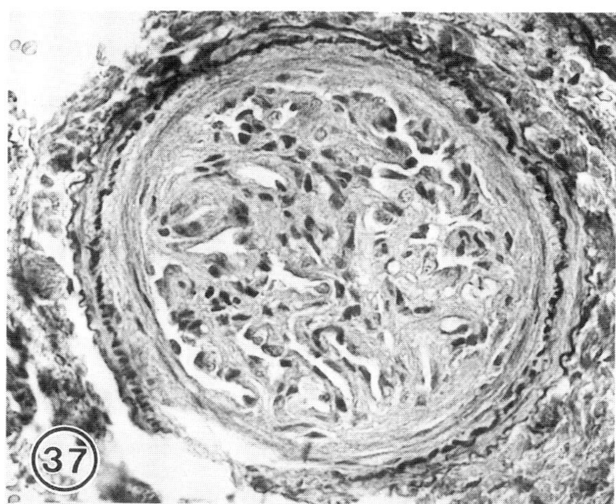

Figure 37 Colander-like lesion mimicking a plexiform lesion. Note that the small vascular channels are confined to the lumen and the media is intact (VvG, × 80).

and not associated with wall destruction and microaneurysm formation (see Fig. 37). The distinction is important, because the plexiform lesions are considered by some investigators essential for the histopathological diagnosis of PPH (2,3). Moreover, plexiform lesions identify a subset of patients with "plexogenic arteriopathy," a type of pulmonary hypertensive arteriopathy that may have a distinct pathogenesis and clinical course (5).

Dilatation or angiomatoid lesions are composed of dilated and tortuous thin-walled channels (see Fig. 27), often located distally to plexiform lesions. They are uncommon and of little diagnostic or hemodynamic significance.

Necrotizing arteritis (see Figs. 19 and 20) may be present in about 30% of cases of PPA (3). It is generally associated with severe pulmonary hypertension and is thought to be the precursor of plexiform lesions (see Fig. 24). Healing of the arteritis is associated with intimal thickening, scarring of the arterial wall, and deposition of calcium and iron salts on elastic laminae (siderosis). Unlike PPA caused by left-to-right shunts, marked segmental necrosis, with infiltration of the arterial wall by neutrophiles and mononuclear inflammatory cells, is rare in PPH (30).

Thrombotic Pulmonary Arteriopathy

The diagnostic features of this type of hypertensive pulmonary arteriopathy are the presence of medial thickening of small muscular arteries and arterioles with EIF, CnLIF, (see Figs. 15 and 16), and colander-like lesions (see Figs. 36 and 37). By definition, CLIF, plexiform, or dilatation lesions must be absent.

As discussed earlier, EIF, CnLIF, and colander-like lesions are considered the result of the mural organization of thrombi or emboli. Thus, thrombotic pulmonary arteriopathy (TPA) is considered by some to be a form of pulmonary hypertension secondary to chronic silent pulmonary embolism (1–3,28,46). However, it is now well established that TPA is present in a high proportion of patients with PPH (see Table 2) in the absence of any clinical or pathological evidence of a source of chronic emboli. Thus, TPA most likely is due to primary in situ thrombosis of small, muscular arteries and not caused by chronic pulmonary embolism (4–6).

Isolated Pulmonary Arteritis

Few cases of PPH have been reported in which the underlying vascular pathology was a primary pulmonary arteritis with secondary obstructive thrombosis (Fig. 38; 4,47,48). Most reported cases were in children (4,47), and the arteritis was not associated with plexiform or dilatation lesions, systemic angiitis, or connective tissue diseases. There may be overlap between isolated arteritis and PPH, because there are cases of PPH in which few plexiform lesions can be found, even though arteritis is the predominant vascular pathology (44; see Figs. 24 and 25). The

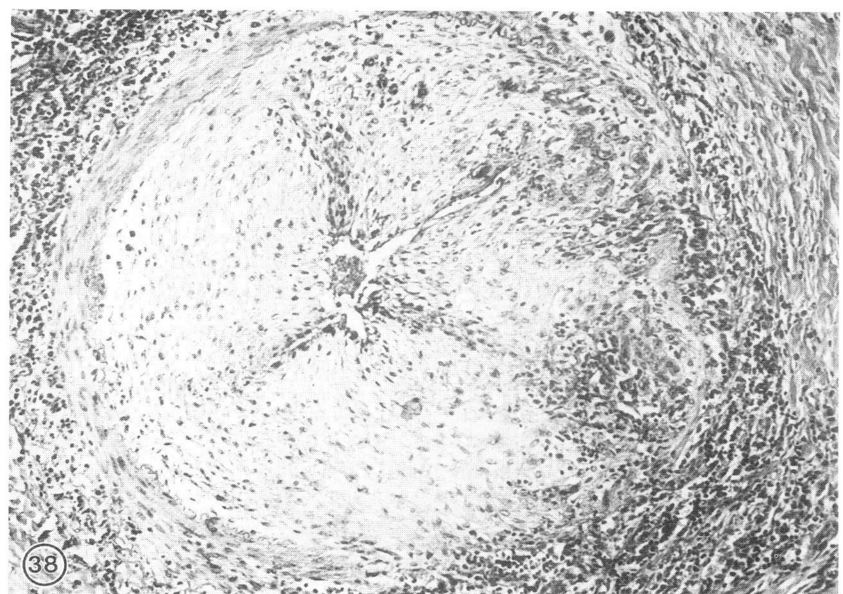

Figure 38 Isolated pulmonary arteritis characterized by mononuclear cell infiltration in the media and adventitia, necrosis of the media, marked intimal thickening and narrowing of the lumen (HE, × 180). (Courtesy Dr. William D. Edwards.)

development of necrotizing arteritis and pulmonary hypertension in rats administered pyrrolizidine alkaloids (49) raises the prospect that the human pulmonary arteritis might be secondary to dietary or other exogenous angiotoxic substances.

B. Pulmonary Veno-occlusive Disease

In a small proportion of patients with PPH, the hypertensive lesions involve primarily the pulmonary veins with occlusive intimal lesions. This entity has been designated pulmonary veno-occlusive disease (PVOD; see Table 2). The disease is rare, usually affecting children, adolescents, and young adults (50–53), and it may be familial (53). It has been observed in patients treated with chemotherapeutic agents (54), oral contraceptives (55), after bone marrow transplantation (56,57), and in patients with HIV infection (42,58).

Pulmonary veno-occlusive disease was so designated because it was thought to be caused by a primary obstructive thrombotic disorder of the pulmonary venules and veins (50,51). The histopathological diagnosis of this disease is based on the presence, within pulmonary veins and venules, of obstructive eccentric fibrous intimal pads and tortuous sinusoidal channels filling long segments of their lumens (see Figs. 28 and 39). Often there is arterialization of pulmonary veins, characterized by the development of a prominent medial muscle coat bounded by internal and external elastic laminae (see Fig. 39). The arterialized veins closely resemble muscular pulmonary arteries, but the uneven thickness of the muscularized media and the discontinuous elastic laminae allow their correct identification (see Figs. 29 and 39). As a consequence of venous flow obstruction, the alveolar capillaries are markedly congested, the interstitial space edematous and the lymphatics dilated (see Fig. 29). Capillary congestion leads to interstitial and alveolar hemorrhages. Breakdown of extravasated red blood cells results in the accumulation of hemosiderin in alveolar macrophages, type II pneumocytes, and elastic laminae of blood vessels. In a lung biopsy, the thickening of the alveolar septa, the associated hyperplasia of type II cells, and the presence of focal lymphocytic infiltrates may be mistaken for interstitial pneumonia. Capillary congestion is sometimes very focal and sharply demarcated and may be confused with the lesions of pulmonary capillary hemangiomatosis (see following section). As in all cases of postcapillary obstruction to venous drainage, there are medial hypertrophy of muscular pulmonary arteries, muscularization of arterioles, and eccentric or concentric nonlaminar fibrosis (EIF or CnLIF). Concentric laminar fibroelastosis (CLIF) or plexiform lesions are usually absent, but, rarely, dilatation lesions and fibrinoid necrosis may occur (3,59,60).

The resemblance of the occlusive intimal lesions in the pulmonary veins

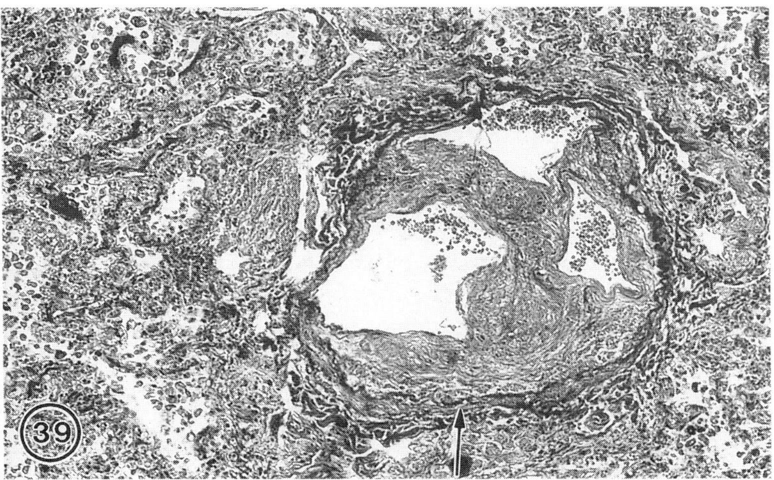

Figure 39 Transverse section of a vein from a case of pulmonary veno-occlusive disease. The lower half of the vessel shows arterialization (arrow), and the lumen is subdivided by irregular fibrous bands into endothelial-lined channels (VvG, × 60).

(and in the arteries) to organized thrombi has led to the belief that PVOD is the result of in situ thrombosis, but no satisfactory explanation for the thrombosis has yet been proposed. The frequent association of the disease with a preceding respiratory viral infection (61) and its occasional unilateral presentation (62) have suggested a viral-induced damage to the venous endothelium. The coexistence of plexogenic arteriopathy and PVOD in cases of pulmonary hypertension associated with HIV infection (41), or following ingestion of denaturated rapeseed oil (36,37), suggests that the arterial lesions in PVOD may not be secondary changes, and that the disease is caused by a variety of angiopathic injuries involving, to a different degree, the entire pulmonary endothelium (52,56,59,63). Thus, this entity should be designated pulmonary occlusive angiopathy (POA), rather than pulmonary veno-occlusive disease.

C. Pulmonary Capillary Hemangiomatosis

Pulmonary capillary hemangiomatosis, an extremely rare condition, is characterized by the proliferation of thin-walled microvessels infiltrating the peribronchial–perivascular interstitium, the lung parenchyma (Figs. 40 and 41) and the pleura. Infiltration of the walls of pulmonary veins of different diameter causes expansion of the media, destruction of the medial elastic fibers, and fibrous luminal obstruction. Because of the occlusion of pulmonary veins by fibrous tissue containing small vascular channels, pulmonary capillary hemangiomatosis may be confused with PVOD (68). Indeed, some authors believe that the two entities overlap (30) and are not two distinct disease processes. Although clinically and radiologically PVOD and PCH cannot be readily distinguished from each other, this can be done by histological examination. In PVOD, the alveolar capillaries are markedly distended and engorged with blood, but only a single capillary is present in each alveolar wall. In contrast, in PCH, two or more capillaries are found in the alveolar walls. Often the lesions are patchy, and the proliferating vessels may form small nodules within the alveolar interstitial space (see Figs. 40 and 41). The thin-walled microvessels are prone to bleeding, resulting in the accumulation of hemosiderin-laden macrophages in the alveolar spaces and, clinically, in hemoptysis. In addition, there is medial and intimal thickening of muscular arteries (see Fig. 40) and muscularization of the arterioles (64–68). In one case of pulmonary capillary hemangiomatosis (PCH), the presence of endothelial nuclear atypia and pleomorphism suggested a neoplastic process (64).

The condition may occur spontaneously, or in families, with an autosomal recessive inheritance pattern (67).

V. Lung Biopsy

Lung biopsy has been advocated to determine the type of pulmonary vascular disease underlying the clinical presentation of pulmonary hypertension and to

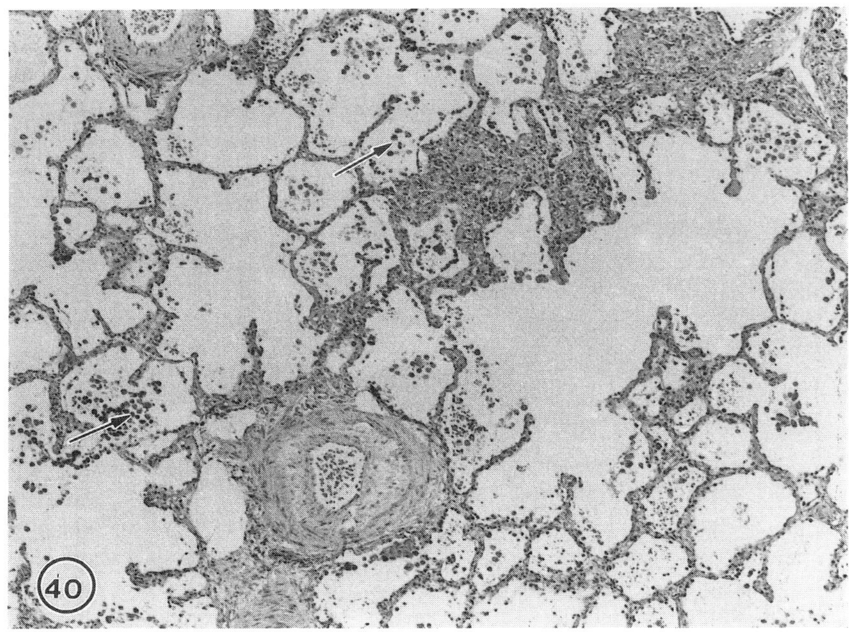

Figure 40 Pulmonary capillary hemangiomatosis characterized by expansion of the pulmonary interstitial space by proliferation of small blood vessels. The muscular arteries show medial and intimal thickening. The black dots in the alveoli (arrows) represent hemosiderin-laden macrophages (HE, × 40).

provide insights into pathogenetic mechanisms (46) that may guide medical therapy.

Because of the need to sample an adequate number of small vessels located in the lung periphery, only open or thoracoscopic lung biopsies are suitable for diagnosis. Transbronchial lung biopsy is of no value, because it does not sample blood vessels adequately, and the few vessels that may be present often show crush artifacts.

Although open-lung biopsy provides a representative sample of vascular pathology (5,69,70), it is now recognized that the histopathology of PPH is heterogeneous (4,5,29), and that thrombotic lesions are also present in plexogenic arteriopathy (5,28,29,45). Thus, lung biopsy is of little value in distinguishing plexogenic from thrombotic arteriopathy. It remains an option in selected cases to establish a diagnosis when confounding factors coexist.

As in every biopsy procedure, there are three key elements for accurate

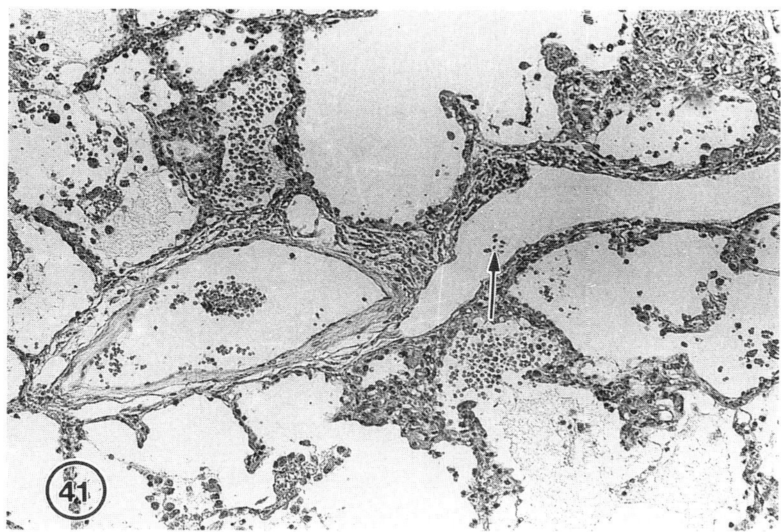

Figure 41 Pulmonary capillary hemangiomatosis. In contrast to PVOD there is intimal fibrosis of a pulmonary vein, but its lumen is widely patent; in its proximity a dilated lymphatic (arrow) (HE, × 40).

diagnosis: (1) good communication between clinicians and pathologist, (2) adequate tissue sample, and (3) the pathologist's experience (69).

The lung microanatomy varies in different lobes or segments, and this should be recognized in selecting a site for biopsy. In the apical segments, there are relatively fewer blood vessels than in the lower lobes, and the vessels may show nonspecific intimal fibrosis. In the tip of the right middle lobe and lingula, the blood vessels may also show nonspecific intimal fibrosis and interstitial fibrosis. These sites should be avoided.

In pulmonary hypertension, the diagnostic pathological changes are found in the muscular pulmonary arteries accompanying small airways 0.5–1.0 mm in diameter (Fig. 42), as well as in the arterioles and veins. Because the muscular arteries and interlobular veins are unevenly distributed, the lung tissue sampled should be a wedge measuring about 2 × 2 × 1.5 cm, and not a thin sleeve of tissue from the edge of a lobe (69). The biopsy tissue should be fixed in a distended state, either under negative pressure or by manual translaveolar infiltration of fixative with a syringe. After adequate fixation, the entire specimen should be sectioned in serial slices, 0.5 cm in thickness, parallel to the plane of surgical resection. The evaluation of the biopsy sample should not be limited to the pulmonary vasculature, but should include all the tissue components (i.e., airways, alveolar walls and

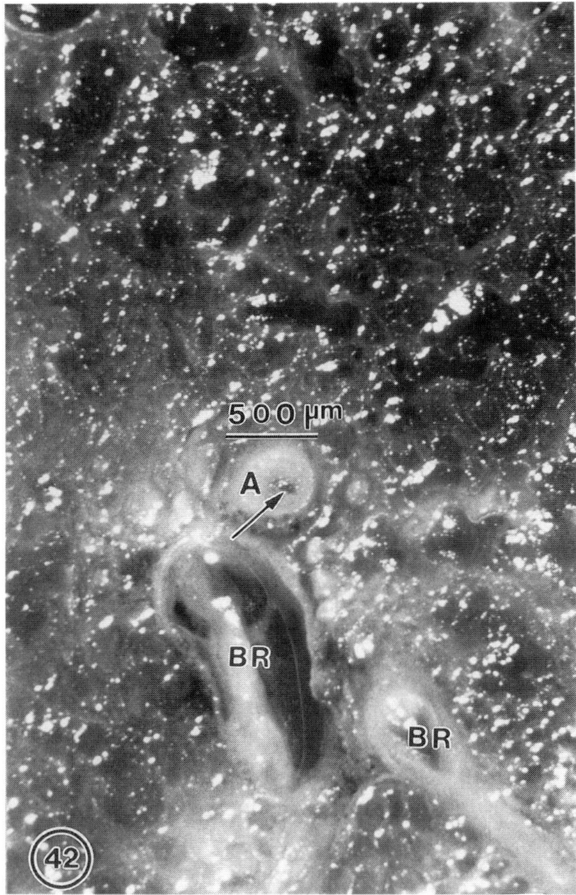

Figure 42 Lung biopsy from a case of PPH. The lung tissue was fixed in distended state with formalin. The cut section reveals a pulmonary artery (A), 0.5 mm in diameter, with markedly thickened wall and small lumen (arrow). BR, bronchiole (×25).

alveoli, lymphatics and pleura). Special attention should be paid to the nature and extent of vascular lesions. Electron microscopy or immunohistochemistry are rarely required for diagnostic purposes.

VI. Grading and Morphometric Analysis

In the early days of cardiac surgery, a grading system was developed to assess the potential reversibility of hypertensive pulmonary arteriopathy in candidates for surgical repair of left-to-right shunts (71). Six grades of histopathological changes were identified; grades 1–3 included potentially reversible lesions, whereas the remaining grades indicated irreversible lesions. Grade 1 indicated medial hypertrophy (thickening), without intimal changes; grade 2 included medial hypertrophy and cellular intimal thickening; and in grade 3 medial hypertrophy and intimal fibrosis. Grade 4 was characterized by the presence of plexiform lesions, and grade 5 by dilatation lesions; grade 6 indicated necrotizing arteritis.

Although this grading system was devised for congenital cardiac defects having pulmonary hypertension from birth, it has been applied indiscriminately to all types of pulmonary hypertension. This was based on the unproved assumption that the vascular lesions in all forms of pulmonary hypertension are uniformly distributed and develop in a well-defined stepwise progression. This does not seem to be true in PPH, since no correlation has been found between grading and either survival or pulmonary artery pressure (5,29,44,70). The lack of correlation between grading and clinical parameters is probably because both the original grading system proposed by Heath and Edwards (71) and its modifications (14,72) are based on the most severe vascular changes and ignore the variability in severity and frequency of each lesion.

Morphometric evaluation of wall thickness (72,73) should provide a better estimate of the severity and extent of vascular pathological changes. However, this technique can be applied only to vessels cut perpendicularly to their long axis and in tissue samples fixed and processed by well-standardized methods. Measurements of ratios of medial and intimal areas to total vascular cross-sectional areas (69,72,74) overcome some of these problems. By this approach intimal thickening in muscular arteries of patients with PPH was correlated inversely with age and survival, whereas medial thickening correlated with response to vasodilators (70). However, the great heterogeneity of the vascular lesions, and the large variability of measurements in individual vessels within the same lung, limit the value of morphometric analysis to large series of patients to obtain statistically significant data.

In clinical practice, the evaluation of a lung biopsy sample for vascular diseases should include a description of the various lesions involving different segments of the pulmonary vasculature and an estimate of their frequency. This approach does not require any special instrumentation and provides more meaningful information to the clinician than a diagnostic label and a grade.

References

1. Hatano S, Strasser T, eds. Primary Pulmonary Hypertension. Report on a WHO Meeting. Geneva: World Health Organization, 1975;7–45.
2. Wagenvoort CA, Wagenvoort N. Primary pulmonary hypertension. A pathologic study of the lung vessels in 156 clinically diagnosed cases. Circulation 1970; 42: 1163–1184.

3. Kay MJ, Heath D. Pathologic study of unexplained pulmonary hypertensin. Semin Respir Med 1985; 7:180–192.
4. Bjornsson J, Edwards WD. Primary pulmonary hypertension: a histopathologic study of 80 cases. Mayo Clin Proc 1985; 60:16–25.
5. Pietra GG, Edwards WD, Kay JM, et al. Histopathology of pulmonary hypertension: a qualitative and quantitative study of pulmonary blood vessels from 58 patients in National Heart, Lung, and Blood Institute, Primary Pulmonary Hypertension Registry. Circulation 1989; 80:1198–1206.
6. Fuster V, Steele PM, Edwards WD, et al. Primary pulmonary hypertension: natural history and the importance of thrombosis. Circulation 1984; 70:580–587.
7. Hasleton PS, Heath D, Brewer D. Hypertensive pulmonary vascular disease in states of chronic hypoxia. J Pathol Bacteriol 1968; 95:431–440.
8. Naeye RL, Dellinger WS. Pulmonary arterial changes with age and smoking. Arch Pathol 1971; 92:284–288.
9. Reid LM. Vascular remodeling. In: Fishman AP, ed. The Pulmonary Circulation Normal and Abnormal. Mechanisms, Management and the National Registry. Philadelphia, University of Pennsylvania Press, 1990:259–282.
10. Magno MG, Fishman AP. Origin, distribution and blood flow of bronchial circulation in anesthetized sheep. J Appl Physiol 1982; 53:272–279.
11. Orell SR, Karnell J, Wahlgren F. Malformation and multiple stenoses of the pulmonary arteries with pulmonary hypertension. Acta Radiol 1960; 54:449–459.
12. Downing SE, Vidone RA, Brandt HM, et al. The pathogenesis of vascular lesions in experimental hyperkinetic pulmonary hypertension. Am J Pathol 1963; 43:739–765.
13. Jones R. Ultrastructural analysis of contractile cell development in lung microvessels in hyperoxic pulmonary hypertension. Fibroblasts and intermediate cells selectively reorganize nonmuscular segments. Am J Pathol 1992; 141:1491–1505.
14. Roberts WC. A simple histologic classification of pulmonary arterial hypertension. Am J Cardiol 1986; 58:385–386.
15. Palmer RMJ, Ferrige AG, Moncada S. Nitric oxide release accounts for the biological activity of endothelium-derived relaxing factor. Nature 1987; 327:524–526.
16. Coflesky JT, Evans JN. Pharmacologic properties of isolated proximal pulmonary arteries after seven-day exposure to in vivo hyperoxia. Am Rev Respir Dis 1988; 138:945–951.
17. Yanagisawa M, Kurihara H, Kimura S, et al. A novel potent vasoconstrictor peptide produced by vascular endothelial cells. Nature 1988; 332:411–415.
18. Nagao T, Vanhoutte PM. Endothelium-derived hyperpolarizing factor and endothelium-dependent relaxation. Am J Respir Cell Mol Biol 1993; 8:1–6.
19. Jones R, Zapol WM, Reid L. Pulmonary artery remodeling and pulmonary hypertension after exposure to hyperoxia for 7 days. A morphometric and hemodynamic study. Am J Pathol 1984; 117:273–285.
20. Hirata Y, Tagaki Y, Futhude Y, et al. Endothelium is a potent mitogen for rat vascular smooth muscle cells. Atherosclerosis 1989; 78:225–228.
21. Wood P. Pulmonary hypertension with special reference to the vasoconstrictive factor. Br Heart J 1959; 21:557–570.

22. Heath D, Smith P. Electron microscopy of hypertensive pulmonary vascular disease. Br J Dis Chest 1983; 77:1–13.
23. Moschowitz E, Rubin E, Strauss L. Hypertension of the pulmonary circulation due to congenital glomoid obstruction of the pulmonary arteries. Am J Pathol 1961; 39: 75–93.
24. Naeye RL, Vennart GP. Structure and significance of plexiform structures. Am J Pathol 1960; 36:593–621.
25. Tandon M, Warnock ML. Plexogenic angiopathy in pulmonary intralobar sequestrations: pathogenetic mechanisms. Hum Pathol 1993; 24:263–273.
26. Saldana ME, Harley RA, Liebow AA, et al. Experimental extreme pulmonary hypertension and vascular disease in relation to polycythemia. Am J Pathol 1968; 52: 935–981.
27. Moser KM, Bloor CM. Pulmonary vascular lesions occurring in patients with chronic major vessel thromboembolic pulmonary hypertension. Chest 1993; 103:685–692.
28. Fujinami M, Morimoto S, Nishikawa T, et al. Primary pulmonary hypertension. Study of eight autopsy cases. Acta Pathol Jpn 1987; 37:401–412.
29. Loyd JE, Atkinson JB, Pietra GG, et al. Heterogeneity of pathologic lesions in familial primary pulmonary hypertension. Am Rev Respir Dis 1988; 138:952–957.
30. Burke AP, Farb A, Virmani R. The pathology of primary pulmonary hypertension. Modern Pathol 1991; 4:269–282.
31. Naeye RL. "Primary" pulmonary hypertension with coexisting portal hypertension. A retrospective study of six cases. Circulation 1960; 22:376–384.
32. Edwards BS, Weir EK, Edwards WD, et al. Coexistent pulmonary and portal hypertension: morphologic and clinical features. J Am Coll Cardiol 1987; 10:1233–1238.
33. Saunders JB, Constable TJ, Heath D, et al. Pulmonary hypertension complicating portal vein thrombosis. Thorax 1979; 34:281–283.
34. Widgren S, Kapanci Y. Menocilbedingte pulmonale Hypertonie. Vorläufige morphologische Ergebnisse über 8 pathologisch-anatomisch untersuchte Fälle. Z Kreislaufforsch 1970; 59:924–930.
35. Pietra GG, Rüttner JR. Specificity of pulmonary vascular lesions in primary pulmonary hypertension. Respiration 1987; 52:81–85.
36. Garcia-Dorado D, Miller DD, Garcia EJ, et al. An epidemic of pulmonary hypertension after toxic rapeseed oil ingestion in Spain. J Am Coll Cardiol 1983; 1:1216–1222.
37. Gomez-Sanchez MA, Saenz De La Calzada C, Gomez-Pajuelo C, et al. Clinical and pathologic manifestations of pulmonary vascular disease in the toxic oil syndrome. J Am Coll Cardiol 1991; 18:1539–1545.
38. Coplan NL, Shimony RY, Ioachim HL, et al. Primary pulmonary hypertension associated with human immunodeficiency viral infection. Am J Med 1990; 89:96–99.
39. Speich R, Jenni R, Opravil M, et al. Primary pulmonary hypertension in HIV infection. Chest 1991; 100:1268–1271.
40. Mette SA, Palevsky HI, Pietra GG, et al. Primary pulmonary hypertension in association with human immunodeficiency virus infection: a possible viral etiology for some forms of hypertensive arteriopathy. Am Rev Respir Dis 1992; 145:1196–1200.

41. Jacques C, Richmond G, Tierney L, et al. Primary pulmonary hypertension and human immunodeficiency virus infection in a non-hemophiliac man. Hum Pathol 1992; 23:191–194.
42. Duchesne N, Gagnon JA, Fouquette B, et al. Primary pulmonary hypertension associated with HIV infection. Can Assoc Radiol J 1993; 44:39–41.
43. Bentur L, Cullinane C, Wilson P, et al. Fatal pulmonary arterial occlusive vascular disease following chemotherapy in a 9-month-old infant. Hum Pathol 1991; 22:1295–1298.
44. Kinare SG, Deshpande J. Primary pulmonary hypertension in India (autopsy study of 26 cases). Indian Heart J 1987; 39:9–15.
45. Wagenvoort CA, Mulder PGH. Thrombotic lesions in primary plexogenic arteriopathy. Similar pathogenesis or complication? Chest 1993; 103:844–849.
46. Wagenvoort CA. Lung biopsy specimens in the evaluation of pulmonary vascular disease. Chest 1980; 77:614–625.
47. Clausen KP, Geer JC. Hypertensive pulmonary arteritis. Am J Dis Child 1969; 118:718–724.
48. Okubo S, Kunieda T, Ando M, et al. Idiopathic isolated pulmonary arteritis with chronic cor pulmonale. Chest 1988; 94:665–666.
49. Lalich JI, Mercov L. Pulmonary arteritis produced in rats by feeding *Crotalaria spectabilis*. Lab Invest 1961; 10:744–750.
50. Heath D, Segel, Bishop J. Pulmonary veno-occlusive disease. Circulation 1966; 34:242–248
51. Wagenvoort CA, Wagenvoort N. The pathology of pulmonary veno-occlusive disease. Virchows Archiv A Pathol Anat 1974; 364:69–79.
52. Hasleton PS, Ironside JW, Whittaker JS, et al. Pulmonary veno-occlusive disease. A report of four cases. Histopathology 1986; 10:933–944.
53. Davies P, Reid L. Pulmonary veno-occlusive disease in siblings: case report and morphometric study. Hum Pathol 1982; 13:911–915.
54. Joselson R, Warnock M. Pulmonary veno-occlusive disease after chemotherapy. Hum Pathol 1983; 13:88–91.
55. Townend JN, Roberts DH, Jones EL, et al. Fatal pulmonary venoocclusive disease after use of oral contraceptives. Am Heart J 1992; 124:1643–1644.
56. Troussard X, Bernaudin JF, Cordonnier C, et al. Pulmonary venoocclusive disease after bone marrow transplantation. Thorax 1984; 39:956–957.
57. Hackman RC, Madtes DK, Petersen FB, et al. Pulmonary venoocclusive disease following bone marrow transplantation. Transplantation 1989; 47:989–992.
58. Pietra GG. Unpublished observations
59. Wagenvoort CA, Wagenvoort N, Takahashi T. Pulmonary veno-occlusive-disease: involvement of pulmonary arteries and review of the literature. Hum Pathol 1985; 16:1033–1041.
60. Heath D, Scott O, Lynch J. Pulmonary veno-occlusive disease. Thorax 1971; 26: 633–674.
61. McDonald PJ, Summer WR, Hutchins GM. Pulmonary veno-occlusive disease. Morphological changes suggesting a viral cause. JAMA 1981; 246:667–671.

62. Pajewski M, Reif R, Manor H, et al. Pulmonary veno-occlusive disease in a unilateral hypertransradiant lung. Thorax 1981; 36:397–399.
63. Moragas A, Hupnet P, Toran N, et al. Morphogenesis of pulmonary veno-occlusive disease in a newborn. Pathol Res Pract 1983; 176:176–184.
64. Wagenvoort CA. Capillary haemangiomatosis of the lung. Histopathology 1978; 2:401–406.
65. Whittaker JS, Pickering CAC, Heath D, et al. Pulmonary capillary haemangiomatosis. Diagn Histopathol 1983; 6:77–84.
66. Magee F, Wright JL, Kay MJ, et al. Pulmonary capillary-hemangiomatosis. Am Rev Respir Dis 1985; 132:922–925.
67. Langleben D, Heneghan J, Batten AP, et al. Familial pulmonary capillary hemangiomatosis resulting in primary pulmonary hypertension. Ann Intern Med 1988; 109:106–109.
68. Tron V, Magee F, Wright L, et al. Pulmonary capillary hemangiomatosis. Hum Pathol 1986; 17:144–1150
69. Pietra, GG. The histopathology of primary pulmonary hypertension. In: Fishman AP, ed. The Pulmonary Circulation: Normal and Abnormal. Mechanisms, Management and the National Registry. Philadelphia, University of Pennsylvania Press, 1990: 459–472.
70. Palevski HI, Schloo BL, Pietra GG, et al. Primary pulmonary hypertension. Vascular structure, morphometry, and responsiveness to vasodilator agents. Circulation 1989; 80:1207–1221.
71. Heath D, Edwards JE. The pathology of hypertensive pulmonary vascular disease. A description of six grades of structural changes in the pulmonary arteries with special reference to congenital cardial septal defects. Circulation 1958; 18:533–547.
72. Yamaki S, Tezuka F. Quantitative analysis of pulmonary vascular disease in complete transposition of the great arteries. Circulation 1976; 54:805–809.
73. Rabinowitch M, Haworth SG, Castaneda AR, et al. Lung biopsy in congenital heart disease: a morphometric approach to pulmonary vascular disease. Circulation 1978; 59:935–981.
74. Yamaki S, Wagenvoort CA. Comparison of primary plexogenic arteriopathy in adults and children. A morphometric study in 40 patients. Br Heart J 1985; 54:428.

3

Insights into the Pathogenesis of Primary Pulmonary Hypertension from Animal Models

MARLENE RABINOVITCH

University of Toronto
The Hospital for Sick Children
Toronto, Ontario, Canada

I. Introduction

Uncovering the pathogenesis of primary pulmonary hypertension (PPH) requires a great deal of detective work. Several features make this a particularly arduous task. For one, patients generally present in a very advanced state of disease in which features of the vascular lesions give few clues to how they might have been initiated (1–3). Second, the disease may have a variety of different etiological triggers, in that it is sometimes, but not always, seen in families (4,5), sometimes, but not always, observed in association with characteristics shared by autoimmune disease (e.g., Raynaud's phenomenon; 6–11), and occasionally, a toxin has been identified that may have induced the disease (12,13). In an attempt to present a unifying hypothesis related to the pathogenesis of PPH, this chapter will focus first on etiological possibilities; second, on common morphological features; and third, on findings in experimental models.

II. Etiological Possibilities

The factors that could result in fixed pulmonary vascular obstructive disease include those that are hemodynamic, hematological, or immune-related. Since similar pulmonary vascular abnormalities develop in patients with congenital heart lesions characterized by increased pulmonary artery blood flow and pressure, it has been proposed that there is abnormal vascular reactivity in the pulmonary circulation that, over many years, leads to the development of fixed structural changes. Several mechanisms could cause altered vasoreactivity leading to profound or sustained pulmonary vasoconstriction. These could include impaired release of a vasodilator, such as prostacyclin (14) or endothelial-derived relaxing factor (EDRF; 15), or alternatively, heightened release or production of a vasoconstrictor (e.g., endothelin; 16), especially if coupled with increased expression of receptors for that vasoconstrictor. The cellular mechanism may be related to a malfunction that is genetic in etiology or acquired secondary to endothelial injury.

There may also be impaired smooth-muscle relaxation as a primary defect or as a result of an injury mechanism. Despite numerous attempts, however, no vasoconstrictive mechanism has been uncovered related to PPH. Moreover, the hypothesis may be unlikely, given that hypoxic vasoconstriction causes pulmonary hypertension that is largely reversible, as it is accompanied by medial hypertrophy, but not the occlusive neointimal formation observed in PPH.

Another possibility is that there is a hypercoagulable mechanism whereby thrombi selectively form and recanalize in small pulmonary arteries. It is frequently difficult in advanced lesions to distinguish those that initially may have had a primary from those with a secondary thrombotic etiology. This is because thrombi will tend to form in partially occluded vessels when there is stasis. Moreover, some patients with PPH do have coagulation disturbances related to increased phospholipid antibodies, production of von Willebrand's factor (18,19) or protein S (20). Increased production of biologically active von Willebrand's factor (vWF) in patients with unexplained pulmonary hypertension (19,20) may predispose to platelet fibrin microthrombi, or may reflect endothelial dysfunction.

The association of Raynaud's phenomenon and autoimmune (collagen vascular) disease with pulmonary hypertension (21) suggests that there may be an immune, or inflammatory component of the pathophysiological process. This is further suggested by studies documenting pulmonary vascular disease in patients with infections such as human immunodeficiency virus (HIV; 22). Furthermore, familial PPH is associated with expression of major histocompatibility complex (MHC) loci, specifically HLADR3, DRw52, DQw2 (6). It is intriguing to speculate that the expression of these antigens predisposes to their interaction with activated T cells, as has been shown in the immune-mediated coronary arteriopathy following transplantation. The mechanism whereby an immune inflammatory reaction can lead to neointimal formation will be described later.

It is also possible that either as a primary abnormality, or as a consequence of endothelial or smooth-muscle cell injury, there may be enhanced growth factor release, activation, receptor availability, and intracellular signaling, leading to induction of smooth-muscle proliferation, migration, and extracellular matrix synthesis. The growth factors that have been implicated in vascular pathobiology include basic fibroblast growth factor (bFGF; 23), platelet-derived growth factor (PDGF; 24), transforming growth factor-β (TGF-β; 25), or insulin-like growth factor-1 (IGF-1; 26). Stimulation of connective tissue synthesis may also be a direct response to enzymatic degradation of matrix components induced by injury to the artery wall.

III. Common Structural Features

If we accept that there may be multiple etiologies that result in PPH, then uncovering the common pathogenetic mechanisms depends on identifying common structural features. Alterations in the endothelial cells appears to precede and accompany almost all forms of pulmonary hypertension (PH) described to date. Abnormalities in endothelial cells associated with pulmonary vascular changes have been described in children with congenital heart defects (27). On scanning electron microscopy, the endothelial cells in normal arteries form neat corduroy-like ridges, whereas those from hypertensive vessels are "cabled" with twisted ridges and deep gullies. It is speculated that these altered surface characteristics may influence interactions between circulating blood elements (e.g., platelets, lymphocytes, neutrophils, and vascular endothelial cells). This could result in adhesion and transendothelial migration of inflammatory cells, increased release of vasoconstrictors and growth factors, and platelet aggregation leading to thrombus formation.

Moreover, the transmission electron microscopic appearance of the endothelial cells indicates heightened metabolic functions, as there is an increased volume proportion of rough endoplasmic reticulum. In addition, there is altered organization of the cytoskeleton, evident from increased numbers of microfilament bundles. These structural abnormalities were associated with functional disturbances (i.e., increased production of vWF; 20). A further ultrastructural abnormality of significance was related to the subendothelium in patients with pulmonary hypertension. It was observed that the internal elastic lamina was fragmented, suggesting that a proteolytic enzyme that degrades elastin, an elastase, might be stimulating the remodeling process.

In congenital heart defects, pulmonary vascular disease is associated with abnormalities in the normal process of growth and remodeling of the peripheral vessels. In childhood PPH, there is also muscularization of normally nonmuscular peripheral arteries and medial hypertrophy of muscular arteries. This process is the result of differentiation, proliferation, and hypertrophy of vascular smooth-muscle cells, and an increase in intercellular connective tissue protein synthesis. Increased expression of growth factors, especially TGF-β_3, has been recently documented in pulmonary vascular lesions in adult patients with PPH (25; Fig. 1). Moreover, even in advanced lesions, there is evidence by in situ hybridization of ongoing synthesis of connective tissue (extracellular matrix) proteins (e.g., collagen, elastin, and fibronectin; 26; Fig. 2). Botney et al. (28), using an antibody that recognizes the proform of collagen, has shown that there is active collagen synthesis in advanced pulmonary vascular lesions from lungs of PPH patients who are transplant candidates.

The role of inflammatory cells in perpetuating the response was further illustrated by documenting, especially in the neointima, colocalization of macrophages in regions where there was marked expression of connective tissue protein synthesis (29,30; Fig. 3). Thus, it would seem that stimulation of connective tissue protein synthesis and cell proliferation and migration is in response to growth factors, as well as cytokines produced by infiltrating inflammatory cells.

IV. Experimental Models

Suffice it to say that, since we do not know the etiology of PPH, it has not been possible to produce a model of this disease. However, there are experimental models that share important pathogenic features of PPH, especially endothelial injury (31), and there is an experimental rat in which the mechanism of development of PPH is inherited (32,33). One of the drawbacks, however, is that, in these experimental models, the severity of the lesions observed is less than that seen in clinical PPH, perhaps because the rate of progression and the severity of the PH results in the animal's more rapid demise.

A purely vasoconstrictive model of pulmonary hypertension has been produced by prolonged indomethacin treatment (34). The fawn-hooded rat manifests, at high altitude (5280 feet; Denver, Colorado), levels of pulmonary artery pressure and resistance twice those of control rats, and this feature is associated with elevated circulating endothelin-1 levels (33). The severe pulmonary hypertension is associated with marked extension of muscle into peripheral arteries, medial hypertrophy of muscular arteries, and reduction in the number of barium-filled arteries. Pulmonary hypertension persists in these rats when backcrossed with normal rats, but is largely alleviated by exposure to 25% oxygen. The mechanism of development of the severe pulmonary hypertension at high altitude is not

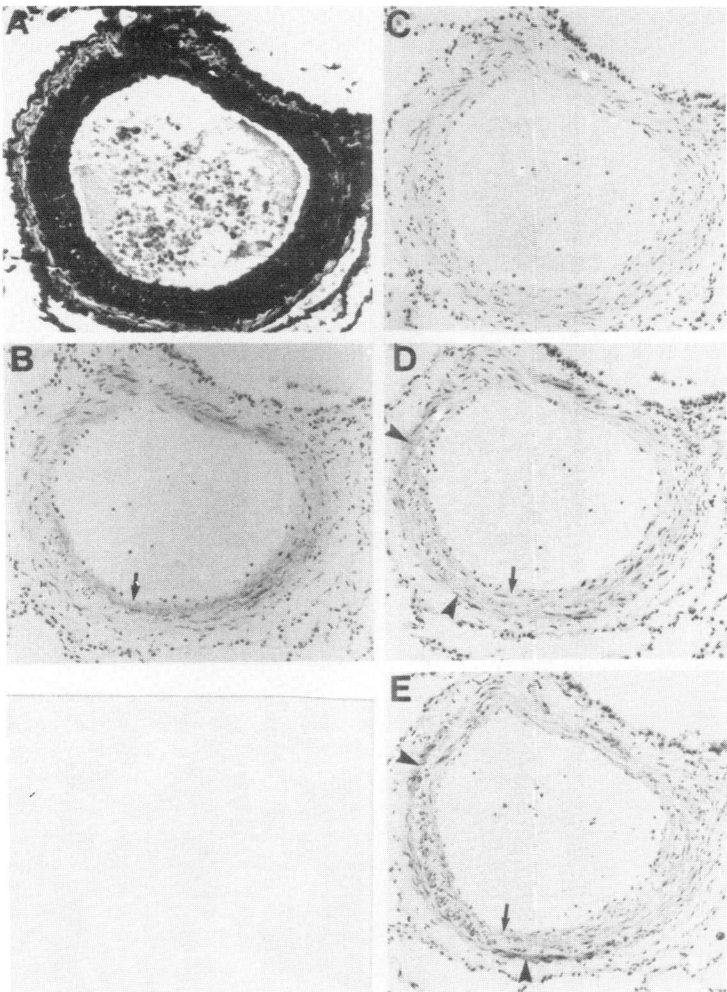

Figure 1 Procollagen and TGF-β immunohistochemistry in hypertensive pulmonary artery taken from lung removed at transplantation. (A) elastic tissue stain; (B) procollagen immunohistochemistry showing evidence of neocollagen synthesis restricted largely to the intimas; (C, D, E) immunohistochemistry with antibodies that detect TGF-β_1, TGF-β_2, and TGF-β_3, respectively. Note the positive immunostaining in the media, as well as the neointima for TGF-β_2 and TGF-β_3. (From Ref. 25.)

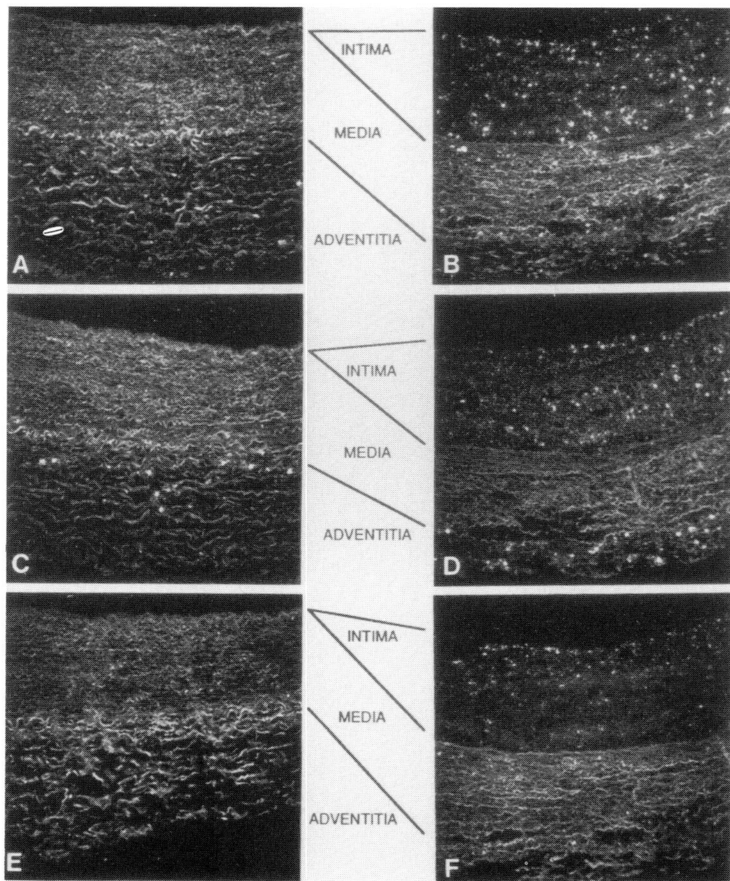

Figure 2 In situ hybridization with probes for (A, B) fibronectin, (C, D) thrombospondin, and (E, F) tropoelastin mRNA, respectively: (A, B, C) pulmonary artery from a control patient; (B, D, E) from a patient with primary pulmonary hypertension. Note the increased hybridization signal for all these matrix proteins in the hypertensive pulmonary artery, fibronectin being predominantly expressed in the neointima; little signal is seen in the control vessel (A). Thrombospondin is seen in the neointima and adventitia of the hypertensive artery (D), but there are only a few cells, presumably macrophages, in the adventitia that express signal in the control vessel (C). There is no expression of tropoelastin mRNA in the control vessel (E), but there is signal in the intima primarily in the hypertensive artery (F). (From Ref. 30.)

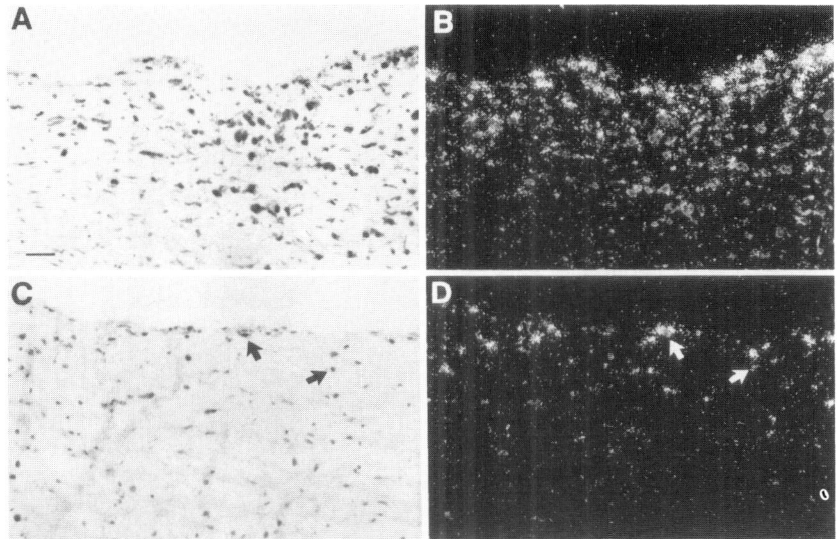

Figure 3 Macrophage immunohistochemistry and procollagen in situ hybridization. Sequential immunohistochemistry in situ hybridization was performed on the same tissue sections of hypertensive lobar pulmonary arteries to evaluate the spatial relationship between macrophages and neointimal cells expressing type I procollagen mRNA. Immunohistochemistry was performed with HAM 36, and in situ hybridization was performed with [^{35}S]-labeled Hf677 antisense cRNA probe. A close relationship is observed between nonfoamy macrophages and procollagen gene expression (A and B; × 400). There is little procollagen gene expression in areas with few macrophages (C and D; × 400). Bright field (A and C), dark field (B and D). (From Ref. 29.)

known, but these animals clearly have a genetic predisposition to acute hyperreactivity to hypoxia.

The sheep air embolization model of pulmonary hypertension is the result of endothelial injury and the rapid induction of an inflammatory response, as evidenced by increases in lung lymph flow (36). After a short exposure, there is muscularization of peripheral arteries, medial hypertrophy of muscular arteries, intimal hyperplasia of preacinar arteries, and a very striking loss of distal arteries (36). Similar changes can be produced with *Escherichia coli* endotoxin administration (37). Since specific induction of inflammatory mediators has not been shown in either model, it is not known how endothelial injury might perpetrate the structural abnormalities. Increased expression of some growth factors has been shown and these include transforming growth factor (TGF)-β, both in situ in small vessels (38) (Fig. 4), and in lung lymph (37), as well as insulin-like growth

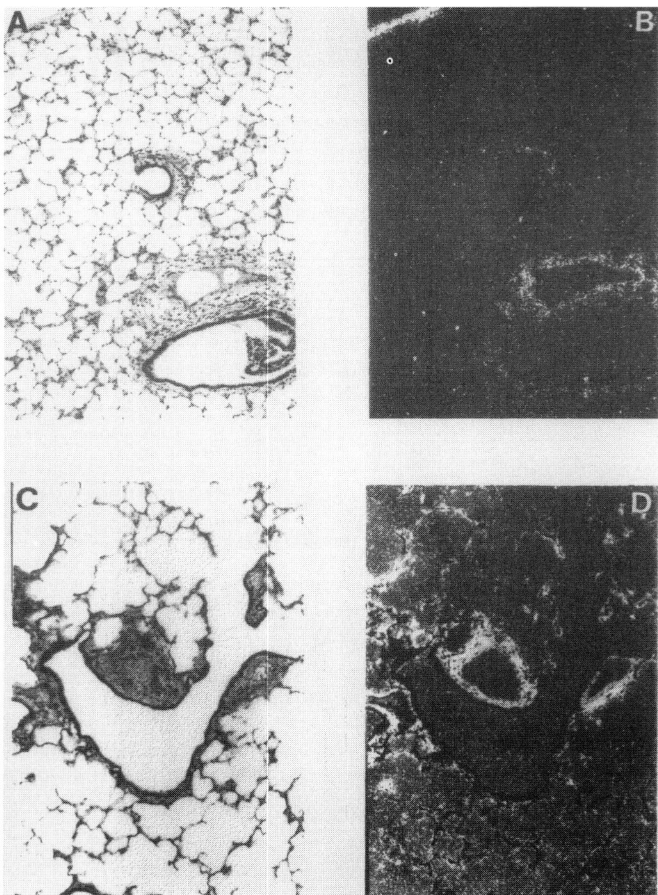

Figure 4 In a control sheep lung in situ hybridization for TGF-β_3 is seen around a muscular artery associated with a large preacinar, but not smaller (respiratory) bronchiole. (A) Light microscopy is shown for orientation, and (B) shows darkfield in situ hybridization. By day 8 after air embolization, (C) the circulation is remodeled and several muscular arteries are present around a terminal bronchiolus shown (for orientation) on light microscopy and (D) are demonstrating intense TGF-β_3 expression by in situ hybridization (dark field). (From Ref. 38.)

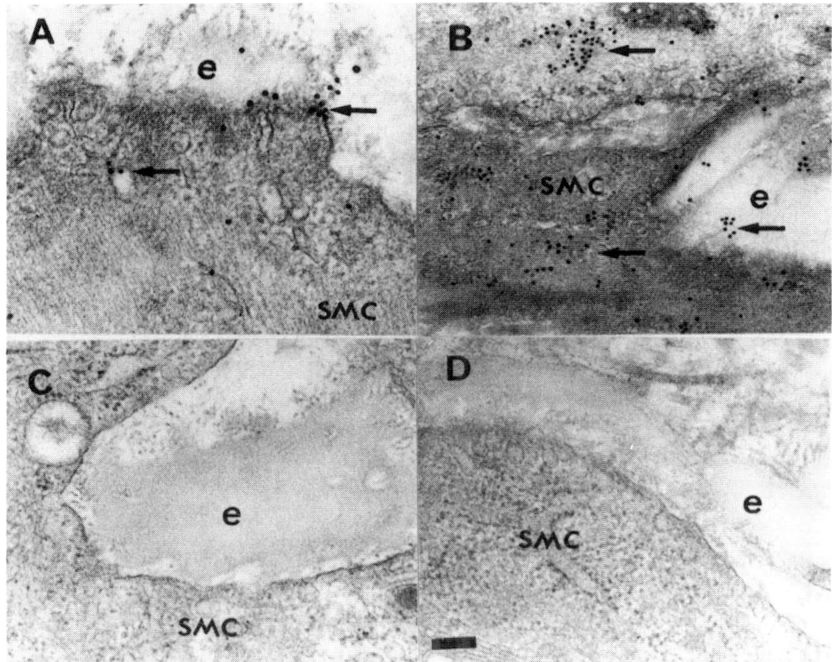

Figure 5 Representative immunoelectron photomicrographs using a polyclonal antibody raised in a rabbit to the adipsin sequence: Cys-Ala-Glu-Ser-Asn-Arg-Arg-Asp. Goat anti-rabbit antibody was conjugated with 15-nm gold particles and hybridized to the adipsin antibody reflecting the antigenic sites (arrows). (A) A smooth-muscle cell (SMC) from a rat pulmonary artery 28 days after injection of monocrotaline shows adipsin antigenic sites related to the cell surface, to secretory vesicles, and in close proximity with elastin (e). (B) The antibody is seen more extensively over the SMC. (C) The antibody has been preabsorbed to an adipsin affinity column and no, or only rare, antigenic sites were apparent on the tissue. (D) The tissue was immunoreacted with normal rabbit serum and there are positive sites (magnification 48, 600 ×). (From Ref. 46.)

factor-1 (39). These growth factors are associated with the induction of connective tissue protein (especially elastin); synthesis and increased elastin peptides are found in the lung lymph of these animals (40). In addition, these may induce other growth-related effects, such as smooth-muscle cell proliferation or migration, either directly or indirectly (e.g., as a result of TGF-β activation of the PDGF B chain).

The rat monocrotaline model of pulmonary hypertension is probably the most extensively studied to date. Monocrotaline is a toxin that has been used to induce structural changes in the pulmonary arteries of rats and associated progres-

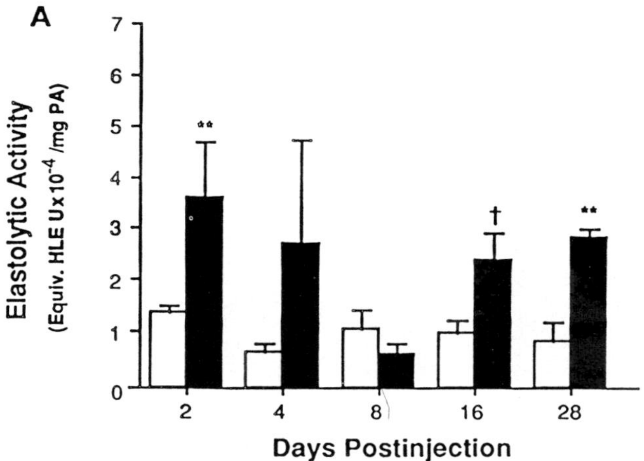
A
Elastolytic Activity
(Equiv. HLE U x 10^{-4} /mg PA)
7
6
5
4
3
2
1
0
**
†
**
2
4
8
16
28
Days Postinjection

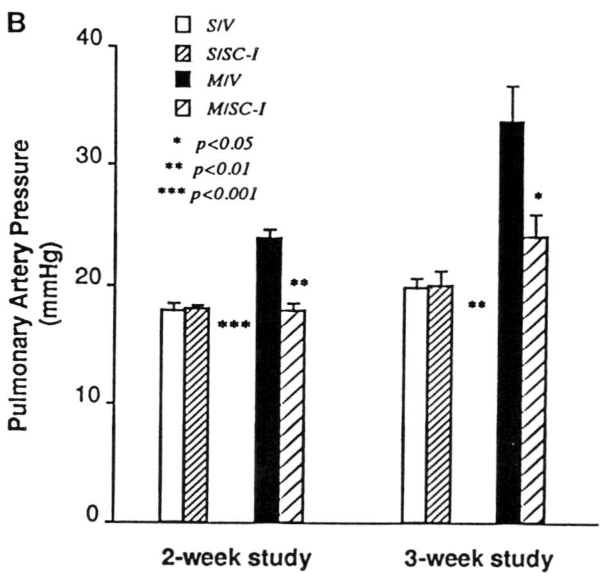
B
S/V
S/SC-I
M/V
M/SC-I
* p<0.05
** p<0.01
*** p<0.001
Pulmonary Artery Pressure
(mmHg)
40
30
20
10
0
***
**
**
*
2-week study
3-week study

sive pulmonary hypertension (31,40–43). The mechanism of action is unknown, but just a single subcutaneous injection of the toxin in a rat results in a cascade of vascular abnormalities that appear to be initiated by endothelial injury seen as early as several days later. There is no increase in pulmonary vascular reactivity, nor does the pulmonary artery pressure rise until 12 days, when there is substantial evidence of vascular changes, including muscularization of distal vessels and medial hypertrophy of muscular arteries. There is a further progressive increase in mean pulmonary artery pressure and associated vascular changes that result in the animal's death 4–6 weeks after injection.

Although there is an increase in ornithine decarboxylase activity and in polyamines (44,45) in association with monocrotaline-induced pulmonary hypertension, it was not known how this reflected the etiological mechanism of vascular differentiation. However, there was high turnover of elastin in the pulmonary artery wall, as judged by synthesis levels that were tenfold higher than values reflecting accumulation of elastin (40). Moreover, the association of breaks in the elastic lamina with early endothelial injury suggested that an elastolytic enzyme might be active in stimulating vascular remodeling (42). There was also increased activity of a serine elastase, expressed both early after injection of the toxin before the development of vascular changes, as well as at a later time point associated with their progression (42). A cause and effect relationship was further established

---

Figure 6 (A) Central pulmonary artery elastolytic activity in adult rats both controls injected with saline (open bars) and experimental animals injected with the toxin, monocrotaline (closed bars). Values are normalized per milligram pulmonary artery (PA) tissue and standardized against a curve generated with human leukocyte elastase (HLE). There is a significant increase in elastase activity only 2 days after injection of the toxin ($p < 0.01$). By 8 days, values are at control level, but with the development of medial hypertrophy at 16 days ($p < 0.054$) and with its progression at 28 days, there is a second rise in elastase activity. The second rise in elastase activity is seen only in the adult monocrotaline rats in which pulmonary artery hypertension is malignant and progressive, but is not seen in hypoxic rats or in rats injected with monocrotaline as infants in which pulmonary hypertension is potentially reversible. (B) Pulmonary artery pressure values are seen in control rats injected with saline and vehicle (S/V) or an elastase inhibitor (S/SC-I), a product of Searle (SC-37698), rats injected with monocrotaline and vehicle (M/V), or monocrotaline and the elastase inhibitor (M/SC-I). A 2-week infusion of the elastase in vitro shows no rise in pulmonary artery pressure in the M/SC-I group when compared with M/V. In the 3-week study, the elastase inhibitor was given for the second 2 weeks of a 3-week experimental period. Pulmonary artery hypertension was significantly reduced in the monocrotaline injected group (M/SC-I) compared with M/V, but values were higher than in S/V or S/SC-I. * denotes *p* values representing differences between saline and monocrotaline or monocrotaline with and without the elastase inhibitor. $*$ denotes *p* values representing differences between saline and monocrotaline or mono crotaline with and without the elastase inhibitor. (From A: Ref 42; B, Ref. 41.)

in studies in which serine elastase inhibitors were administered that effectively prevented the rise in elastase in the arterial wall, the vascular changes, and the pulmonary hypertension (41,43; Fig. 5). Moreover, using elastase inhibitors to inhibit the second rise in elastase activity retarded the progression of vascular disease. Subsequent molecular and biochemical studies have identified a relationship between this enzyme and the serine proteinase, adipsin, and have localized the source of the enzyme primarily to the smooth-muscle cells of the vessel wall (46; Fig. 6).

The mechanism of activation and release of elastase may be related to infiltration of a serum factor, or to release of an endothelial factor into the

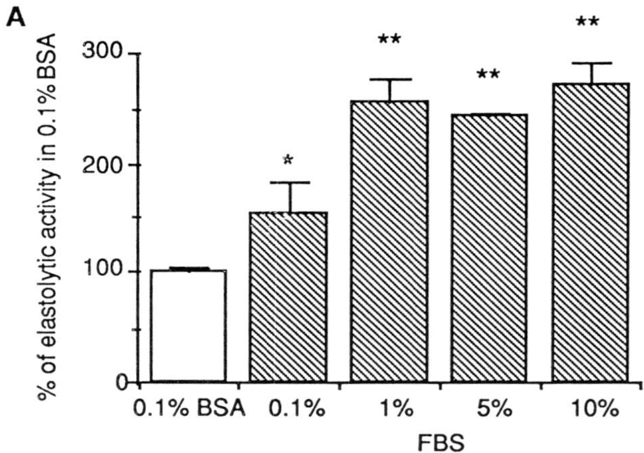

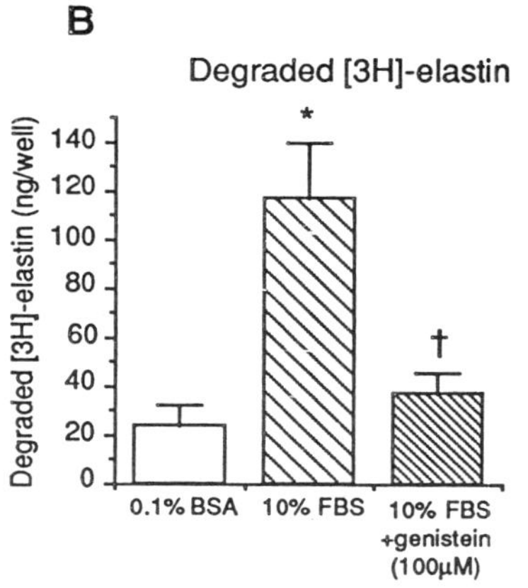

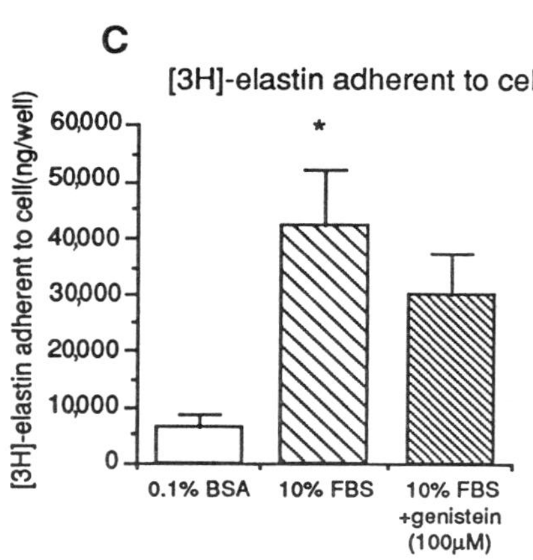

subendothelium when there is endothelial injury (47). Serum stimulation leads to the increased activity of elastase from pulmonary artery smooth-muscle cells, and the mechanism appears to involve increased binding of elastin to the elastin-binding protein on smooth-muscle cell surfaces and to tyrosine kinase activity (47; Fig. 7).

The increased activity of elastase in the monocrotaline-injected rat seems critical to the pathophysiological evolution of the disease process. We have speculated on how increased activity of an elastolytic enzyme might stimulate the remodeling process (Fig. 8). First, elastase could activate or induce the release of growth factors normally stored in the extracellular matrix in an inactive form, such as bFGF and TGF-β (48–50). These growth factors are known to induce smooth-muscle hypertrophy and proliferation and increases in connective tissue protein (e.g., collagen and elastin) synthesis (50,51). Continued elastase activity will also induce connective tissue protein synthesis through release of elastin peptides (52). Elastase activity could cause migration of smooth-muscle cells in two ways; first, perhaps by removing a physical barrier; and second, by changing the cell extracellular matrix-signaling processes so that a new constellation of gene products would be produced, providing the smooth-muscle cells with the machinery necessary to switch from the contractile to motile phenotype (49,53,54).

Models of systemic vascular pathobiology might also shed light on the pathophysiology of PPH. We have investigated the pathogenesis of accelerated coronary arteriopathy in piglets after heterotopic heart transplantation (55–63). The process is related to immune and inflammatory mechanisms. There is an increased expression of MHC II antigens on donor coronary artery endothelial cell surfaces (55), as well as of the adhesion molecules, VCAM-1 and ICAM-1, early after heart transplantation (63). There is also evidence of up-regulation of cytokines, interleukin (IL)-1β and tumor necrosis factor (TNF)-α, and increased accumulation of the extracellular matrix component fibronectin. By culturing coronary artery endothelial and smooth-muscle cells, we were able to show that

---

Figure 7 (A) Serum induction of elastolytic activity in fetal lamb pulmonary artery (PA) smooth-muscle cells (SMC). The data are represented as an increase in elastolytic activity over that under serum-free conditions (i.e., 0.1% bovine serum albumin; BSA). There was significant elastolysis with a fetal bovine serum (FBS) concentration of only 0.1% ($^*p < 0.05$) and maximum activity was evident with a concentration of 1% ($^{**}p < 0.01$), with no further increase observed using 5 or 10% FBS. Values represent mean ±SE of three separate assays. (B) Effect of genistein on elastase activity and serum-induced elastin adhesion to smooth-muscle cells (SMC). Ten percent FBS induced both elastin adhesion and elastolytic activity, compared with 0.1% BAS ($^*p < 0.01$) (A and B). Serum-induced elastolytic activity was, however, significantly inhibited by genistein (100 μ*M*) ($^{\dagger}p < 0.01$) (A) without a significant reduction in elastin adhesion to SMC (C). Values are mean ± standard error of three separate assays. (From Ref. 47.)

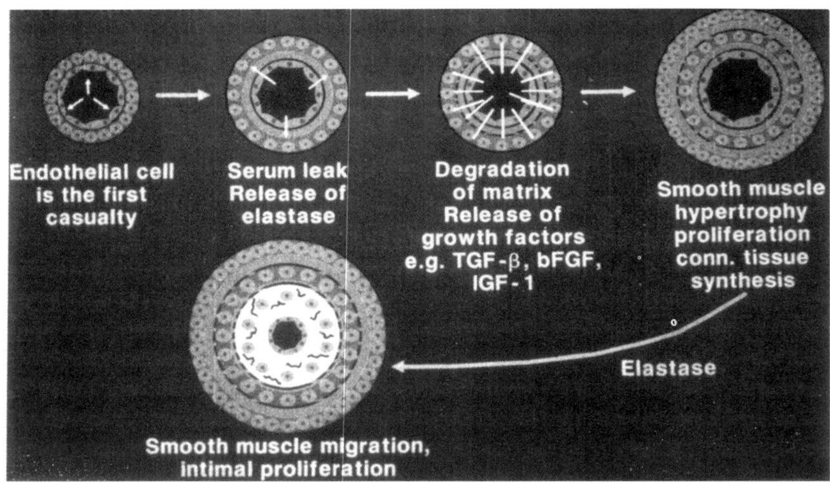

Figure 8 We have speculated as to how a stimulus might induce activity of an elastolytic enzyme and how this might stimulate the remodeling process. The process of progressive pulmonary hypertension involves a series of switches in the smooth-muscle cell phenotype (i.e., differentiation of muscle from nonmuscle precursor cells, smooth-muscle cell hypertrophy, and proliferation accounting for medial hypertrophy, and smooth-muscle cell migration resulting in neointimal formation). In response to a stimulus, such as high flow and pressure, the first "casualty" could be the endothelial cell. As a result of structural and functional alterations in endothelial cells, some of the barrier function would be lost; allowing a leak into the subendothelium of a serum factor normally excluded from this region. The serum factor could induce activity of an endogenous vascular elastase. This enzyme released from precursor or mature smooth muscle cells would activate growth factors normally stored in the extracellular matrix in a inactive form, such as basic fibroblast growth factor and transforming growth factor-β, which are known to induce smooth-muscle hypertrophy and proliferation and increases in connective tissue protein (e.g., collagen and elastin) synthesis. This would result in the differentiation of precursor cells to mature smooth muscle related to the muscularization of normally nonmuscular small peripheral arteries. In the muscular arteries, the release of growth factors would result in hypertrophy of the vessel wall. Continued elastase activity would cause migration of smooth-muscle cells in two ways, first perhaps by removing a physical barrier and also by so changing the cell extracellular matrix-signaling processes that a new constellation of gene products would be produced, thereby providing the smooth-muscle cells with the machinery necessary to switch from the contractile to motile phenotype. (From Ref. 65.)

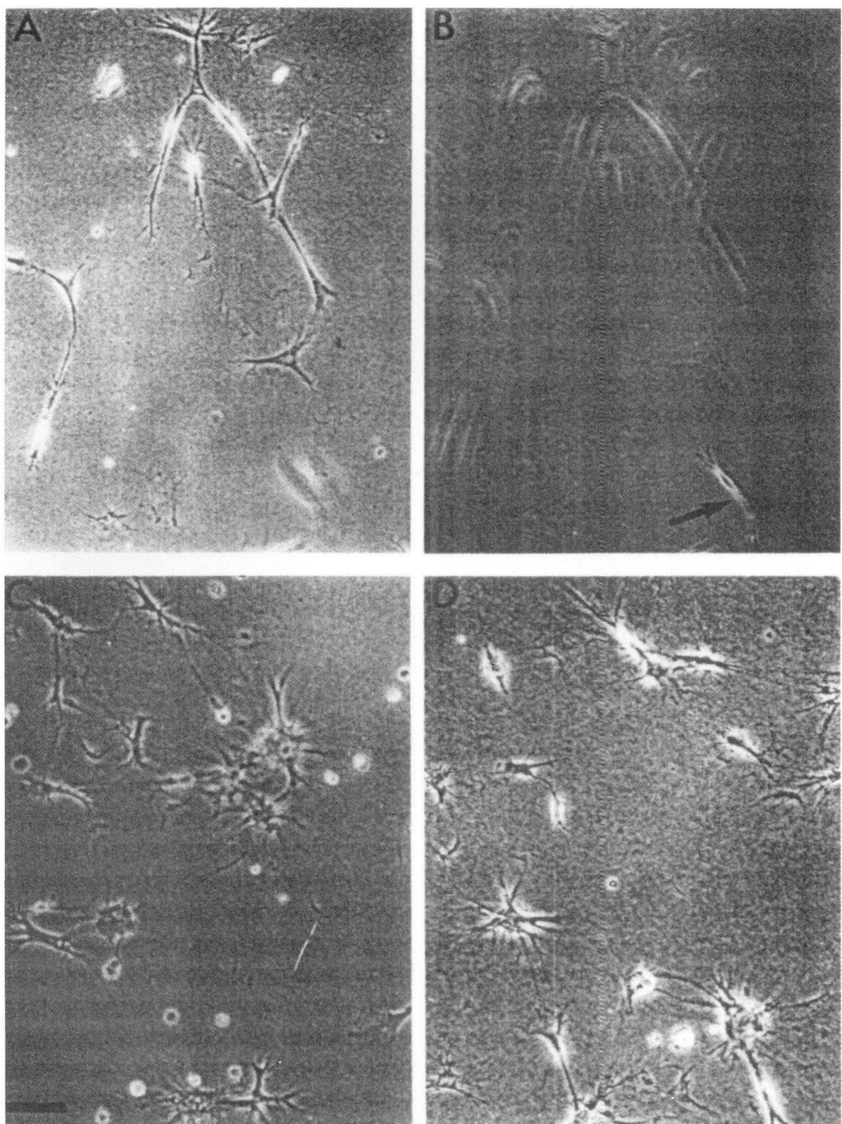

Figure 9 DA and Ao smooth-muscle cells on collagen (2 mg/ml) gels: (A) DA smooth muscle cells 2 days following seeding onto the surface of collagen gels. The cells exhibit a spindle-like elongated morphology, and the majority of cells are visible on the surface of the gels. The arrow in B indicates the outline of a cell that has migrated below the surface of the gel. By focusing into the gel at a depth of 250 μm (B), this cell comes clearly into focus. (C) Ao cells, 2 days following seeding onto the surface of the gel, exhibit a flattened, stellate morphology. In the presence of antibodies against fibronectin (1:100), DA smooth-muscle cells (D) also display a more flattened, stellate appearance. (From Ref. 54.)

there was induction of fibronectin synthesis by up-regulation of endogenous IL-1β in both endothelial and smooth-muscle cells. Moreover, there was likely reciprocal coinduction of tumor necrosis factor and IL-1β in the coronary arteries.

From this information, we were able to show that TNF receptor blockade effectively reduced by 50% the number of vessels with neointimal formation and the severity of the lesions in the affected vessels (57). Moreover, expression of adhesion molecules, induction of fibronectin, and infiltration of T cells were reduced, as judged by immunostaining of the tissue. We speculated that the increased subendothelial accumulation of fibronectin might have a dual role. We had previously demonstrated that increased production of fibronectin accounts for the enhanced migration seen in smooth-muscle cells cultured from the ductus, compared with the aorta (54; Fig. 9). In addition to directing a change in smooth-muscle cell phenotype, perhaps the increased production of fibronectin might also serve to traffic smooth-muscle cells into the subendothelium (64). This is based on interactions between peptides in fibronectin (RGD and CS-1) and receptors on lymphocytes ($\alpha4\ B_1$ and $\alpha5\ B_1$, respectively). With an in vitro endothelial smooth-muscle cell coculture system, CS-1 peptides effectively blocked transendothelial migration of lymphocytes following IL-1-mediated up-regulation of smooth-muscle cell fibronectin (59). Moreover, injection of CS-1 peptides also proved effective in reducing, by greater than 50%, the number of vessels with intimal proliferation and the severity of the lesions (62). It is of further interest that, in the donor compared with the host coronary arteries, there is also increased fragmentation of elastin associated with a fourfold or greater increase in elastase activity (61). This enzyme, similar to the endogenous vascular elastase found in pulmonary hypertension, is expressed as a 20-kDa serine elastase on a substrate gel. We have further preliminary evidence that cytokines may induce the release of this elastase and that the elastase may play an integral role, through the release of elastin peptides, in the upregulation of fibronectin.

It is possible that, if immune mediation plays a role in the pathogenesis of PPH, then mechanisms similar to those described in the coronary arteries in graft arteriopathy may be operational. Thus, further studies should be directed at exploring the possible influence of transendothelial lymphocyte migration and cytokine expression. Also, uncovering the molecular mechanisms regulating fibronectin as well as elastase expression in the pathobiology of vascular disease should provide highly targeted therapeutic strategies.

References

1. Wagenvoort CA, Wagenvoort N. Primary pulmonary hypertension: a pathological study of the lung vessels in 136 clinically diagnosed cases. Circulation 1970; 42:1163–1184.

2. Pietra GG, et al. Histopathology of primary pulmonary hypertension: a qualitative and quantitative study of pulmonary blood vessels from 58 patients in the National Heart, Lung and Blood Institute Primary Pulmonary Hypertension Registry. Circulation 1989; 80:1198–1206.
3. Rich S, et al. Primary pulmonary hypertension: a national prospective study. Ann Intern Med 1977; 107:216–223.
4. Puolijoki HJ, et al. Unexplained severe pulmonary hypertension in two brothers. Eur Respir J 1990; 3:349–53.
5. Morse JH, et al. Familial pulmonary hypertension: immunogenetic findings in four Caucasian kindreds. Am Rev Respir Dis 1992; 145:787–792.
6. Barst RJ, et al. Evidence for the association of unexplained pulmonary hypertension in children with the major histocompatibility complex. Circulation 1992; 85:249–58.
7. Lloyd JE, et al. Familial primary pulmonary hypertension. Clinical patterns. Am Rev Respir Dis 1984; 129:194–197.
8. Rich S, et al. Antinuclear antibodies in primary pulmonary hypertension. J Am Coll Cardiol 1986; 8:1307–1311.
9. Padeh S, et al. Primary pulmonary hypertension in a patient with systemic-onset juvenile arthritis. Arthritis Rheum 1991; 34:1575–1579.
10. Gladman DD. Increased frequency of HLA-DRw52 in systemic sclerosis. Arthritis Rheum 1990; 33:R35.
11. Asherson RA, et al. Pulmonary hypertension in a lupus clinic: experience with twenty-four patients. J Rheum 1990; 17:1292–1298.
12. Gomez-Sanchez MA, et al. Clinical and pathologic manifestations of pulmonary vascular disease in the toxic oil syndrome. J Am Coll Cardiol 1991; 18:1539–1545.
13. Fishman AP. Dietary pulmonary hypertension. Circ Res 1974; 35:657–660.
14. Christman BW, et al. An imbalance between the excretion of thromboxane and prostacylin metabolites in pulmonary hypertension. N Engl J Med 1992; 327:70–75.
15. Dinh Xuan AT, et al. Impairment of endothelial dependent pulmonary artery relaxation in chronic obstructive lung disease. N Engl J Med 1991; 324:1539–1547.
16. Stewart DJ, et al. Increased plasma endothelin-1 in pulmonary hypertension; marker or mediator of disease. Ann Intern Med 1991; 114:464–496.
17. Luchi ME, et al. Primary idiopathic pulmonary hypertension complicated by pulmonary arterial thrombosis. Association with antiphospholipid antibodies. Arthritis Rheum 1992; 35:700–705.
18. O'Sullivan J, et al. Protein S deficiency: early presentation and pulmonary hypertension. Arch Dis Child 1992; 67:960–961.
19. Geggel RL. von Willebrand factor abnormalities in primary pulmonary hypertension. Am Rev Respir Dis 1987; 135:294–299.
20. Turner-Gomes SO, et al. Abnormalities in von Willebrand factor and antithrombin III after cardiopulmonary bypass operations for congenital heart disease. J Thorac Cardiovasc Surg 1992; 103:87–97.
21. Winters WL, et al. "Primary" pulmonary hypertension with Raynaud's phenomenon. Arch Intern Med 1964; 114:822–830.
22. Polos PG, et al. Pulmonary hypertension and human immunodeficiency virus infection. Two reports and a review of the literature. Chest 1992; 101:474–478.

23. Lindner V, et al. Role of basic fibroblast growth factor in vascular lesion formation. Circ Res 1991; 63:106–113.
24. Pierce GF, et al. Platelet-derived growth factor β and transforming growth factors induce in vivo and in vitro tissue repair activities by unique mechanisms. J Cell Biol 1989; 109:429–440.
25. Botney MD, et al. Vascular remodeling in primary pulmonary hypertension. Potential role for transforming growth factor β. Am J Pathol 1994; 144:286–295.
26. Perkett EA, et al. Insulin-like growth factor 1 and pulmonary hypertension induced by continuous air embolization in sheep. Am J Respir Cell Mol Biol 1992; 6:82–87.
27. Boudreau N, Rabinovitch M. Developmentally regulated changes in extracellular matrix in endothelial and smooth muscle cells in the ductus arteriosus may be related to intimal proliferation. Lab Invest 1991; 64:187–199.
28. Botney MD, et al. Active collagen synthesis by pulmonary arteries in human primary pulmonary hypertension. Am J Pathol 1993; 143:121–129.
29. Liptay MJ, et al. Neointimal macrophages colocalize with extracellular matrix gene expression in human atherosclerotic pulmonary arteries. J Clin Invest 1993; 91: 588–594.
30. Botney MD, et al. Extracellular matrix protein gene expression in atherosclerotic hypertensive pulmonary arteries. Am J Pathol 1992; 140:357–364.
31. Rosenberg HC, Rabinovitch M. Endothelial injury and vascular reactivity in monocrotaline pulmonary hypertension. Am J Physiol 1988; 255:H1484–H1491.
32. Stelzner TJ, et al. Increased lung endothelin-1 production in rats with idiopathic pulmonary hypertension. Am J Physiol 1992; 262(5 Pt 1):L614–L620.
33. Sato K, et al. Factors influencing the idiopathic development of pulmonary hypertension in the fawn hooded rat. Am Rev Respir Dis 1992; 145:793–797.
34. Meyrick BO, et al. Pulmonary hypertension and increased vasoreactivity caused by repeat indomethacin in sheep. J Appl Physiol 1985; 59:443–452.
35. Meyrick BO, Brigham KL. Acute effects of *Escherichia coli* endotoxin on the pulmonary microcirculation of anesthetized sheep: structure, function relationships. Lab Invest 1983; 48:458–470.
36. Perkett EA, et al. Continuous air embolization into sheep causes sustained pulmonary hypertension and increased pulmonary vasoreactivity. Am J Physiol 1988; 132: 444–454.
37. Perkett EA, et al. Transforming growth factor-β activity in sheep lung lymph during the development of pulmonary hypertension. J Clin Invest 1990; 86:1459–1464.
38. Perkett EA, Pelton RW, Meyrick B, Gold LI, Miller DA. Expression of transforming growth factor beta mRNA and proteins in pulmonary vascular remodelling in the sheep embolization model of pulmonary hypertension. Am J Respir Cell Mol Biol 1994; 11:16–24.
39. Perkett EA, et al. Sequences of structural changes and elastic peptide release during vascular remodelling in sheep with chronic pulmonary hypertension induced by air embolization. Am J Pathol 1991; 139:1319–1332.
40. Todorovich-Hunter L, et al. Altered elastin and collagen synthesis associated with progressive pulmonary hypertension induced by monocrotaline: a biochemical and ultrastructural study. Lab Invest 1988; 58:184–195.

41. Ye C, Rabinovitch M. Inhibition of elastolysis by SC-37698 reduces development and progression of monocrotaline pulmonary hypertension. Am J Physiol 1991; 261: H1255–H1267.
42. Todorovich-Hunter L, et al. Increased pulmonary artery elastolytic activity in adult rats with monocrotaline-induced progressive hypertensive pulmonary vascular disease compared with infant rats with nonprogressive disease. Am Rev Respir Dis 1992; 146:213–223.
43. Shemie S, Rabinovitch M. The effect of alpha-1 antitrypsin inhibition of early elastase release on the pathophysiology of progressive pulmonary hypertension. Am Rev Respir Dis 1993; 147:A–495.
44. Olson JW, et al. Prolonged activation of rat lung ornithine decarboxylase in monocrotaline-induced pulmonary hypertension. Biochem Pharmacol 1984; 3:3633–3637.
45. Olson JW, et al. Polyamines and the development of monocrotaline-induced pulmonary hypertension. Am J Physiol 1984; 247:H682–H685.
46. Zhu L, et al. The endogenous vascular elastase which governs development and progression of monocrotaline-induced pulmonary hypertension in rats is a novel enzyme related to the serine proteinase adipsin. J Clin Invest 1994; 94:1163–1171.
47. Kobayashi J, et al. Serum-induced vascular smooth muscle cell elastolytic activity through tyrosine kinase intracellular signalling. J Cell Physiol 1994; 160:121–131.
48. Taipale J, et al. Release of transforming growth factor-β1 from the pericellular matrix of cultured fibroblasts and fibrosarcoma cells by plasmin and thrombin. J Biol Chem 1992; 267:25378–25384.
49. Sato Y, Rifkin DB. Inhibition of endothelial cell movement by pericytes and smooth muscle cells: activation of a latent transforming growth factor-β1-like molecule by plasmin during co-culture. J Cell Biol 1989; 109:309–315.
50. Klagsburn M, Edelman ER. Biological and biochemical properties of fibroblast growth factor. Arteriosclerosis 1989; 9:269–278.
51. Quaglino D, et al. Transforming growth factor β stimulates wound healing and modulates extracellular matrix gene expression in pig skin. Lab Invest 1990; 63:317–319.
52. Foster JA, et al. Pulmonary fibroblast, an in vitro model of emphysema. Regulation of elastin gene expression. J Biol Chem 1990; 265:1444–1449.
53. Madri JA, William SK. Capillary endothelial cell cultures: phenotypic modulation by matrix components. J Cell Biol 1983; 97:153–165.
54. Boudreau N, et al. Fibronectin, hyaluronan and a hyaluronan binding protein contribute to increased ductus arteriosus smooth muscle cell migration. Dev Biol 1991; 143:235–247.
55. Clausell N, et al. Increased interleukin-1β and fibronectin expression are early features of the development of the post-cardiac transplant coronary arteriopathy in piglets. Am J Pathol 1993; 142:1772–1786.
56. Clausell N, Rabinovitch M. Upregulation of fibronectin synthesis by interleukin-1β in coronary artery smooth muscle cells is associated with the development of the post-cardiac transplant arteriopathy in piglets. J Clin Invest 1992; 92:1850–1858.
57. Molossi S, et al. Coronary artery endothelial interleukin-1β mediates enhanced fibronectin production related to post-cardiac transplant arteriopathy in piglets. Circulation 1993; 88:248–256.

58. Clausell N, et al. In vivo blockade of tumor necrosis factor-α in cholesterol-fed rabbits after cardiac transplant inhibits acute coronary artery neointimal formation. Circulation 1994; 89:2768–2779.
59. Molossi S, Elices M, Arrhenius T, Rabinovitch M. Lymphocyte transendothelial migration toward smooth muscle cells in interleukin-1β stimulated cocultures is related to fibronectin interactions with α4β1 and α5β1 integrins. J Cell Physiol 1995; 164:620–633.
60. Molossi S, Clausell N, Rabinovitch M. Reciprocal induction of tumor necrosis factor-α and interleukin-1β activity mediates fibronectin synthesis in coronary artery smooth muscle cells. J Cell Physiol 1995; 163:19–29.
61. Oho S, Rabinovitch M. Post-cardiac transplant arteriopathy in piglets is associated with fragmentation of elastin and increased activity of a serine elastase. Am J Pathol 1994; 145:202–210.
62. Molossi S, Elices M, Arrhenius T, Diaz R, Coulber C, Rabinovitch M. Blockade of very late antigen-4 integrin binding to fibronectin with CS1 peptide reduces accelerated coronary arteriopathy in rabbit cardiac allografts. J Clin Invest 1995; 95: 2601–2610.
63. Molossi S, Clausell N, Sett S, Rabinovitch M. ICAM-1 and VCAM-1 expression in accelerated cardiac allograft arteriopathy and myocardial rejection are influenced differently by cyclosporine-A and tumor necrosis factor-α blockade. J Pathol 1995; 176:175–182.
64. Ager A, Humphries MJ. Use of synthetic peptides to probe lymphocyte-high endothelial cell interactions: lymphocytes recognize a ligand on the endothelial surface which contains the CS1 adhesion motif. Intern Immunol 1991; 2:921–928.
65. Rabinovitch M. Elastase, remodeling of the extracellular matrix, and pulmonary hypertension. Semin Respir Crit Care Med 1994; 15:199–206.

4

Pathophysiology of Primary Pulmonary Hypertension: From Physiology to Molecular Mechanisms

NORBERT F. VOELKEL and RUBIN M. TUDER

University of Colorado Health Sciences Center
Denver, Colorado

E. KENNETH WEIR

University of Minnesota
and Department of Veterans Affairs Medical Center
Minneapolis, Minnesota

"The end is where we start from."
T. S. Eliot

I. Introduction

Our understanding of the pathogenesis and pathophysiology of so-called primary pulmonary hypertension has advanced rather slowly during the last decade, to a large degree because of lack of information about the early stages of the disease process. Primary pulmonary hypertension (PPH) remains a diagnosis of exclusion, which is reflected in the clinically useful term "unexplained pulmonary hypertension." Thus, primary pulmonary hypertension is an unexplained disease restricted to the vessels of the lung. All hemodynamic studies of patients with PPH show high pulmonary arterial pressure and resistance to blood flow through the lung circulation. High shear stress in the system occurs, in principle either because of a dramatic change in the vasomotor tone or in the geometry of the vessels. It follows then that the categorical lines of pathophysiological investigation continue to focus on vascular tone regulation and on vascular remodeling.

Vessels are semistable systems undergoing continuous remodeling, under the influence of shear stress, of dietary factors, or of oxidant stress. It appears that the vascular endothelium is the integrator of the factors prevailing in the pathophysiological milieu and that endothelial cell biology is of great importance in vascular remodeling. The endothelium provides a permeability barrier and generates factors that control the contractile machinery of the smooth-muscle cells.

The endothelial cells can produce, bind, and amplify signals that affect vascular tone and cause cell proliferation and differentiation. Growth factors, cytokines, and hormones interact with specific membrane receptors and trigger a cascade of intracellular signals, resulting in activation or repression of various genes (1). One hypothesis that is developed in this chapter is that vasoconstriction (shear stress) and cell proliferation use overlapping signaling processes that result in common intracellular events. Therefore, vasoconstriction and vascular remodeling constitute two linked phenomena in the lung circulation. A second hypothesis is that only *susceptible* individuals—those with a genetic disposition—develop severe forms of pulmonary hypertension including PPH. The following schematic (Fig. 1) integrates the important components of this model hypothesis. The model is open and unbiased, assigning a primary or initiating role to either vasoconstriction or proliferation. The model further considers that *progressive* disease results from a vicious cycle in which shear stress and vasoproliferation are mutually enhancing. Although, as stated, we lack information on the vascular morphological changes in early PPH, pathologists continue to operate with the concept of early and advanced lesions (2,3).

What factors are critically involved in the development and maturation of the vascular lesions? Do inflammatory cells and inflammatory mediators participate? We expect that the answer to these questions could result in new therapeutic approaches in patients with PPH.

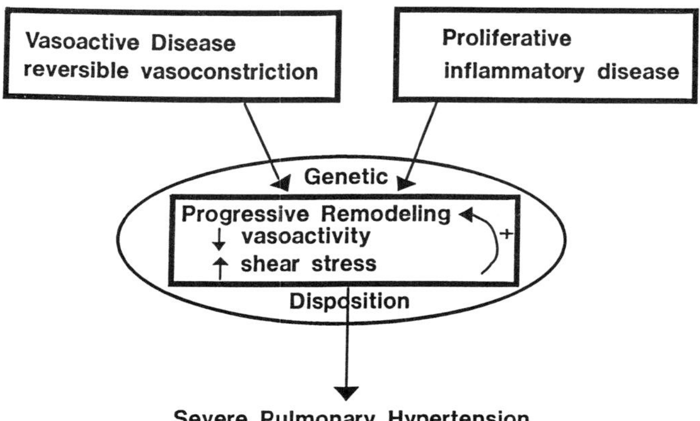

Figure 1 Schematic display of the initially important factors and how they interact in the development of severe pulmonary hypertension.

II. Vasoconstriction in Primary Pulmonary Hypertension

There are three elements that combine to cause the increased pulmonary vascular resistance present in PPH. These are vasoconstriction, remodeling of the wall of the pulmonary vessels, and thrombosis in situ. The latter two can readily be appreciated on light microscopy. Vasoconstriction is best demonstrated by observing the effect of vasodilators.

In their classic 1951 paper describing the clinical features of PPH, Dresdale et al. (4) reported that the α-adrenergic blocker, tolazoline could "lower the blood pressure in the lesser circulation and increase the blood flow significantly." From this observation they concluded that, "the increased vascular resistance in some instances was due to increased vascular tone and not due to organic changes." Paul Wood drew a similar conclusion when he reported that bolus injections of acetylcholine reduced pulmonary artery pressure in five out of six patients with PPH (5).

Early histological studies of the small pulmonary arteries in lung tissue obtained from patients who died as a result of PPH suggested that, in some cases, "increased tonus of the small pulmonary arteries with contraction of the terminal arterial segments is an important possibility" (6). These reports described medial hypertrophy of the small pulmonary arteries (6–8) and wrinkling of the elastic laminae (7). The changes were interpreted to mean that vasoconstriction had led to increased thickness of the muscular media. This conclusion has been supported by the correlation of hemodynamic and histologic data. In one instance, in 1969, a 12-year-old boy with PPH showed a pulmonary vasodilator response to acetylcholine, isoproterenol, and tolazoline (9). He died because a catheter perforated the right ventricle. Histological examination demonstrated medial hypertrophy of the small pulmonary arteries, with minimal intimal fibrous thickening. The authors contrasted the fixed intimal fibrous obstruction reported in other cases of PPH with the medial hypertrophy in this patient and commented that the latter "would be expected to respond with a fall in pulmonary arterial pressure under appropriate vasodilatory stimulus." In these early papers, evidence was provided that pulmonary vasoconstriction is partly responsible for the resistance to blood flow in PPH. An association between PPH and the systemic vasospastic condition, Raynaud's phenomenon, was also well recognized before 1964 (10).

Wagenvoort and Wagenvoort observed that, in infants with PPH, the most prominent histological feature is medial hypertrophy (8). With increasing age, intimal fibrosis and plexiform lesions are seen more commonly. This sequence suggests that vasoconstriction may be important early in PPH, whereas irreversible obstructive changes occur later. Pharmacological testing has provided parallel information supporting this hypothesis (11). Prostacyclin and nifedipine were administered to nine patients with PPH between the ages of 9 months and 23 years. The youngest patients demonstrated the greatest pulmonary vasodilatation in

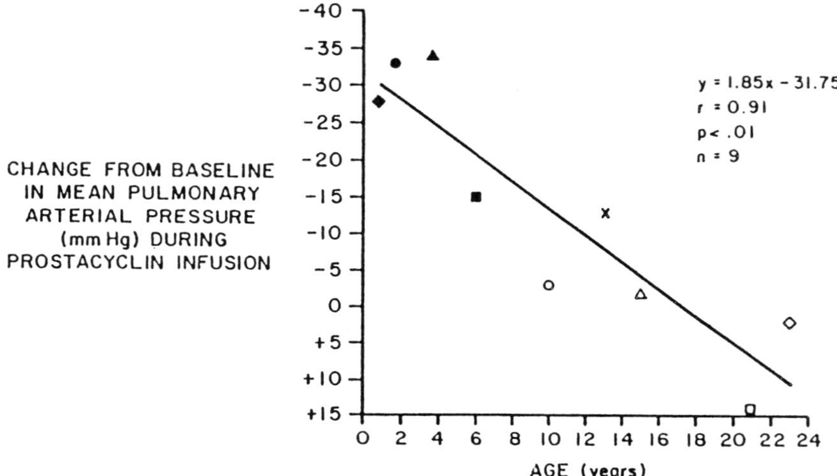

Figure 2 Relation between age of the patient and the change from baseline in mean pulmonary arterial pressure with prostacyclin infusion. Significant inverse correlation ($r = 0.91$, $p < 0.01$) indicates that prostacyclin produces a greater fall in pulmonary arterial pressure in younger patients with primary pulmonary hypertension than in the older ones. (From Ref. 11.)

response to these drugs (Fig. 2). Two patients died. They were nonresponders and had severe intimal disease.

Palevsky et al. (12) reported on both pulmonary vasodilator responses and pulmonary vascular histology in 19 adult patients. The area of the media correlated best with the changes in hemodynamics caused by vasodilators; medial hypertrophy was associated with vasodilatation. In the three patients who had a lung biopsy and a subsequent autopsy, the mean cross-sectional area of the artery wall did not change. However, the medial area decreased, whereas the intimal area increased. In one patient who had sequential vasodilator challenges there was an associated loss of responsiveness to vasodilators (12). Again, these changes imply that vasoconstriction and medial hypertrophy may be superseded over time by intimal fibrosis.

The foregoing discussion indicates that, in selected cases, vasoconstriction can play a major role in the pathophysiology of PPH. How often is vasoconstriction an important factor? Reeves et al. (13) reviewed the literature prior to 1986 and found that, of 117 PPH patients having acute vasodilator challenges, 45% reduced their pulmonary vascular resistance more than 30%. In the prospective Primary Pulmonary Hypertension Registry, vasodilators reduced the total pulmonary resistance more than 20%, together with a fall in the resistance ratio (total pulmonary resistance/total systemic resistance) in 30% of patients (14). In these two reports a variety of vasodilators were used. When high-dose calcium channel blockers were given orally, 26% of patients responded with a fall in both pulmonary artery pressure and resistance of over 20% (15). The number of patients who show a vasodilator response to calcium channel blockers over a period of months or years is not so relevant as a measure of preexisting vasoconstriction, because these agents, like several other vasodilators, can also inhibit cellular proliferation. Clearly, the percentage of acute responders varies somewhat according to the hemodynamic criteria used for success. However, these papers indicate that, in approximately a third of PPH patients, vasoconstriction is still an important factor at the time of cardiac catheterization. Catheterization is performed on average 2 years after the recognition of symptoms (16). It is unknown how long the onset of the disease precedes the recognition of symptoms, but it seems likely that vasoconstriction may be a significant factor in a greater percentage of patients close to the onset.

III. Mechanisms of Vasoconstriction

Theoretically, there are many mechanisms by which pulmonary vasoconstriction might be elicited (Fig. 3). The more plausible mechanisms in the etiology of PPH include an increase in circulating vasoconstrictors [e.g., serotonin (5-hydroxytryptamine) or thromboxane], a decrease in endothelium-derived dilating factors

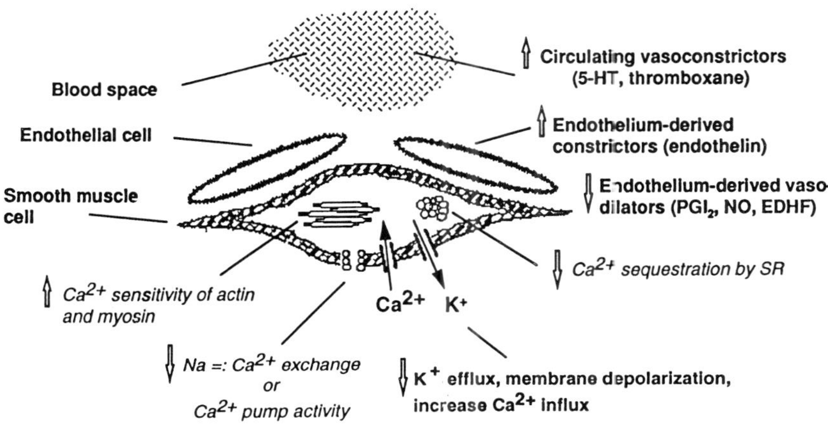

Figure 3 Mechanisms that might increase pulmonary vascular tone. The mechanisms that are more likely to be involved in primary pulmonary hypertension are in bold print, those that are less likely are in italics.

(e.g., prostacyclin, nitric oxide, or EDHF), an increase in endothelium-derived constricting factors (e.g., endothelin) or, finally, a change in ion channel activity, giving rise to calcium influx through the voltage-dependent calcium channel.

A. Circulating Vasoconstrictors

Serotonin (5-Hydroxytryptamine)

A possible role for serotonin (5-hydroxytryptamine; 5-HT) in the pathogenesis of PPH has been high-lighted by Herve and colleagues (17). Serotonin causes contraction of isolated pulmonary arteries (18). It is markedly elevated in the plasma of patients with primary pulmonary hypertension (24±8 SEM n*M*/L compared with less than 2 n*M*/L in controls) (17). In several of these patients the elevation of 5-HT persisted after heart–lung transplantation, indicating that the increased 5-HT levels are not secondary to the pulmonary hypertension. It seems unlikely that high levels of 5-HT alone could cause primary pulmonary hypertension, as patients with carcinoid tumors, which secrete enough 5-HT to damage heart valves, do not develop pulmonary hypertension. Abnormal platelet interaction with 5-HT may be an indication that endothelial or smooth-muscle handling of 5-HT is also abnormal in these patients. Alternatively, the abnormal platelet interaction with 5-HT might be only a genetically linked marker for some other etiological agent. The latter explanation seems less plausible, because ketanserin, a 5-HT antagonist, reduced pulmonary artery pressure and resistance in a single patient with an elevated plasma 5-HT level, platelet storage pool disease, and pulmonary hypertension (19).

The hypothesis that increased plasma levels of 5-HT could contribute to the development of pulmonary hypertension, is strengthened by the observation that the fawn-hooded rat, which has platelet storage disease and elevated plasma 5-HT, develops pulmonary hypertension at the relatively low altitude of Denver (barometric pressure about 630 mmHg) (20,21). A parallel model in the systemic vasculature is provided by the report that, in the setting of coronary endothelial injury and stenosis in the dog, vasoconstriction and neointimal proliferation occur. The vasoconstriction can be inhibited by the 5-HT receptor antagonists, ketanserin and LY53857 (22). This experiment was interpreted to mean that platelet aggregation caused 5-HT release, which then stimulated vasoconstriction.

Thromboxane

Thromboxane is a potent vasoconstrictor that is derived mainly from platelet activation. Measurement of the thromboxane metabolite thromboxane B_2 (TxB_2) has been used to assess platelet activation. In 1980 and 1985, case reports of children with PPH were published in which plasma levels of TxB_2 were markedly increased (23,24).

Prolonged administration of the thromboxane synthesis inhibitor permagrel (CGS 13080) has been reported to reduce pulmonary vascular resistance in five of ten patients with PPH (16). These observations might have indicated an etiological role for thromboxane in PPH; however, a more recent study demonstrated that 24-hr urinary excretion of 11-dehydro-thromboxane B_2 is high, not only in patients with PPH, but also in patients with pulmonary hypertension secondary to collagen vascular disease, Eisenmenger's syndrome and other causes (25,26). Thus, although thromboxane may be a contributing cause of vasoconstriction in PPH and other forms of pulmonary hypertension, it is probably a secondary player, being elevated as a result of platelet activation, which is itself precipitated by endothelial dysfunction and thrombotic abnormalities.

Thrombin activity is increased in PPH patients, giving rise to increased plasma concentrations of fibrinopeptide A, and plasminogen activator inhibitor-1 activity may also be elevated (19 of 27 patients) (27). Decreased fibrinolytic activity (tissue plasminogen activator; t-PA) has been observed in thromboembolic as well as in PPH patients (28). Although cross-linked fibrin degradation products are detected only occasionally in PPH (27), they can cause experimental pulmonary vasoconstriction through the generation of thromboxane (29).

B. Reduction of Endothelium-Derived Vasodilators

The normal pulmonary vascular endothelium produces prostacyclin, nitric oxide (NO), and perhaps a hyperpolarizing factor. The primary or secondary loss of these vasodilators could promote vasoconstriction. The acute loss of cyclooxygenase metabolites does not increase pulmonary vascular resistance under normoxic circumstances in the anesthetized dog (30). Similarly NO synthase inhibition in the isolated perfused rat lung (31) or in the conscious dog does not cause pulmonary vasoconstriction (32), and removal of the endothelium in small pulmonary arteries from the cat does not increase resting tension (33). However, when a vasoconstrictor stimulus is present, such as hypoxia, inhibition of these endogenous vasodilators increases the vasoconstriction (30,31). In the fetus and neonate, NO synthase inhibition also causes vasoconstriction (34,35). It seems that when significant vascular tone is present or is induced, the endogenous endothelial dilators oppose it, if the endothelium is functioning normally. Nitric oxide production by the isolated perfused lung, which cannot be detected in control, normoxic rats, is easily measured in lungs from rats with chronic hypoxic pulmonary hypertension (36).

The histological appearance of intimal proliferation or fibrosis in PPH makes it evident that endothelial function cannot be normal when these changes are present. Early in the disease a vasodilator response to endothelium-dependent vasodilators may still be seen. In 1960 Samet et al. (37) reported an impressive vasodilator response to acetylcholine in a 44-year-old woman with PPH. Three years after the initial catheterization, a comparable dose of acetylcholine had no effect on pulmonary artery pressure or cardiac output (38). The authors ascribe this change to "progressive pulmonary vascular disease." A similar lack of response to the endothelium-dependent vasodilators, acetylcholine, calcitonin gene-related peptide, and substance P was more recently described in PPH patients, who did show pulmonary vasodilatation in response to a non–endothelium-dependent vasodilator, nicardipine (39). Impairment of endothelium-dependent relaxation has also been reported from in vitro studies of the pulmonary arteries of patients with end-stage chronic obstructive lung disease (COLD) (40) and from hemodynamic studies in 2 of 13 patients with COLD and pulmonary hypertension (41).

In both primary and several secondary forms of pulmonary hypertension, the urinary excretion of 6-ketoprostaglandin $F_{1\alpha}$ (a stable metabolite of prostacyclin) is diminished (Fig. 4) (25,26). This indicates a reduced endothelial capacity for prostacyclin synthesis. The impaired ability of the endothelium to generate nitric oxide or prostacyclin is probably not the primary cause of vasoconstriction in PPH, as similar deficits in endothelial-derived relaxing factor

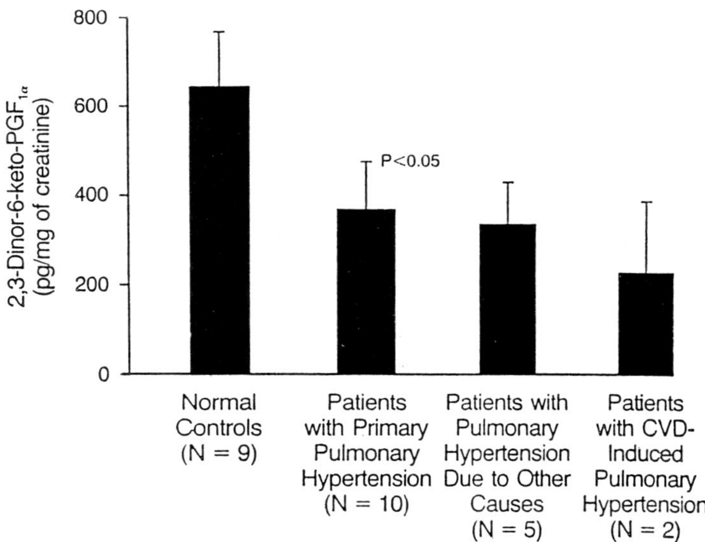

Figure 4 Mean (±SEM) urinary excretion of 2,3-dinor-6-keto-PGF$_{1\alpha}$, a metabolite of prostacyclin, in normal controls and in three groups of patients with primary or secondary pulmonary hypertension. Patients with primary pulmonary hypertension excreted less of the metabolite than did normal controls ($p < 0.05$). CVD denotes collagen vascular disease. (From Ref. 25.)

(EDRF) responses and in 6-keto-$PGF_{1\alpha}$ are present in other less severe forms of pulmonary hypertension. However, the lack of these endogenous vasodilators must contribute to the development of pulmonary hypertension. Certainly the "replacement" of endogenous nitric oxide by inhaled nitric oxide (42,43), the infusion of prostacyclin (44,45), or both together (46), are logical approaches to the treatment of the "vasoconstriction" element of PPH.

C. Increase of Endothelium-Derived Vasoconstrictors

As illustrated in Figure 3, the endothelium also generates vasoconstrictor substances, such as the endothelins. The endothelins are a family of three 21-amino acid peptides. Endothelin 1 (ET-1) is produced in endothelial cells as preproendothelin 1 (over 200 amino acids), which is converted to big-ET-1 (38 amino acids), and that is metabolized to the active peptide, ET-1. Endothelin-1 is generally considered to be a potent vasoconstrictor (47,48); however, at low doses in the preconstricted pulmonary vascular bed, it can act as a vasodilator (49). This may be because it causes the release of nitric oxide and prostacyclin (50). A recent study in which ET-1 was genetically reduced in mice found a surprising increase in systemic arterial pressure, again indicating that ET-1 may have a physiological vasodilator effect (51).

Through its action on the ET_A receptor in smooth muscle cells, ET-1 stimulates calcium entry through the voltage-gated calcium channels (52) and also causes the release of calcium from intracellular stores (53). There is some evidence to suggest that it might be involved in the pathophysiology of the pulmonary hypertension that occurs in the fawn-hooded rats, mentioned earlier (54), and in chronic experimental, hypoxic pulmonary hypertension (55,56). An increase in ET-1 mRNA, ET-1 peptide, and ET_A receptor mRNA was observed in the lungs of rats exposed to hypoxia (10% oxygen) for 2 days (55). In addition, the ET_A receptor antagonist, BQ123, markedly inhibited the increase in pulmonary artery pressure and resistance caused by a 2-week exposure to hypobaric hypoxia (380 mmHg)(56). In 13 children undergoing cardiac catheterization (only 1 of whom had PPH), the severity of the pulmonary pressor response to acute hypoxia correlated with the normoxic plasma levels of ET-1 (57). The ET-1 levels were higher in those children who had pulmonary hypertension at baseline, but it was not apparent if the ET-1 levels were the result of the pulmonary hypertension, or if the ET-1 caused the pulmonary hypertension. If ET-1 contributes to the vasoconstriction, ET-1 expression can be inhibited by NO (57) and by prostacyclin (25,26). Conversely, if endothelial dysfunction reduces the production of NO and prostacyclin, ET-1 expression may be increased.

In 1991, Stewart et al. (58) reported that ET-1 plasma levels were elevated in patients with either primary or secondary pulmonary hypertension. They pointed out that, although ET-1 levels are reduced during passage across the lung in patients without pulmonary hypertension, they are unchanged in those with secondary pulmonary hypertension, and they are actually increased in PPH. This suggests that ET-1 is normally taken up or metabolized in the pulmonary vasculature, but that there is a net production of ET-1 from the pulmonary vascular endothelium of PPH patients. More recently, the same group published the finding that ET-1-like immunoreactivity is more marked in the endothelium of muscular arteries in PPH patients, compared with those with secondary pulmonary hypertension (Fig. 5; 59). This study also provided direct evidence of increased expression of ET-1 mRNA and prepro-ET-1 mRNA in the endothelium of patients with pulmonary hypertension. Taken together, these observations indicate enhanced local production of ET-1 in the pulmonary vascular endothelium in pulmonary hypertension, especially in PPH patients. This could be a primary abnormality in PPH, or, as discussed earlier, it could be secondary to the escape of ET-1 expression from NO and prostacyclin inhibition. In either event, ET-1 is likely to contribute to the vasoconstrictive component of PPH. A parallel in the systemic circulation is the increased ET-1 serum levels seen in patients with primary Raynaud's phenomenon, which increases markedly with cold exposure, concomitantly with the fall in digital arterial pulsatility (60).

D. Decreased Potassium Efflux and Membrane Depolarization

The classic model of pulmonary vasoconstriction is that stimulated by acute hypoxia. Recent work suggests that hypoxic vasoconstriction could provide clues for the vasoconstriction in PPH. Since the first detailed description of hypoxic pulmonary vasoconstriction (HPV) by von Euler, in 1946 (61), a number of characteristics have become apparent: it can occur in isolated pulmonary arterial smooth-muscle cells (62), it requires extracellular calcium [being blocked by Ca^{2+} channel blockers (63) and enhanced by calcium channel agonists (64,65), it involves smooth-muscle membrane depolarization (66), and it occurs within 7 sec of the onset of hypoxia in the perfused lung (67).

What might give rise to the membrane depolarization? Potassium channels are essential in the control of smooth-muscle membrane potential. The K^+ channel blockers, such as tetraethylammonium (TEA) and 4-aminopyridine (4-AP), inhibit the outward K^+ current, depolarize the membrane, permit Ca^{2+} influx through the voltage-dependent Ca^{2+} channels, and increase tension in pulmonary artery rings (68) and pulmonary artery pressure in perfused lungs (69).

Inhibition of the outward K^+ current by hypoxia is an attractive hypothesis to explain the onset of HPV. In the carotid body type 1 cell, hypoxia inhibits the K^+ current, depolarizing the membrane, and leading to an increase in the influx of extracellular Ca^{2+} (70). Similarly, hypoxia inhibits whole-cell K^+ current and depolarizes the membrane in freshly isolated pulmonary artery smooth-muscle cells (Fig. 6; 68) and in cultured pulmonary artery smooth-muscle cells (71). In

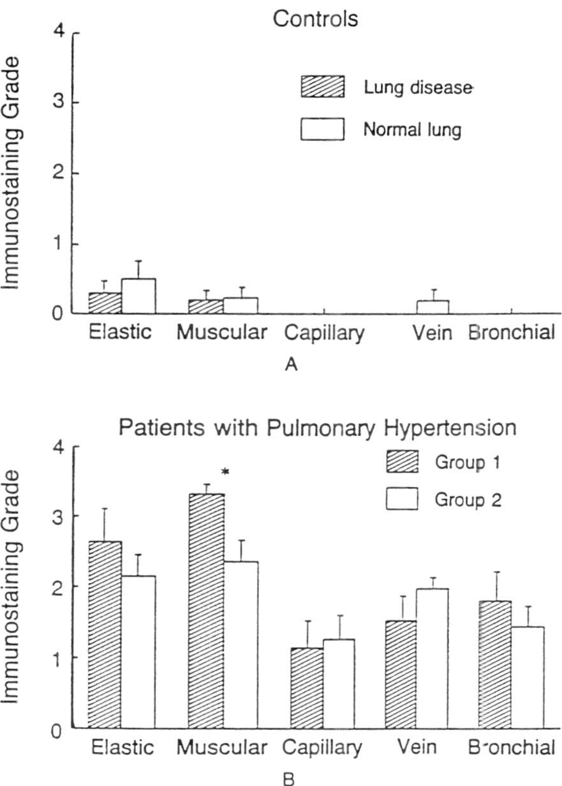

Figure 5 Mean (± SEM) level of endothelin-1-like immunoreactivity in vascular endothelium of lung tissue from (A) two groups of controls and (B) two groups of patients with pulmonary hypertension. The patients with pulmonary hypertension were further subdivided according to morphological and clinical criteria into those with the plexogenic form of PPH (group 1) and those with secondary pulmonary hypertension (group 2). Endothelin-1-like immunoreactivity was assessed in the endothelium of elastic and muscular pulmonary arteries, capillaries, pulmonary veins, and bronchial vessels. The level of endothelin-1-like immunoreactivity was significantly greater in the patients with pulmonary hypertension than in the controls in all vessels. The asterisk indicates $p = 0.003$ for the comparison between groups. (From Ref. 59.)

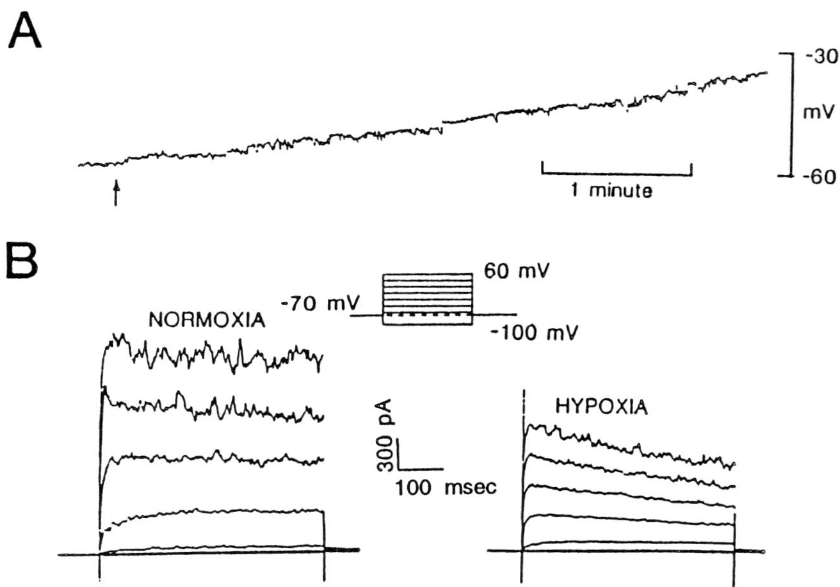

Figure 6 Effect of hypoxia on membrane potential and voltage-dependent K^+ currents in pulmonary artery smooth-muscle cells. (A) effect of hypoxia on membrane potential in pulmonary artery smooth-muscle cell. Start of hypoxia: arrow. (B) Family of currents elicited by voltage steps before and after 5-min exposure to hypoxia. (From Ref. 68.)

these studies hypoxia failed to reduce the K^+ current in either renal or mesenteric vascular smooth-muscle cells.

The mechanism of HPV is relevant to PPH as a model of vasoconstriction. In addition, as shown in Figure 7, the pulmonary artery pressure of some PPH patients can be significantly altered by changes in the inspired oxygen tension. This does not necessarily indicate that the vasoconstriction of PPH and HPV share a common mechanism. However, we have recently found that aminorex, an anorexigenic agent that produces a clinical syndrome identical with PPH, also inhibits an outward potassium current in pulmonary vascular smooth-muscle cells.

IV. The Vascular Lesions

Generally, at the time when the patients with (unexplained) PPH come to clinical attention, the catheter studies reveal severe pulmonary hypertension and—if an

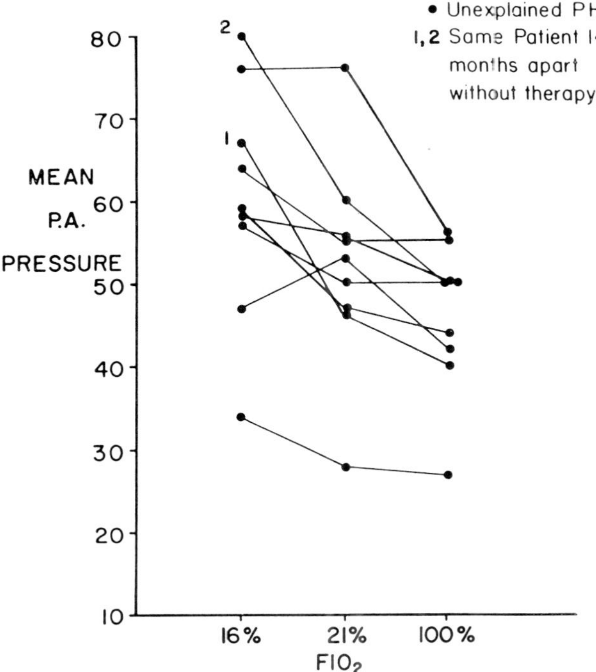

Figure 7 Increased inspired oxygen tension reduces pulmonary artery pressure in patients with unexplained pulmonary hypertension.

open-lung biopsy is obtained—the pulmonary vasculature is abnormal. Frequently, some of the small arteries show bizarre scar deformations, the muscle layers contain large amounts of glycosaminoglycans, and the adventitia is enlarged by layers of collagen and elastin (Fig. 8). A detailed description of the vascular lesions and their relative incidence in individual cases of PPH is found in Chapters 2 and 6. It is unclear whether the form of the vascular lesion and the frequency at which the lesions occurs in the lung are linked to the hemodynamic condition of the patient. Whereas two recent studies of PPH patients (72) and of patients with familial PPH (73) conclude that there is no single pathognomonic vascular lesion of PPH, there is the consensus that plexiform lesions are frequently present in the lungs of PPH patients [in 28–51% of the cases; in Wagenvoort's series (8) in 71% of the cases, and in the lungs of patients with PH due to congenital heart diseases in 10 of 11 cases (74)]. The survival time of patients after diagnosis of PPH is shorter when plexiform lesions are present (72) than in patients who have thrombotic lesions. The plexiform lesions are perhaps present

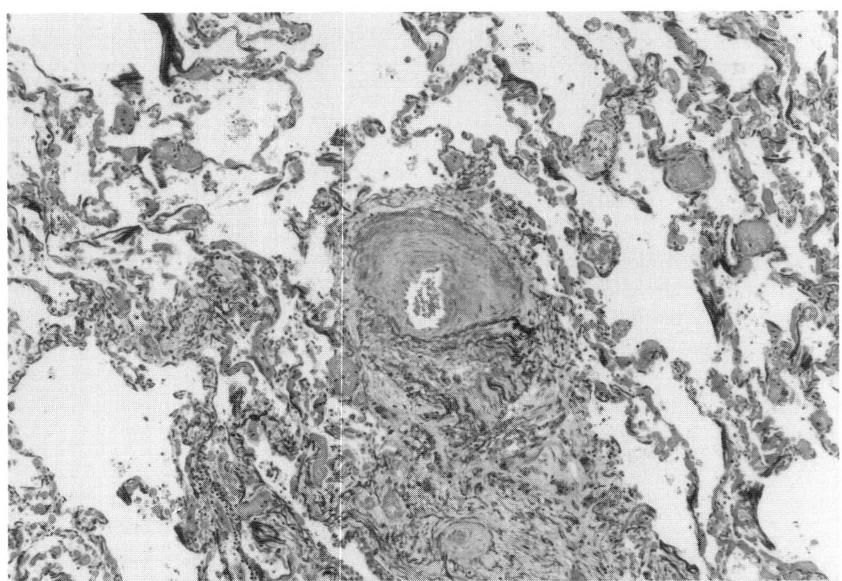

Figure 8 Pentachrome stain of a lung section from a patient with primary pulmonary hypertension. The small artery is embedded in a vast amount of collagen and contains "ground substance."

in younger patients and associated with higher pulmonary artery pressures (12,72). However, a wide range of pulmonary artery pressures is observed inpatients with plexiform lesions (Fig. 9). Whether plexiform lesions are markers of disease severity or of rapidly progressive disease is still unclear.

How do the lung vessels get to this point of obstructive and restrictive disease? Shear stress, hypoxemia, ischemia–reoxygenation, inflammatory cells—and mediators—as well as certain drugs and toxins, can damage the endothelial layer of resistance vessels. The schematic in Figure 10 has at its center the injury and repair of the vascular wall, in particular of the endothelium. Whereas these factors all *can* cause vascular injury, the pathophysiologist is uncertain whether endothelial damage actually *does* occur in *all* cases at some stage of the disease development. Another assumption is that the disease process begins and ends within the vascular wall—as may well be true early in the course of vasoconstrictive pulmonary hypertension. If one considers that alveolar macrophages are increased in lungs of PPH patients (3) and that macrophages are secretory cells, then the possibility arises that parenchyma cells could secret growth factors that target vessels that are altered because of intense vasoconstriction (shear stress) or cell injury.

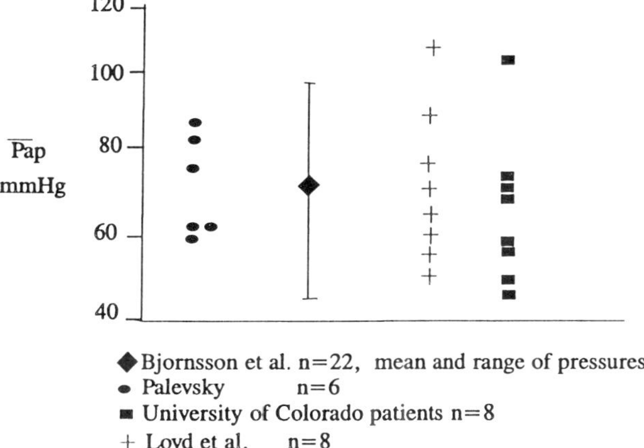

Figure 9 In patients with primary pulmonary hypertension and histologically documented plexiform lesions there is a wide range of pulmonary artery pressures. This indicates that the pulmonary artery pressure does not predict whether plexiform lesions are present and that plexiform lesions may be present when the pulmonary artery pressure is comparatively low.

V. Endothelial Cell Injury and Dysfunction

Vascular endothelial cells exhibit a complex set of responses to shear stress. Mechanotransduction involves activation of extracellular matrix receptors, such as members of the integrin family (75), activation of ion channels (76,77), alteration of the activities of adenylate cyclase and of protein kinase C(PKC), all activities related to cell proliferation. Thus, mechanical stress conceivably can activate a cell proliferation program, even without injury. The direct evidence for

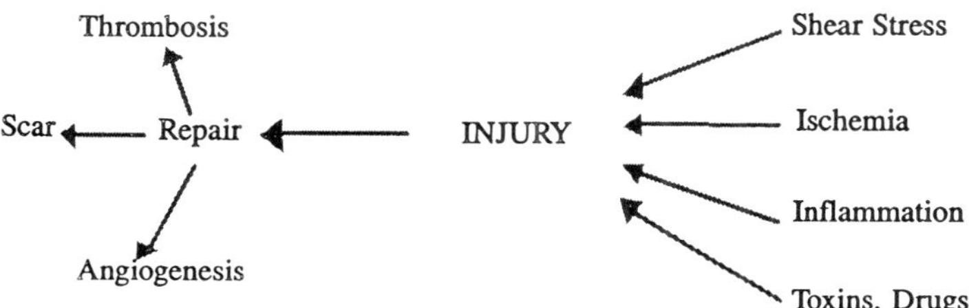

Figure 10 Vascular injury in severe pulmonary hypertension may have many causes. One needs to consider that the repair process is exuberant and prolonged.

endothelial injury in severe pulmonary hypertension comes mostly from animal models. Indirect evidence comes from three clinical studies. Dinh-Xuan et al. (78) studied endothelium-dependent relaxation in vitro obtained from patients with end-stage chronic obstructive lung disease (many with cystic fibrosis) and with Eisenmenger's syndrome (40). These arteries showed intimal thickening and had an impaired dilator response to acetylcholine. Although the authors did not provide pulmonary artery pressure measurements, one can assume that the patients had some degree of pulmonary hypertension.

In a second study factor VIII antigen and the ristocetin cofactor was measured in six patients with PPH (79). The ristocetin factor was elevated relative to the factor VIII antigen. Also, as pointed out earlier, urinary levels of the thromboxane metabolite 11-dehydrothromboxane B_2 were increased and the levels of 2,3-dinor-6-keto-$PGF_{1\alpha}$, the prostacyclin metabolite, were decreased in patients with PPH (25,26). It is not known whether the patients in the latter studies had plexiform lesions or not, but in the aggregate, the data support the notion of a dysfunctional pulmonary endothelium in PPH. If one considers the histological evidence, one wonders whether the endothelial blebs or endothelial swelling described in a previous study (80) are sufficient findings, since fixation and tissue processing are perhaps important factors influencing the endothelial cell morphological appearance.

On the other hand, endothelial damage in the clinical setting may be rather innocuous, manifested by functional, not structural, changes. Yet, the traditional interpretation of endothelial lesions in PPH is expressed as follows: "Regardless of the type of the intimal lesion, the cellular elements are almost exclusively smooth muscle cells and myofibroblasts, and they are presumably derived from the media" (81). Figure 11 perhaps challenges this concept, as it demonstrates intense factor VIII staining of cells of a plexiform lesion, yet a relative absence of staining for muscle-specific actin. Many of the factor VIII-positive cells are also stained positively with an antibody against vimentin, a cytoskeletal protein. Thus, this example demonstrates findings consistent with actively proliferating endothelial cells.

VI. Muscular Hypertrophy

Virtually all patients with severe pulmonary hypertension show varying degrees of muscularization of small pulmonary arteries, and occasionally, patients are being reported in whom media hypertrophy is the only detectable vascular lesion (12).

This lesion is perhaps the "appropriate" vascular response to shear stress, since it fortifies the vessel wall. It is found in virtually all the animal models of pulmonary hypertension and is felt to be the result of vasoconstriction ("work

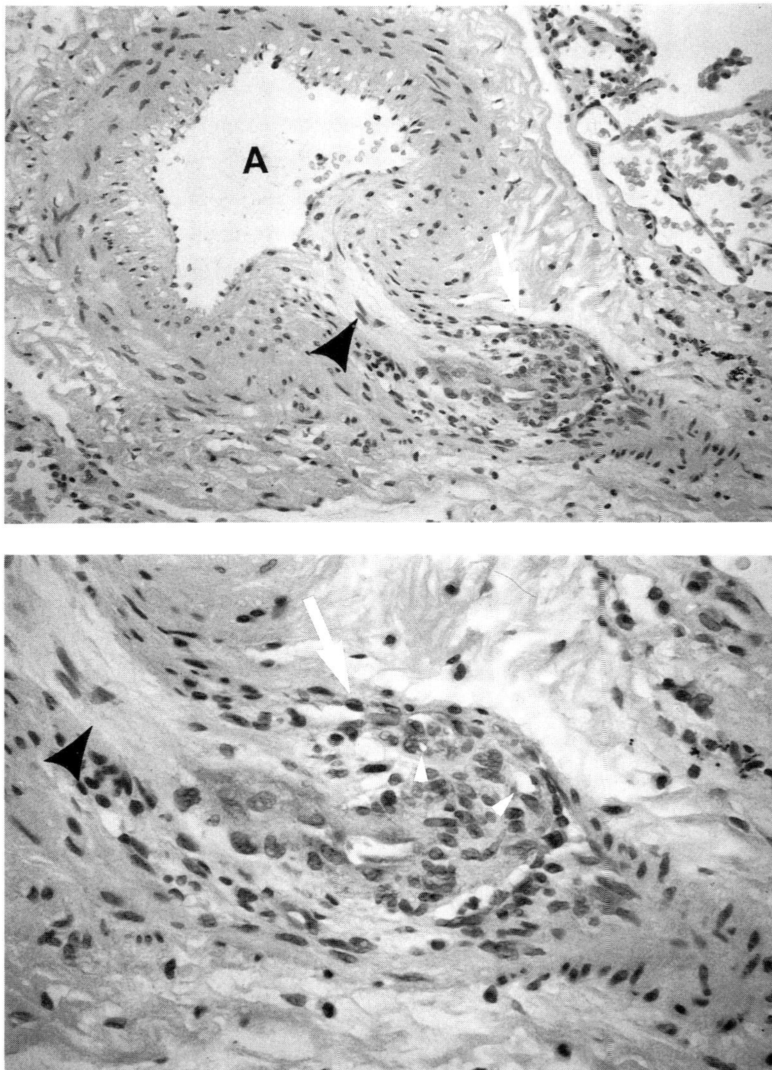

Figure 11 Plexiform lesions (arrow) at a branching site of a medium-sized artery. Note the obliteration of the vascular lumen by a loose connective tissue proximal to the plexiform lesion (black arrowhead). High magnification of the plexiform lesion. Multiple vascular channels are lined by plump endothelial cells (white arrowhead) in between the vascular channels, a cluster of cells form a solid mass, with focal vacuolization suggestive of early blood vessel formation (arrow).

hypertrophy''). Palevsky et al. (74) suggest that a high diastolic pulmonary artery pressure in PPH patients may be indicative of pronounced medial hypertrophy. Indeed, contracted vessels were found in 24 of 26 patients in a histological examination of specimens from PPH patients. One possibility is that vasoconstrictors that double as growth factors are released locally in the lungs or gain access to the vascular muscle cells from the blood. This possibility of dual-function mediators has been discussed in recent animal experimental studies during which prolonged treatment with platelet-activating factor (PAF) antagonists inhibited lung vessel remodeling and pulmonary hypertension. The PAF antagonists used had no detectable hemodynamic actions and are not Ca^{2+} antagonists (82,83).

A. Adventitial Fibrosis

The adventitia of small pulmonary arteries in the lungs of patients with pulmonary venous hypertension is thickened (2) and contains large amounts of collagen and elastin. Little attention has yet been paid to the adventitial changes in the small pulmonary arteries of patients with PPH. The extent of this appositional growth of the adventitia can be demonstrated with the pentachrome-staining technique (see Fig. 7); it may be due to the phenotypically altered secretory smooth-muscle cells (1,84). The growth of adventitial collagen leads to loss of vascular motility, causing a restrictive arteriopathy. Whether the adventitial alterations in PPH are part of only end-stage lesions, or evolve in concert with intimal and medial thickening, has not been systematically investigated. Whether during the pulmonary vascular remodeling process there are growth factor concentration gradients across the artery wall—one directed from the injured intima toward the adventitia and another gradient from lung parenchyma cells (that express growth factors, such as VEGF or endothelin) toward the adventitia—is unknown.

B. Inflammation

Although inflammation as part of the vasculopathy of PPH has been appreciated in various publications throughout the history of the disease (Table 1), starting with Arrillaga, in 1913 (85), pathologists continue to detect features of typical arteritis, which are indeed present in approximately one-third of the cases in the series of PPH patients described by Bjornsson et al. (86; Table 2). Wagenvoort and Wagenvoort (2) have reviewed earlier literature on PPH and state: "Polymorphonuclear or more often mononuclear inflammatory cells are seen regularly in or around plexiform lesions. Though this has been denied by some authors, it may suffice to point out that others have used the term anastomositis to stress the rather common finding of this inflammatory reaction." In addition, in recent years a new concept of "intravascular inflammation" has been emerging. After careful morphological studies of the lungs of smokers and the lungs of patients with chronic obstructive lung disease Hale et al. (87) and Wright et al. (88) described arterial intimal

Table 1 Pathogenesis of Primary Pulmonary Hypertension: Evolution of a Thought Process

Author	Date	Observation
Romberg	1891	Sclerosis of the lung artery
Arrillaga	1913	Pulmonary vessel arteritis
Wood	1957	The vasoconstrictive factor
Blount	1967	PPH: thromboembolism
Wagenvoort	1970	PPH not explained by thromboembolism
Reeves et al.	1979	Vasoconstriction important
Stenmark et al.	1987	Importance of cell proliferation in severe PH

thickening that correlated with the degree of airway inflammation, and Selby et al. (89), found vascular neutrophil retention in the lungs of patients with chronic obstructive disease. What is not known is whether the patients who accumulate intravascular neutrophils in their lungs are also the patients who develop arterial intimal thickening.

Animal model studies demonstrate that lung intravascular inflammatory cells that form intravascular aggregates *can* release constrictor mediators with cell growth potential (90), that lung vascular remodeling follows vascular granulocyte sequestration, and that neutrophil depletion attenuates the pulmonary hypertension (91). Increased numbers of alveolar macrophages in the parenchyma and periarterial clusters of lymphocytes in patients with plexogenic pulmonary hypertension were found in the series of patients reported by Caslin et al. (3). The significance of this finding for the pathogenesis of PPH is unclear; however, alveolar macrophages and lymphocytes are cytokine-secreting cells that may be part of the injury—or the repair—process. Neointimal macrophages in large pulmonary arteries from PPH patients have been described (92), and some of these cells show a positive immunostaining pattern for transforming growth factor-β (TGF-β; 93).

Table 2 Arteritis in PPH

Author (Ref.)	*n*	Arteritis associated with plexiform lesions (% of cases)	Arteritis without plexiform lesions (*n*)
Bjornsson and Edwards (86)	80	36	3
Loyd et al. (73)	23	21	—
Fanburg (208)			1
Pietra (72)	58		—

Recently Hales (94) discussed the case of a woman with severe rheumatoid arthritis and severe pulmonary hypertension (pulmonary artery systolic/diastolic pressure 82/32 mmHg) without plexiform lesions, but with medial and intimal thickening of the arteries and lymphocytic infiltration of the adjacent respiratory bronchioles. Schwarz et al. (95) reported the lung histology of a male patient in whom bronchiolitis obliterans was the only manifestation of rheumatoid arthritis. In the latter patient obvious pulmonary vascular involvement, with profound medial thickening was present. In both patients, the remarkable common features were the association of pulmonary hypertension with lymphocyte accumulation in the perivascular or bronchial spaces. Given the well-known association of collagen vascular disease and PPH, these examples, although perhaps anecdotal, may give rise to a greater awareness of the hypothesis that severe pulmonary hypertension, including PPH, may be preceded and accompanied by inflammation. Tuder et al., (96) analyzed ten cases with PPH and plexiform lesions and found, in all cases, frequent macrophages and T and B lymphocytes at the perimeter of plexiform lesions, (see Fig. 7). The role of T lymphocytes in atherogenesis has recently been addressed (97).

C. Angiogenesis

Clusters of dilated arteries forming "vein-like branches" have been described in the lungs of patients with PPH (98), and the rare form of PPH called pulmonary capillary hemangiomatosis (99). In the latter disorder, thin-walled vessels (with their lumen occluded) form sheets around pulmonary veins and arteries. Angiogenesis in the lungs from rats treated with monocrotaline has recently been reported (100). One wonders which of the many angiogenesis factors are involved in the formation of these lesions. A vascular sprout, perhaps an early plexiform lesion is shown in Figure 12.

D. Immune Disorders and Primary Pulmonary Hypertension

The association of PPH and autoimmune disorder has been known for some time and has been reviewed (101). Antinuclear antibodies (ANA) have been reported to be present in the sera of patients with PPH (102,103), and anti-Ku antibodies were found in 23% of PPH patients (103). However, Morse et al. (104) examined patients with familial PPH and found several PPH patients who lacked autoantibodies, but tested positive for the human leukocyte antigen (HLA) class II alleles that accompany autoimmune disorders. Eight of 15 patients with familial PPH had HLA-DRw52, whereas another subset expressed a different MHC class II haplotype (HLA-DR4). The Ku autoantigen has been shown to bind to double-stranded DNA in vitro and may play a role in gene expression (105).

Although PH is being reported in patients with systemic lupus erythematosus (106–109), the incidence of severe PH in patients with SLE is unknown.

Quismorio et al. (110) found two cases in their SLE clinic of 400, and a recent report by Cervera et al. (111), on 1000 cases of SLE, did not mention the occurrence of pulmonary vascular disease. In Asherson's series of 22 patient with SLE and PH (106), the manifestation of PH occurred between 2 and 11 years after the onset of SLE, 15 had Raynaud's syndrome, 12 were positive for antiphospholipid antibodies (lupus anticoagulant and cardiolipin antibodies). Immune complex deposits in the walls of pulmonary arteries (intima and media) and small collections of lymphocytes surrounding arterioles have been reported by Quismorio et al. (110). Less-recognized features of lung disease in SLE are pulmonary hemorrhage (112) and small vein angiitis associated with massive pulmonary hemorrhage (113). Pulmonary hemorrhage with hemosiderin-laden macrophages are a very frequent finding characterizing the lesions in the lungs of patients with PPH (3). Is there perhaps a connection between parenchyma hemorrhage, extravasation of plasma and blood cell products, and pulmonary vascular remodeling? Plexogenic pulmonary arteriopathy has also been described in polymyositis (114).

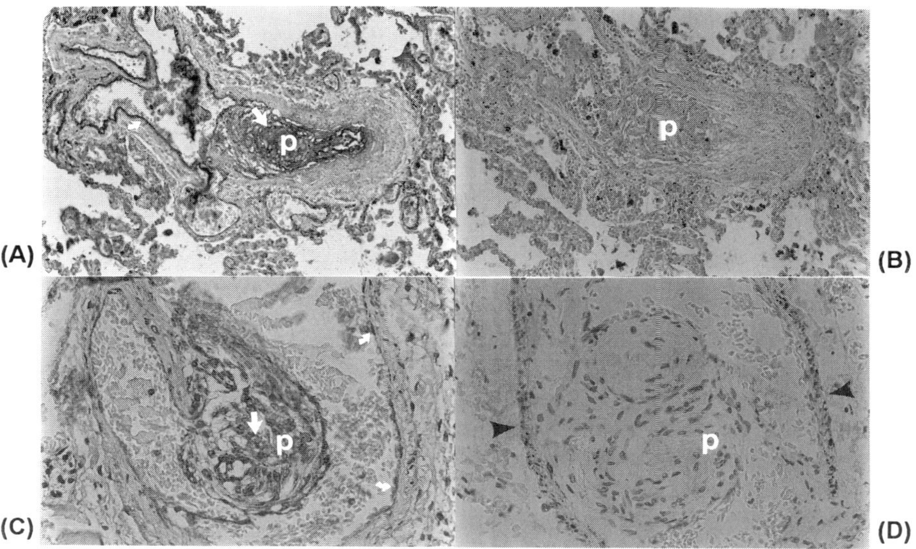

Figure 12 Serial sections of plexiform lesions (p) immunostained with Factor VIII-related antigen (A and C) or muscle-specific antigen (B and D). Note the cells within the plexiform lesions express factor VIII r.Ag, including the cells in between the blood vessel channels (white arrows). Only the smooth muscle cells react with the anti-smooth muscle-specific antibody (black arrowheads), whereas only the lining of the pulmonary artery reacts with the factor VIII r.Ag (curved arrow).

An association of thyroid autoimmune disease has been recognized in the series of PPH patients described by Rawson and Woske (115). Badesch et al. (116) described four female patients with hypothyroidism and severe PH. The four patients had low-titer positive ANA, two had Raynaud's syndrome. Another recent case of hypothyroidism and PPH has been reported by Martas (117). The association between PPH and hypothyroidism is of importance because it suggests that autoimmune disorders, other than collagen vascular diseases, can perhaps cause pulmonary vascular disease in susceptible individuals; alternatively, thyroid insufficiency might alter pulmonary vasculature.

The link between autoimmune (including collagen vascular disorders) diseases and PPH remains unclear. One possibility is the manifestation of a localized immune response that follows lung vascular injury. However, since many patients with PPH and with familial PPH do not develop autoantibodies, it is perhaps more likely that two genetic dispositions converge in these patients: one disposition for the development of autoimmune disease and a second disposition to develop severe PH.

E. Severe Pulmonary Hypertension in Patients with the Acquired Immune Deficiency Syndrome

We have found in the recent literature reports of 26 cases of severe (primary) pulmonary hypertension associated with human immunodeficiency virus (HIV) infection. Some of these patients had plexiform lesions (118–120). In two further patients, studied by Mette et al. (121), histochemistry, DNA in situ hybridization, and polymerase chain reaction studies did not reveal direct vascular HIV infection. Thus, the mechanisms involved in the development of severe PH in an overall very small subset of HIV-infected patients worldwide is unclear. Several working hypotheses come to mind. Since HIV is apparently not present in the vascular wall, indirect mechanisms are to be considered. First, the visceral changes could be induced by cytomegalovirus (CMV) infection rather than HIV infection. A CMV infection of cultured endothelial cells results in mitogen production (122). Kamer et al. (123) describe release of β-fibroblast growth factor (FGF) and arterial smooth-muscle cell proliferation when smooth muscle cells are incubated with conditioned (CMV-infected) endothelial cell medium. Another possibility is that activation of the immune system early in the HIV infection leads to a vasculitis or to macrophage activation and production of mitogens which, in turn, could activate transcription factors (like NF-κB) involved in cell growth regulation. Louis et al. (124) obtained hemodynamic data in five HIV-associated PPH patients out of a population of 2793 seropositive HIV patients and found mean pulmonary artery pressure values varying from 38 to 90 mmHg. Acute vasodilation was attempted with the Ca^{2+} entry blocker nifedipine; two of the patients responded with syncope and a small decrease in pulmonary vascular resistance. From this limited trial in a small group of patients, one might postulate that vascular cell proliferation is perhaps the primary pathognomonic element, rather than vasoconstriction in this form of PH. Pulmonary veno-occlusive disease has recently been described in a 2-year-old boy with HIV infection (125).

F. Drug-Induced Severe Pulmonary Hypertension

The medical community was first alerted to the problem of drug-induced PH when from 1967 to 1970 there was a 20-fold increase in the incidence of PPH in three European countries owing to the intake of the appetite depressant aminorex fumarate (Menocil; 126). Although the aminorex-induced disease was virtually indistinguishable from spontaneously occurring PPH, these patients may differ in one very important aspect (i.e., in survival of the disease). Frank et al. (127) reported on nine patients with aminorex-induced disease, who had all survived for more than 20 years. Gurtner (128) compared the survival times of PPH patients who had taken aminorex ($n = 71$) and those with spontaneous forms of the disease ($n = 36$) and reported the median survival time to be 12 years in the aminorex group and 4.5 years in the spontaneous group. When the hemodynamics were revaluated in 20 surviving aminorex patients at 10 years after diagnosis, 12 patients had a significant decrease of the mean pulmonary artery pressure (approximately a 50% decrease). Apparently, after cessation of the drug intake in a group of these patients, the disease was not progressive. A second class of appetite depressants, fenfluramine or dexfenfluramine and methyl-3-(trifluromethyl benzene-enthanamine hydrochloride) has recently been reported to cause severe PH in four cases (129,130). Unfortunately, investigations were unsuccessful in their attempts to use appetite depressants and create an animal model of pulmonary hypertension. Thus, the mechanism of action of the appetite depressants and their role in the development of PPH is not understood. Precisely because aminorex does not "work" in animals and, furthermore, because only 1:1000 women who consumed this amphetamine-like agent did actually develop PPH, we postulate a "pulmonary hypertension gene," or a genetic constellation as the sine qua non of severe (primary) pulmonary hypertension. Rarely, have other drugs, in particular chemotherapeutic agents, been invoked in the pathogenesis of severe PH (131). Pulmonary veno-occlusive disease has been reported in two patients with Hodgkin's lymphoma who had received chemotherapy (132). Mitomycin C reportedly caused PH and hemolytic anemia (133), but the overall incidence of PH in patients receiving mitomycin must be small. Mitomycin, like the monocrotaline pyrrole that causes a form of inflammatory hypertension in rats (82,83,134), is an effective DNA cross-linking agent. The latter aspect may contribute to the endothelial cell damage in the monocrotaline PH model (135).

G. Thrombosis in Primary Pulmonary Hypertension

Blood clotting is a host defence mechanism that is parallel with the inflammatory and repair responses that help protect the integrity of the vessel after injury (136).

Platelets, leukocytes, endothelial cells, and the clotting cascade interact after activation (which includes the rapid establishment of new surface properties). The proenzymes factors VII, X, and XII have an EGF-like domain. Tissue factor, a normal constituent of nonvascular cell surface and stimulated monocytes, initiates clotting (136) by binding to factor VII. The participation of platelet membranes and alterations of endothelial cell surface charges may be critically involved. Protein C and heparin, which is localized on endothelial cells of the microvasculature, slow clotting. On the other hand, visceral injury prompts platelets to marginate, their adherence likely mediated by von Willebrand's factor. Leukocytes and monocytes interact with both the activated platelets and endothelial cells through P-selectin and express their tissue factor, contributing to the first phase of wound healing. Exuberant wound healing may involve constituents of the renin–angiotensin system that (in vitro) is contained within endothelial cells. In experimental animal studies, inhibitors of the angiotensin-converting enzyme inhibit myointimal proliferation after vessel injury (137).

The increase in plasminogen activator after angiotensin system inhibition also leads to endothelial cell expression of the proto-ocogen c-*src* (138). Future therapies may be directed toward elevation of endothelial cell c-*src* activity in vivo, or toward a decrease in thrombin receptor number or activity (139). Lastly, neointimal smooth-muscle cells express thrombomodulin (140); however, immunohistological localization of thrombomodulin to remodeled vessels of lungs from PPH patients has not yet been attempted.

The shear stress itself or injury (caused by intravascular inflammation) of the lung vessels generates a thrombogenic surface. The consensus is that, in most cases of PPH, thrombotic lesions are secondary, but rather frequently occurring, complicating events. The Wagenvoorts in their important study of 156 clinically diagnosed cases of PPH (8) found a combination of thromboembolism with characteristic lesions of PPH in 6 cases; Loyd et al. (73) found evidence of thrombosis in 18 of the 23 cases with familial PPH, and most recently, Wagenvoort and Mulder (141) found thrombotic lesions in the specimens of 67 of 78 adult patients with PH of any cause. Organized thrombi were frequent and were related to the duration of the illness, rather than to the stage of the disease. This recent study affirms that thrombotic lesions are not essential for the development of PPH, but also that thrombotic events are part of the problem in the vast majority of patients. It is likely that endothelial injury and mediators that double as mitogens and procoagulants provide the common pathogenetic denominator in the development of both plexogenic and thrombotic lesions.

A small number of patients with PPH have been evaluated with clotting-screening studies in a few clinical studies. Inglesby et al. (142) described abnormal fibrinolysis in familial PPH. These data were not supported by the study of Tubbs et al. (143), whereas Eisenberg et al. (27) found elevation of plasminogen activator inhibitor-1 activity in 19 of 27 patients with PPH and elevation of fibrinopeptide A in all of patients studied (61% of the patients had values that were at least five times normal). Increased plasma concentrations of fibrinopeptide A are consistent with the presence of a procoagulant activity and the increase of the plasminogen activator inhibitor-1 activity with inadequate fibrinolytic activity of the plasma. Whereas this study does not contain any site-specific information, the data may complement the available histological information. Longitudinal studies in patients with and without anti-coagulation therapy are clearly needed. Herve et al. (19) reported the case of a 46-year-old man with an inherited platelet storage disease who had high plasma serotonin and pulmonary hypertension (mean pulmonary artery pressure 52 mmHg) characterized by plexiform lesions. Ketanserin, a serotonin receptor blocker, caused a clear decrease in pulmonary vascular resistance. Whether platelet abnormalities occur frequently in patients with advanced PPH is not known. However, this index case illustrates the potential for platelet release products to participate in the development of lung vascular disease. Whether platelet dysfunction is a causative factor in the genetic model of the fawn-hooded rat (20,144) that spontaneously develops systemic and pulmonary hypertension is unknown.

VII. Cellular and Molecular Biology

The cells of the pulmonary vessels respond to shear, ischemia, inflammation toxins, and drugs, with a spectrum of responses that lead to altered vascular reactivity, alteration of coagulation and fibrinolysis, cell growth, and cell–cell interactions. A myriad of adhesion proteins, cytokines, growth and differentiation factors are present in the vessel wall (1,59,145), with the potential to act and interact. Gradually, the complexity of the signal transduction pathways in endothelial cells responding to shear stress is emerging. The following schematic (Fig. 13), adapted from a review (77), illustrates how mechanical surface forces can be transmitted to the cytoskeleton and activate ion channels, generate prostacyclin and EDRF, and stimulate protein phosphorylation reactions and gene expression (fundamentally the transcription of mRNA from a DNA molecule). In the following discussion, this schematic will serve several purposes. One purpose is to appreciate the redundancy of the vascular cell system (i.e., the existence of several options that the cells have available to respond). The investigators hope that the pathogenically important tissue-specific chain of signaling events—those that define inflammation, vascular immune responses, and angiogenesis—will eventually emerge. In the following we shall review the most pertinent and accepted paradigms guiding our knowledge of vascular cell growth. Some of these paradigms are now being examined in experimental models of pulmonary hypertension and in lung vascular cells. Immunostaining techniques and in situ hybridization methods are being used to map normal and hypertensive lung vessels and to

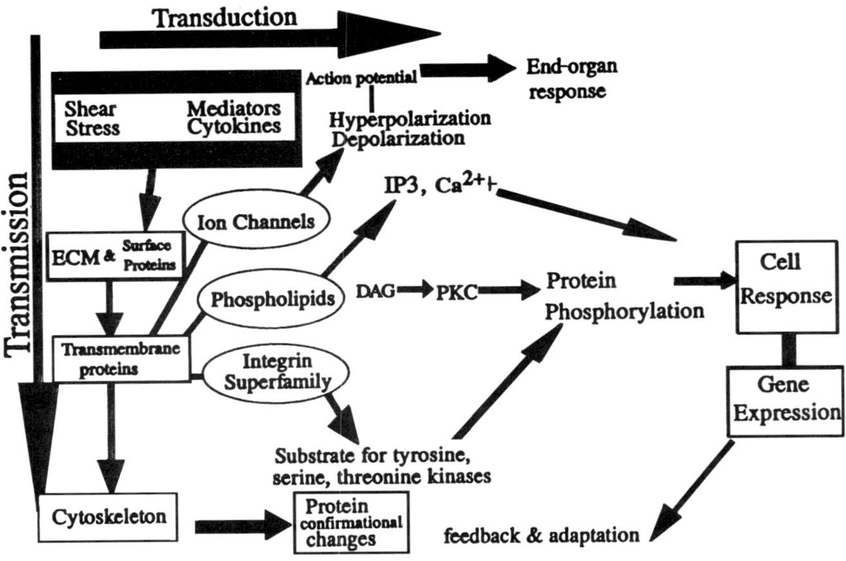

Figure 13 This schematic combines shear stress and cell-derived mediation, suggesting shared signaling pathways that lead to acute vascular responses (for example, vasoconstriction) and to alteration of gene expression (the formation of phenotypically altered, remodeled cells): ECM, extracellular matrix; IP3, inositol triphosphate; DAG, diacylglycerate; PKC, protein kinase C.

localize cytokines, their receptors, and eventually, oncogenes and protein kinases in pulmonary vascular lesions (59,146,147).

A. Cytokines and Growth Factors

In pulmonary vascular remodeling, certain mediators are likely to act simultaneously as inflammatory agents and as regulators of cell growth (Fig. 14). It is likely that in normal lung vessels many of these chemotactic, vasoactive, and proliferative factors are not expressed, and that their production is up-regulated in pulmonary hypertensive vessels.

Interleukin-1

Interleukin-1α (IL-1α) is produced by many inflammatory cells and also by endothelial and vascular smooth-muscle cells. Voelkel et al. (147) demonstrated, using immunostaining and in situ hybridization, the presence of IL-1α and low-level expression of IL-1α mRNA in lungs from monocrotaline-treated rats, and that treatment of the rats with the interleukin receptor blocker IL-1ra inhibited the

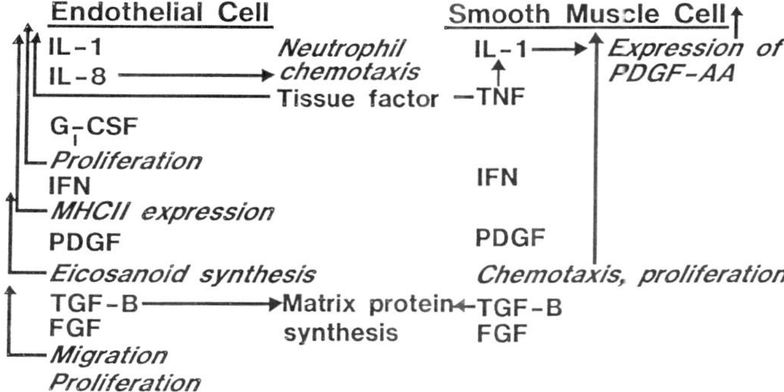

Figure 14 This schematic shows some of the possible cell–cell interactions and the resulting cytokine-dependent cellular responses. Endothelial cells and smooth-muscle cells in the injured vascular wall may form a functional unit.

development of chronic pulmonary hypertension. The authors concluded that the action of IL-1α in promoting pulmonary vascular remodeling was likely indirect. Interleukin-1 has several diverse effects, from the stimulation of PAF production, to c-*fos* proto-oncogene expression (148) and activation of the transcription factor NF-κB, which is implicated in many endothelial cell activation processes (149).

Transforming Growth Factor-β

Transforming growth factor-β (TGF-β) consists of a family of three isoforms: TGF-β_1, β_2, and β_3 and plays an important role in embryonal development and in repair following tissue injury, initiating chemotaxis of neutrophils, control and production of cytokines, synthesis of endothelin, and induction of angiogenesis (150). It is generated by platelets, endothelial cells, and smooth-muscle cells, and opposes many of the actions of IL-1. Perkett et al. (151) localized TGF-β1, β2, and β3 to lung vessels of sheep (which were made pulmonary hypertensive by chronic air embolization), and also showed induction of TGF-β3 mRNA in vascular smooth-muscle cells by TGF-β1 (152). Defective regulation on TGF-β production in the vessels of pulmonary hypertensive patients appears to be an attractive hypothesis that could explain the arterial muscularization and exuberant production of extracellular matrix proteins (150). Botney et al. (153) used immunostaining to localize TGF-β in the pulmonary arteries of calves, made pulmonary hypertensive during high-altitude hypoxia, and found a decrease of TGF-β_1 in remodeled arteries. However, in histological sections of lung tissue from patients with PPH, TGF-β_2 and β_3 immunoreactivity was present in nearly all hypertensive arteries (20–500 μm diameter), whether procollagen staining was present or not. The TGF-β_3 staining was also present in normal human lung vessels and in macrophages situated in the neointima (93). The importance of these findings for the understanding of the pathogenesis of PPH is presently unclear, partly because the antibody staining may not distinguish between latent or "active" forms of TGF-β and because TGF-β in situ may bind to a natural inhibitor, the proteoglycan decorin (154). Yet, as more information becomes available about the regulation of the three TGF-β receptors types (155), the role of TGF-β in ion channel regulation (156), and in regulation of the nitric oxide synthase (NOS), functional data and localization studies may perhaps establish a role for the various TGF-β isoforms in severe PH.

Platelet-Derived Growth Factor

Platelet-derived growth factor, in particular the PDGF BB isoform, is a potent muscle cell mitogen. Direct gene transfer of recombinant PDGF-B leads to expression of PDGF in arteries (that can be demonstrated immunohistochemically) and to intimal hyperplasia (157). Alternatively, antibodies directed against PDGF can inhibit intimal hyperplasia following experimental vascular injury (158). To our knowledge, PDGF has not yet been investigated in lung vessels from hypertensive patients. Localization studies of PDGF and its receptors in lungs from PPH patients will likely provide important information because this family of cationic mitogens is synthesized by many cells, including alveolar macrophages; its production is stimulated by thrombin with TGF-β; and it can cause profound alterations of arachidonic acid metabolism (159). Intracellularly, PDGF causes alkalinization by activation of the Na^+/H^+-exchange, an effect that is attenuated by heparin (160).

Vascular Endothelial Growth Factor

Vascular endothelial growth factor (VEGF), a family of four dimeric glycoproteins, is secreted from macrophages and vascular smooth-muscle cells, causes an increase in vascular permeability, and is an endothelial cell-specific mitogen, likely to play a multifunctional role in vascular remodeling (161–163). This angiogenic factor is present in pulmonary alveolar cells and lymphoid centers of the lung parenchyma (164), it releases von Willdebrand's factor, and binds to specific receptors on proliferating endothelial cells (165), and to heparin sulfate proteoglycans in the extracellular matrix. From these storage sites, VEGF can be released and may become available for endothelial cells (166). In an animal model, treatment with antibodies against VEGF inhibited the growth of tumor-induced angiogenesis (167); angiogenesis also has been inhibited by the anti-trypanosoma agent suramin that binds VEGF (168). Tuder et al. (169) assessed the distribution of VEGF and of VEGF mRNA in the lung tissue obtained from a patient with PPH. The VEGF mRNA was ubiquitously distributed in the "hypertensive" lung and was increased by Northern blot hybridization when compared with a normal human lung sample. It may play an important role in pulmonary vascular remodeling, since gene expression is greatly enhanced by hypoxia (170). Agents, such as heparin or suramin, might be useful therapeutically in treating VEGF-related intimal proliferation.

Insulin-like Growth Factor

Insulin-like growth factor I (IGF-1), may play a role in the vascular-remodeling process in the lungs; it has mitogenic activity when added in vitro to pulmonary artery smooth-muscle cells (171); it stimulates elastin synthesis in bovine pulmonary arterial smooth muscle cells (172); and it is released into the lymph draining from the lungs of sheep during air embolization injury (173). Assessment of the importance of IGF in pulmonary vascular remodeling awaits experiments designed to block IFG synthesis and action; such experiments are of interest because of the synergistic effect of IGF with those of PDGF and with agonists that stimulate the activity of protein kinase C (PKC), such as PAF.

Endothelin

Endothelin is produced in the lung by endothelial and bronchial epithelial cells. Endothelin-1 has been measured in peripheral venous blood obtained from 13 patients with PPH and 12 with Eisenmenger's syndrome. Patients with PPH had values that were roughly three times normal (174). These data, coupled with the report by Giaid et al. (59), which demonstrated increased expression of endothelin-1 in pulmonary arteries from patients with PPH, are compelling and suggest that endothelin may participate in the pathogenesis of PPH. The distribution of endothelin-1 by immunostaining of lung tissue from PPH patients resembles the distribution pattern of factor VIII in the vascular lesions described recently by Tuder et al. (96,169). Both factor VIII and endothelin-1 staining may reflect the proliferative activity of the remodeling endothelium. Certainly, endothelin can have autocrine activity. The expression of the endothelin receptor gene is increased in hypoxic lungs (54). A selective endothelin receptor antagonist that inhibits the ET_A receptor with high affinity for endothelin-1 has recently been shown to inhibit acute hypoxic vasoconstriction and endothelin-induced proliferation of cultured human pulmonary artery smooth muscle cells and to reduce the pulmonary hypertension in chronically hypoxic rats (175,176,176a).

Eicosanoids

Arachidonic acid metabolites, derived either by the cyclooxygenase or the 5-lipoxygenase pathway, have been implicated in lung vascular tone control (177,178) and also in lung vascular remodeling (179). The recent discovery of a second gene for cyclooxygenase (*COX-2*) (180) that can be induced by inflammatory stimuli, including endotoxin and IL-1, has rekindled the interest in lung vascular lipid mediator research. The synthesis of the important endogenous pulmonary vasodilator prostacyclin (PGI_2) is decreased in pulmonary arteries form neonatal calves with hypoxia-induced pulmonary hypertensin and in cultured endothelial cells derived from such hypertensive pulmonary arteries (181, 182). This deficiency in endogenous PGI_2 synthesis may it may reflect endothelial dysfunction, a decrease in the vessel number owing to remodeling, or suicide inhibition of the key enzyme prostacyclin synthase (183). As mentioned, Christman et al. (25,26) measured a stable urinary metabolite of prostacyclin and found a decrease in the amount of excreted PGI_2 metabolite in patients with PPH. In view of such an apparent deficit in the synthesis of an important pulmonary vasodilator, it is of interest that a retrovirus-mediated transfer with prostaglandin H synthase cDNA led to enhanced PGI_2 synthesis by cultured endothelial cells (184). Conceptually, a similar strategy might be possible with the aim to restore the PGI_2 synthesis of hypertensive, remodeled lung vessels. Thus, early in the development of severe pulmonary hypertension, inflammatory reactions (intra- and perivascular) may generate prostaglandins, thromboxane, and leukotrienes, with chemotactic, vasoactive, and proliferative properties, whereas late in the disease, the PGI_2 synthesis deficit may enhance proliferation of vascular cells. Cyclooxygenase inhibitors have not been tested systematically in patients with PPH (a low-dose regimen would be expected to affect thromboxane—but not PGI_2 synthesis), although there is a single report of IV ibuprofen treatment of a patient with pulmonary hypertension caused pulmonary embolism. Treatment reportedly decreased the systolic pulmonary artery pressure from 92 to 24 mmHg (185).

B. Oncogenes, Hormone Receptors, Phosphorylation

As pointed out in the Introduction, shear stress and mitogens may use common intracellular events that ultimately lead to changes in gene expression brought about by specific transcription factors, the activity of which is modulated by phosphorylation. Shear appears to translocate protein kinase C (PKC) to the endothelial cell plasma membrane and causes phospholipase C (PLC) and mitogen-activated protein (MAP) kinase activation which, in turn, can cause gene expression (for example, of the gene encoding the PDGF B chain) (186). The MAP kinases constitute a family of enzymes that are thought to function as intermediaries between membrane signals and the nucleus. These kinases and other kinases are part of a gigantic cellular switch board. Figure 15 illustrates that cytokine and growth factor receptors, as well as hormone receptors and oncogens, can function as kinases (switches) involved in cell growth and differentiation. The key event accomplished by cascades of kinase switches is the transfer of phos-

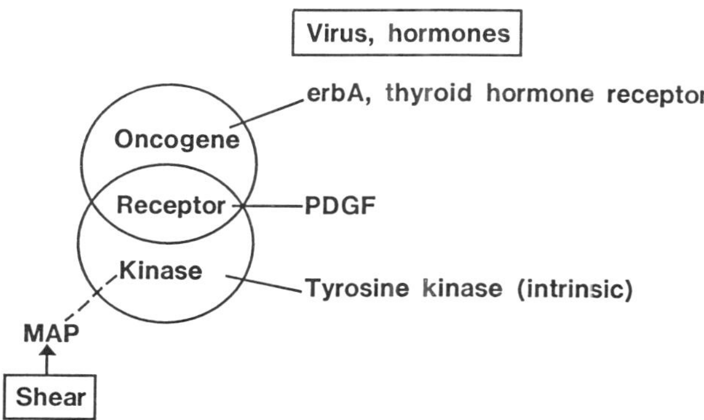

Figure 15 Oncogenes (viral genes), hormones, such as steroid and thyroid hormones, and shear stress can activate kinases and initiate the important phosphorylation reactions involved in vascular cell growth. Growth factor receptors often do double duty as kinases, and oncogenes can be involved in autocrine cell signaling.

phate groups from ATP to specific amino acids (serine, tyrosine, or threonine) of target proteins (187).

In reference to the protein kinase C pathway, Dempsey and co-workers (171,188,189), examined in model systems the effect of hypoxia on aspects of pulmonary vascular remodeling. Multiple signals (including increase of intracellular calcium, activation of PLA_2, PLC, or PLD) lead to activation of PKC (190). Hypoxia stimulates the translocation of PKC in bovine pulmonary artery smooth-muscle cells (188). Hypoxia-induced growth of pulmonary artery smooth-muscle cells may require a priming step that involves a Ca^{2+}-dependent PKC isoform activation. It will be important to identify the biologically relevant priming events (factors) that trigger PKC activation in hypertensive pulmonary arteries. Interestingly PDGF, but not IGF-1, primes bovine pulmonary artery cells PKC and promotes cell growth (191).

On the receptor level, there are important differences in the coupling and postreceptor events. Some receptors, like angiotensin receptors, are coupled by G-proteins to phospholipase (PLC), whereas the PDGF receptor doubles as a tyrosine kinase that is attached to a PLC and to a GTPase-activating protein (GAP). There, at the level of the PDGF receptor/kinase, is a point at which virally transmitted signals can be processed, since the v-*sis* oncogene encodes a protein (c-*sis*) highly analogous to the B chain of PDGF (192). In contrast, lipophilic hormone (steroid hormones and thyroid hormones) responses are mediated by an array of intracellular receptors that compose a large superfamily of transcription factors. Upon binding of the steroid hormone (H) to its receptor (Fig. 16), a heat-

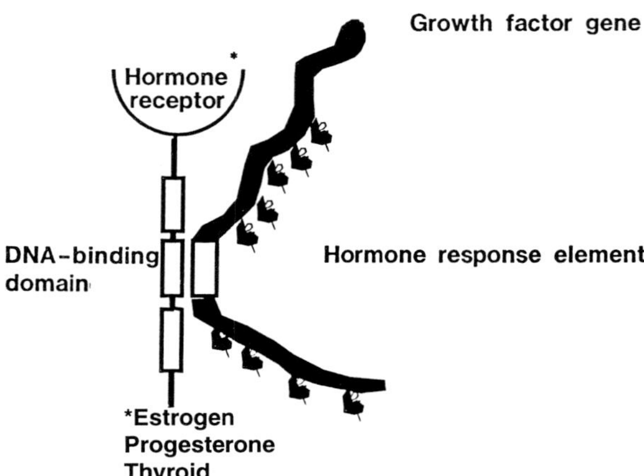

Figure 16 This schematic shows the binding of a (steroid) hormone receptor with its DNA-binding domain to a hormone response element initiating gene transcription.

shock protein (HSP) is released and the receptor is phosphorylated and attaches itself to specific hormone response elements (HRE) located in various gene promoters, both positive and negative. Effects on gene expression by glucocorticoids have been reported (193). Binding of such activated receptors for progesterone to one HRE increases the binding of further progesterone receptors to a second HRE manifold. One particular transcription factor family, called AP-1, mediates hormone-dependent expression as well as repression of many genes involved in control of cell proliferation, such as the vimentin gene (194). These molecular mechanisms may have importance in the well-appreciated, but not well-understood, sex hormone control of lung vascular remodeling. Another important transcription factor is NFκ B. Its binding activity can be induced in most cell types in response to phorbol esters, cytokines, and virus infection (such as HIV infection; 192).

In summary, the molecular mechanisms now being unraveled in the various models of cell growth and transformation are likely also involved in the exuberant proliferative events that characterize the remodeling of vessels in PPH. A detailed understanding of these molecular events may lead to specific therapeutic interventions.

VIII. Synopsis of the Pathophysiology in PPH

The hemodynamic profile of the typical patient with severe, unexplained (primary) pulmonary hypertension has been previously thoroughly described and reviewed (13,195). Briefly, the pulmonary artery pressure is high, the cardiac output is low, and cannot be increased by exercise. Vasodilator administration in the heart catheter laboratory to assess "the residual vasodilator potential" of the lung circulation quite frequently demonstrates a significant, acute (20–30%) reduction in pulmonary vascular reactivity (13). In the NIH registry study of PPH patients (14), a mean decrease in total pulmonary vascular resistance of 7.4 Wood units was observed. In combined acute vasodilator trials in a multicenter cohort of 95 patients with PPH the resistance fell from 32.5 to 25.1 Wood units. Prostacyclin was tested in 24 of these patients and had the most impressive effect on the cardiac output. The effects of prolonged therapy on hemodynamics and survival of PPH were not addressed in the NIH study. In a recent publication, Groves et al. (196) reported data obtained in 44 patients during a 7-year study period of an acute prostacyclin trial that was followed by extended Ca^{2+} antagonist treatment. Five patients had sustained clinical and hemodynamic response from Ca^{2+} channel blocker treatment, 8 different patients did not. The results of this University of Colorado cohort study shows that 7 patients survived 4.8–10.2 years on long-term Ca^{2+} antagonist treatment, whereas 7 patients were alive for 2.6–6.4 years following heart–lung transplantation (6 patients died 0.1–1.2 years following transplantation). However, 8 of the patients with a significant acute prostacyclin vasodilation (26–60% decrease in pulmonary vascular resistance) did not survive 1 year following the heart catheterization. Two patients who had a respectable decrease in pulmonary vascular resistance at 8 weeks of continued diltiazem treatment (−41 and −36%) died at 0.7 and 1.4 years, respectively after their heart catheterization. One of these two patients, a 30-year-old woman still demonstrated a diltiazem response after 1 year of diltiazem therapy. It appears that the disease that we call unexplained (primary) pulmonary hypertension displays a spectrum of disease activities, with a rapidly progressive form on one end and perhaps a slower evolving variant on the other end. Although a low cardiac output and an elevated right atrial pressure are statistical predictors of short survival in the University of Colorado cohort study, 6 patients at the initial catheterization had mean right atrial pressures of 20 mmHg or greater, yet 50% of these patients survived more than 2 years.

We currently know of no marker of disease activity; we can also not predict which patient will develop right ventricular failure, as demonstrated by a subgroup of long-term survivors in the European aminorex patient group. Research is necessary to develop and validate markers of disease activity that (127,128) relate to the relentless vascular cell proliferation. Biochemical markers of lung cell proliferation must be found. It is now clear that a second intravascular event can contribute to the progression of the disease, that is in situ thrombosis (as discussed earlier). The third component is the reserve—or lack there of—of the right ventricular myocardium to withstand the chronic pressure overload. Again, we do not understand—on the molecular level—why the myocardium fails in some patients and does not fail (at the same pulmonary artery pressure elevation) in others. This unpredictable behavior may be due to the right-sided ischemia, since the right ventricular myocardium performs flawlessly shortly following single lung transplantation. If the disease severity in the individual patient is indeed a compilation of these factors: proliferative activity, secondary in situ thrombosis, and right ventricular myocardial failure, then a therapy directed toward each of these three "progression factors" might prolong survival. Short of lung transplantation, which clearly will not be an option for all patients with PPH, a combination drug therapy, rather than a therapy that relies exclusively on Ca^{2+} entry blockade—may have merits. Targeting the failing myocardium of the right ventricle in patients with PPH may be justified, given emerging information on the alterations of contractile proteins in the pressure overloaded heart. Procollagen synthesis is increased in the myocardium (197), an excess of microtubules in stress-hypertrophied cardiocytes and polymerized tubulin may contribute to the contractile dysfunction (198), and alteration of the myocardial β-adrenergic receptor signal transduction may be important (199). In patients with PPH and failing right ventricles, Bristow et al. (199) found, in right heart samples obtained by endomyocardial biopsies, a marked decrease in the β_1-adrenergic receptor density and a marked decrease in the activity of stimulated adenylate cyclase. Thus, it appears that there is increasing evidence for *local* myocardial (membrane and intracellular) mechanisms to be involved in the pathophysiology of the pressure-overloaded right ventricle. A question of potential therapeutic interest is whether the defect in the catalytic subunit of the right ventricular cardiocyte adenylate cyclase can be "repaired" or bypassed. A β-adrenergic receptor desensitization is typically observed in states of increased sympathetic tone, as under conditions of chronic hypobaric hypoxia (200).

Gibbs et al. (201) monitored pulmonary artery pressures in patients with chronic heart failure and with PPH and found in several patients a sleep-related increase in pulmonary hypertension. Since rapid eye movement (REM) sleep is associated with profound sympathetic activation (202), the nocturnal worsening of PH in some patients could be due to diurnal variations in sympathetic activity. Whether sleep-disordered breathing occurred in any of these reported PPH patients with nocturnal worsening of the PH is not known. Regardless, this first pilot study suggests that in some patients with PPH there can be a substantial increase in pulmonary artery pressure during the night, perhaps because of vasoconstriction triggered by activity of the autonomic nervous system.

IX. Summary and Outlook

This review illustrates how our concepts about this severe pulmonary vascular disease have evolved and taken us from a thorough description of the hemodynamics, the vasoconstrictive factor of Paul Wood (195), to the cellular and molecular events that control cell growth in the vessels. The application of immunostaining and in situ hybridization techniques aided by PCR technology will undoubtedly lead to an understanding of the dynamic processes that we call pulmonary vascular remodeling. Endothelial dysfunction in the pulmonary vasculature may result in increased platelet activation, with associated release of 5-HT and thromboxane; and in the reduction of endothelium-derived vasodilator substances, such as nitric oxide and prostacyclin. One important question related to the pathophysiology of PPH is whether the increase of 5-HT or thromboxane, or the decrease in nitric oxide or prostacyclin, might be a primary defect, with the other changes occurring secondary to induced endothelial cell dysfunction. A rise in pulmonary vascular smooth-muscle cell cytosolic calcium will cause vasoconstriction, regardless of which of the mechanisms, illustrated in Figure 2, is responsible for that rise. At present, the roles of 5-HT and endothelin appear the most interesting, and it remains to be determined whether they relate to the gating of the potassium channel, the membrane potential, or the release of intracellular calcium. The principle clinical challenge continues to be the early diagnosis of PPH. Another important challenge to meet is the discovery of markers of disease activity and disease progression. We attempted to provide immunohistological evidence that emphasizes the important role of endothelial cell proliferation in the pathogenesis of PPH. We wonder whether nonvascular lung cells participate in the lung vascular remodeling. For example, chronic hypoxia causes substantial airway epithelial cell proliferation (203): are these cells, sending growth signals to the vessels? New forms of treatment are likely as a consequence of our better understanding of vascular biology. Ornithine decarboxylase inhibitors have been effective as inhibitors of pulmonary vascular remodeling in animal models (204,205). Supplementation of the precursor of nitric oxide (NO), L-arginine, in the diet of chronically hypoxic rats (206), has restored the impaired endothelium-dependent vasodilation. Treatment strategies based on the NO paradigm are currently being designed and available for clinical testing. Since NO amplifies calcium-induced gene transcription and could potentiate protein kinase phosphorylation of cytoplasmic proteins, long-term NO treatment of patients with PPH may be problematic.

Finally, ion channels, in particular K^+ channels, are receiving increasing attention in the context of pulmonary vasomotor tone regulation (68,69). The design of specific K^+ channel drugs may be further warranted, since K^+ channel activity alone may be involved in mitogenesis (207), and in pulmonary vascular remodeling.

Acknowledgments

The authors wish to thank Nancy Hart and Maxine Denton for invaluable secretarial help. This work has been supported by a Grant in Aid 92015300 from the

American Heart Association and by an Academic Vascular Award from the National Institutes of Health.

References

1. Ross R. The pathogenesis of atherosclerosis: a perspective for the 1990s. Nature 1993; 362:801–809.
2. Wagenvoort CA, Wagenvoort N. Pathology of Pulmonary Hypertension. New York: John Wiley & Sons, 1977.
3. Caslin AW, Heath D, Madden B, Yacoub M, Gosney, JR, Smith P. The histopathology of 36 cases of plexogenic pulmonary arteriopathy. Histopathology 1990; 16:9–19.
4. Dresdale DT, Schultz M, Michtom RJ. Primary pulmonary hypertensin: clinical and hemodynamic study. Am J Med 1951; 11:686–705.
5. Wood P. The vasoconstrictive factor in pulmonary hypertension: Br Heart J 1957; 19:279–292.
6. Whitaker W, Heath D. Idiopathic pulmonary hypertension: etiology, pathogenesis, diagnosis and treatment. Prog Cardiovasc Dis 1958; 1:380–396.
7. Wade G, Ball J. Unexplained pulmonary hypertension. Q J Med 1957; 26:83–119.
8. Wagenvoort CA, Wagenvoort N. Primary pulmonary hypertension: a pathologic study of the lung vessels in 156 clinically diagnosed cases. Circulation 1970; 42:1163–1184.
9. Rao BNS, Moller JH, Edwards JE. Primary pulmonary hypertension in a child: response to pharmacologic agents. Circulation 1969; 40:583–587.
10. Winters WL Jr, Joseph RR, Learner N. Primary pulmonary hypertension and Raynaud's phenomenon. Arch Intern Med 1964; 114:821–830.
11. Barst RJ. Pharmacologically induced pulmonary vasodilation in children and young adults with primary pulmonary hypertension. Chest 1986; 89:497–503.
12. Palevsky HI, Schloo BL, Pietra GG. Primary pulmonary hypertension: vascular structure, morphometry and responsiveness to vasodilator agents. Circulation 1989; 80:1207–1221.
13. Reeves JT, Groves BM, Turkevich D. The case for treatment of selected patients with primary pulmonary hypertension. Am Rev Respir Dis 1986; 134:342–346.
14. Weir EK, Rubin LJ, Ayres SM, Bergofsky EH, Brundage BH, Detre KM, Elliott CG, Fishman AP, Goldring RM, Groves BM, Kernis JT, Koerner SK, Levy PS, Pietra GG, Reid LM, Rich S, Vreim CE, Williams GW, Wu M. The acute administration of vasodilators in primary pulmonary hypertension. Am Rev Respir Dis 1989; 140: 1623–1630.
15. Rich S, Kaufmann E, Levy PS. The effect of high doses of calcium-channel blockers on survival in primary pulmonary hypertension. N Engl J Med 1992; 327:76–81.
16. Rich S, Hart K, Kieras K, et al. Thromboxane synthetase inhibition in primary pulmonary hypertension. Chest 1987; 91:356–360.
17. Herve P, Launay JM, Drouet L, et al. (1988). Significance of high plasma serotonin in primary pulmonary hypertension (abstrt). Am Rev Respir Dis 1990; 137:106.
18. McGoon MD, Vanhoutte PM. Aggregating platelets contract isolated canine pulmonary arteries by releasing 5-hydroxytryptamide. J Clin Invest 1984; 74:828–833.

19. Herve P, Drouet L, et al. Primary pulmonary hypertension in a patient with a familial platelet storage pool disease: role of serotonin. Am J Med 1990; 89:117–120.
20. Sato K, Webb S, Tucker A, et al. Factors influencing the idiopathic development of pulmonary hypertension in the fawn hooded rat. Am Rev Respir Dis 1992; 145: 793–797.
21. Ashmore RC, Rodman DM, Sato K, et al. Paradoxical constriction to platelets by arteries from rats with pulmonary hypertension. Am J Physiol 1991; 260:H1929–1934.
22. Willerson JT, Eidt JF, McNatt J, et al. Role of thromboxane and serotonin as mediators in the development of spontaneous alterations in coronary blood flow and neointimal proliferation in canine models with chronic coronary artery stenoses and endothelial injury. J Am Coll Cardiol 1991; 17:101B–110B.
23. Watkins WD, Peterson MB, Crone RK, et al. Prostacyclin and prostaglandin E_1 for severe idiopathic pulmonary artery hypertension. Lancet 1980; 1:1083.
24. Barst RJ, Stalcup SA, Steeg CN, et al. Relation of arachidonate metabolites to abnormal control of the pulmonary circulation in a child. Am Rev Respir Dis 1985; 131:171–177.
25. Christman BW, McPherson CD, Newman JH, et al. An imbalance between the excretion of thromboxane and prostacyclin metabolites in pulmonary hypertension. N Engl J Med 1992; 327:70–75.
26. Christman BW, Newman JH, Loyd JE, et al. Thromboxane and prostacyclin metabolites in pulmonary hypertension (letter). N Engl J Med 1992; 327:1458.
27. Eisenberg PR, Lucore C, Kaufman L, et al. Fibrinopeptide A levels indicative of pulmonary vascular thrombosis in patients with primary pulmonary hypertension. Circulation 1990; 82:841–847.
28. Huber K, Beckmann R, Frank H, et al. Fibrinogen, t-PA and PAI-1 plasma levels in patients with pulmonary hypertension. Am J Respir Crit Care Med 1994; 150: 929–933.
29. Seeger W, Neuhof H, Hall J, et al. Pulmonary vasoconstrictor response to soluble fibrin in isolated lungs: possible role of thromboxane generation. Circ Res 1988; 62:651–659.
30. Weir EK, McMurtry IF, Tucker A, et al. Prostaglandin synthetase inhibitors do not decrease hypoxic pulmonary vasoconstriction. J Appl Physiol 1976; 41:714–718.
31. Archer SL, Tolins JP, Weir EK, et al. Hypoxic pulmonary vasoconstriction is enhanced by inhibition of the synthesis of an endothelium derived relaxing factors. Biochem Biophys Res Commun 1989; 164:1198–1205.
32. Nishiwaki K, Nyhan DP, Rock P, et al. N^{ω}-Nitro-L-arginine and pulmonary vascular pressure-flow relationship in conscious dogs. Am J Pathol 1992; 262:H1331–1337.
33. Marshall C, Marshall BE. Hypoxic pulmonary vasoconstriction is not endothelium dependent. Proc Soc Exp Biol Med 1992; 201:267–270.
34. Abman SH, Chatfield BA, Hall SL, et al. Role of endothelium-derived relaxing factor during transition of pulmonary circulation at birth. Am J Pathol 1990; 259: H1921–1927.
35. Fineman JR, Chang R, Soifer SJ. EDRF inhibition augments pulmonary hypertension in intact newborn lambs. Am J Physiol 1992; 262:H1365–1371.

36. Archer S, Hampl V, McKenzie Z, et al. Role of endothelial-derived nitric oxide in normal and hypertensive pulmonary vasculature. Semin Respir Crit Care Med 1994; 15:179–189.
37. Samet P, Bernstein WH, Widrich J. Intracardiac infusion of acetylcholine in primary pulmonary hypertension. Am Heart J 1960; 60:433–439.
38. Samet P, Bernstein WH. Loss of reactivity of the pulmonary vascular bed in primary pulmonary hypertension. Am Heart J 1963; 66:197–199.
39. Uren NG, Ludman PF, Crake T, et al. Response of the pulmonary circulation to acetylcholine, calcitonin gene-related peptide, substance P and oral nicardipine in patients with primary pulmonary hypertension. J Am Coll Cardiol 1992; 19:835–841.
40. Dinh-Xuan A, Higenbottam T, Clelland M. Impairment of endothelium-dependent pulmonary-artery relaxation in obstructive lung disease. N Engl J Med 1991; 324: 1539–1547.
41. Adnot S, Kouyoumdjian C, Defouilloy C, et al. Hemodynamic and gas exchange responses to infusion of acetylcholine and inhalation of nitric oxide in patients with chronic obstructive lung disease and pulmonary hypertension. Am Rev Respir Dis 1993; 148:310–316.
42. Pepke-Zaba J, Higenbottam TW, Dinh-Xuan AT, et al. Inhaled nitric oxide as a cause of selective pulmonary vasodilation in pulmonary hypertension. Lancet 1991; 338: 1173–1174.
43. Kinsella JP, Neish SR, Shaffer E, et al. Low-dose inhalational nitric oxide in persistent pulmonary hypertension of the newborn. Lancet 1992; 340:819–820.
44. Rubin LJ, Groves BM, Reeves JT, et al. Prostacyclin-induced acute pulmonary vasodilation in primary pulmonary hypertension. Circulation 1982; 66:334–338.
45. Rubin LJ, Mendoza J, Hood M, et al. Treatment of primary pulmonary hypertension with continuous intravenous prostacyclin. Ann Intern Med 1990; 112:485–491.
46. Ivy DD, Wiggins JW, Badesch DB, et al. Nitric oxide and prostacyclin treatment of an infant with primary pulmonary hypertension. Am J Cardiol 1994; 74:414–416.
47. Inoue A, Yanagisawa M, Kimura S, et al. The human endothelin family: three structurally and pharmacologically distant isopeptides predicted by the separate genes. Proc Natl Acad Sci USA 1989; 86:2863–2867.
48. Eddahibi S, Raffestin B, Braquet P, et al. Pulmonary vascular reactivity to endothelin-1 in normal and chronically pulmonary hypertensive rats. J Cardiovasc Pharmacol 1991; 17:S358–361.
49. Hasunuma K, Rodman DM, O'Brien RF, et al. Endothelin-1 causes pulmonary vasodilation in rats. Am J Physiol 1990; 259:H48–H54.
50. de Nucci G, Thomas R, D'Orleans-Juste P, et al. Pressor effects of circulating endothelin are limited by its removal in the pulmonary circulation and by the release of prostacyclin and endothelium-derived relaxing factors. Proc Natl Acad Sci USA 1988; 85:9797–9800.
51. Kurihara Y, Kurihara H, Suzuki H, et al. Elevated blood pressure and craniofacial abnormalities in mice deficient in endothelin-1. Nature 1994; 368:703–710.
52. Goto K, Kasuya Y, Matsuki N, et al. Endothelin activates the dihydropyridine-sensitive, voltage-dependent Ca^{2+} channel in vascular smooth muscle. Proc Natl Acad Sci USA 1989; 86:3915–3918.

53. Wallnofer A, Weir S, Ruegg U, et al. The mechanism of action of endothelin-1 as compared with other agonists in vascular smooth muscle. J Cardiovasc Pharmacol 1989; 13(Suppl 5):23–31.
54. Stelzner TJ, O'Brien RF, Yanagisawa M, et al. Increased lung endothelin-1 production in rats with idiopathic pulmonary hypertension. Am J Physiol 1992; 262:L614–L620.
55. Li H, Elton TS, Chen YF, et al. Increased endothelin receptor gene expression in hypoxic rat lung. Am J Physiol 1994; 266:L553–L560.
56. Bonvallet ST, Zamora MR, Hasunuma K, et al. BQ123, an ET_A-receptor antagonist, attenuates hypoxic pulmonary hypertension in rats. Am J Physiol 1994; 266:H1327–H1331.
57. Kourembanas S, McQuillan LP, Leung GK, et al. Nitric oxide regulates the expression of vasoconstrictors and growth factors by vascular endothelium under both normoxia and hypoxia. J Clin Invest 1993; 92:99–104.
58. Stewart DJ, Levy RD, Cernacek P, et al. Increased plasma endothelin-1 in pulmonary hypertension: marker or mediator of disease? Ann Intern Med 1991; 114:464–469.
59. Giaid A, Yanagisawa M, Langleben D, et al. Expression of endothelin-1 in the lungs of patients with pulmonary hypertension. N Engl J Med 1993; 328:1732–1739.
60. Zamora MR, O'Brien RF, Rutherford RB, et al. Serum endothelin-1 concentrations and cold provocation in primary Raynaud's phenomenon. Lancet 1990; 336:1144–1147.
61. von Euler U, Liljestrand G. Observations on the pulmonary arterial blood pressure in the cat. Acta Physiol Scand 1946; 12:301–320.
62. Madden J, Vadula M, Kurup V. Effects of hypoxia and other vasoactive agents on pulmonary and cerebral artery smooth muscle cells. Am J Physiol 1992; 263:L384–L393.
63. McMurtry I, Davidson A, Reeves JT, et al. Inhibition of hypoxic pulmonary vasoconstriction by calcium antagonists in isolated rat lungs. Circ Res 1976; 38:99–104.
64. McMurtry I. BAY K 8644 potentiates and A23187 inhibits hypoxic vasoconstriction in rat lungs. Am J Physiol 1985; 249:H741–H746.
65. Tolins M, Weir K, Chesler E, et al. Pulmonary vascular tone is increased by a voltage-dependent calcium channel potentiator. J Appl Physiol 1986; 60:942–948.
66. Madden J, Dawson C, Harder D. Hypoxia induced activation in small isolated pulmonary arteries from the cat. J Appl Physiol 1985; 59:113–118.
67. Jensen K, Mico A, Czartolomna J, et al. Rapid onset of hypoxic vasoconstriction in isolated lungs. J Appl Physiol 1992; 72:2018–2023.
68. Post J, Hume J, Archer S, et al. Direct role for K^+ channel inhibition in hypoxic pulmonary vasoconstriction. Am J Physiol 1992; 18:C882–C890.
69. Hasunuma K, Rodman D, McMurtry I. Effects of K^+ channel blockers on vascular tone in the perfused rat lung. Am Rev Respir Dis 1991; 144:884–887.
70. Lopez-Barneo J, Benot A, Urena J. O_2 sensing and the electrophysiology of arterial chemoreceptor cells. NIPS 1993; 8:191–195.
71. Yuan X-J, Goldman W, Tod M. Ionic currents in rat pulmonary and mesenteric arteriolar myocytes in primary culture and subculture. Am J Physiol 1993; 264: L107–L115.

72. Pietra GG, Edwards WD, Kay JM, et al. Histopathology of primary pulmonary hypertension. Circulation 1989; 80:1198–1206.
73. Loyd JE, Atkinson JB, Pietra CG, Virmani R, Newman JH. Heterogenity of pathologic lesions in familial primary pulmonary hypertension. Am Rev Respir Dis 1988; 38:952–957.
74. Yaginuma G, Mohri H, Takahashi T. Distribution of arterial lesions and collateral pathways in the pulmonary hypertension of congenital heart disease: a computer aided reconstruction study. Thorax 1990; 45:586–590.
75. Wang N, Butler JP, Ingber DE. Mechanotransduction across the cell surface and through the cytoskeleton. Science 1993; 260:1124–1128.
76. Davies PF. How do vascular endothelial cells respond to flow? NIPS 1989; 4:22–25.
77. Davies PF, Tripathi SC. Mechanical stress mechanisms and the cell. Circ Res 1993; 72:239–245.
78. Dinh-Xuan AT, Cremona G, Pepke Zaba, et al. Impairment of pulmonary artery endothelium-dependent relaxation in chronic obstructive lung disease is not due to dysfunction of endothelial cell membrane receptors nor to L-arginine deficiency. Br J Pharmacol 1993; 109:587–591.
79. Geggel RL, Carvalho ACA, Hoyer LW, Reid LM. von Willebrand factor abnormalities in primary pulmonary hypertension. Am Rev Respir Dis 1987; 135:294–299.
80. Anderson EG, Simon G, Reid L. Primary and thrombo-embolic pulmonary hypertension: a quantitative pathological study. J Pathol 1973; 110:273.
81. Edwards WD. Pathology of pulmonary hypertension. Cardiovasc Clin 1987; 18: 321–355.
82. Ono S, Voelkel NF. PAF receptor blockade inhibits lung vascular changes in the rat monocrotaline model. Lung 1992; 170:31–40.
83. Ono S, Westcott JY, Voelkel NF. PAF antagonists inhibit pulmonary vascular remodeling induced by hypobaric hypoxia in rats. J Appl Physiol 1992; 73:1084–1092.
84. Mecham RP, Whitehouse LA, Wrenn DS, et al. Smooth muscle-mediated connective tissue remodeling in pulmonary hypertension. Science 1987; 237:423–426.
85. Arrillaga FC. Sclerose de l'artere plumonaire secondaire a certains estats pulmonaires chroniques. Arch Mal Coeur 1913; 6:518.
86. Bjornsson J, Edwards WD. Primary pulmonary hypertension: a histopathologic study of 80 cases. Mayo Clin Proc 1985; 60:16–25.
87. Hale KA, Niewoehner DE, Cosio MG. Morphologic changes in the muscular pulmonary arteries: relationship to cigarette smoking, airway disease and emphysema. Am Rev Respir Dis 1980; 122:273–278
88. Wright JL, Lawson L, Pare PD, et al. The structure and function of the pulmonary vasculature in mild chronic obstructive pulmonary disease. Am Rev Respir Dis 1983; 128:702–707.
89. Selby C, Drost E, Lannan S, Wraith PK, Macnee W. Neutrophil retention in the lungs of patients with chronic obstructive pulmonary disease. Am Rev Respir Dis 1991; 143:1359–1364.
90. Voelkel NF, Czartolomna J, Simpson J, Murphy RC. FMLP causes eicosanoid-dependent vasoconstriction and edema in lungs from endotoxin-primed rats. Am Rev Respir Dis 1992; 145:701–711.

91. Perkett EA, Brigham KL, Meyrick B. Granulocyte depletion attenuates sustained pulmonary hypertension and increased pulmonary vasoreactivity caused by continuous air embolization in sheep. Am Rev Respir Dis 1990; 141:456–465.
92. Liptay MJ, Parks WC, Mecham RP, Roby J, Kaiser LR, Cooper JD, Botney M. Neointimal macrophages co-localize with extracellular matrix gene expression in human atherosclerotic pulmonary arteries. J Clin Invest 1993; 91:588–594.
93. Botney M. Vascular remodeling in primary pulmonary hypertension: what role for transforming growth factor-beta. Semin Respir Crit Care Med 1994; 15:215–222.
94. Hales C. Case records of the Massachusetts General Hospital. N Engl J Med 327: 873–880.
95. Schwarz MI, Lynch DE, Tuder R. Bronchiolitis obliterans the lone manifestation of rheumatoid arthritis? Eur Respir J 1994; 7:817–820.
96. Tuder RM, Groves B, Badesch DB, Voelkel NF. Exuberant endothelial cell growth and elements of inflammation are present in plexiform lesions of pulmonary hypertension. Am J Pathol 1994; 144:275–285.
97. Ross R. The role of T lymphocytes in inflammation. Proc Natl Acad Sci USA 1994; 91:2879.
98. Wagenvoort CA, Wagenvoort N. Pulmonary vascular bed: normal anatomy and responses to disease. In: Moser KM, ed. Pulmonary Vascular Disease. Lung Biology in Health and Disease. Vol. 14, New York: Marcel Dekker, 1979.
99. Kay JM, Heath D. Pathologic study of unexplained pulmonary hypertension. Semin Respir Med 1985; 7:180–192.
100. Schraufnagel DE. Monocrotaline-induced angiogenesis. Am J Pathol 1990; 137: 1083–1090.
101. Voelkel NF, Weir EK. Etiologic mechanisms in primary pulmonary hypertension. In: Weir EK, Reeves JT, eds. Pulmonary Vascular Physiology and Pathophysiology. Lung Biology in Health and Disease. Vol. 38, New York: Marcel Dekker, 1989.
102. Rich S, Kieras K, Hart K, Groves BM, Stobo JD, Brundage BH. Antinuclear antibodies in primary pulmonary hypertension. J Am Coll Cardiol 1986; 8:1307–11.
103. Isern RA, Yaneva M, Weiner E, Parke A, Rothfield N, Dantzker D, Rich S, Arnett FC. Autoantibodies in patients with primary pulmonary hypertension: association with anti-Ku. Am J Med 1992; 93:307–311.
104. Morse JH, Barst RJ, Fotino M. Familial pulmonary hypertension: immunogenetic findings in four Caucasian kindreds. Am Rev Respir Dis 1992; 145:787–792.
105. Chou CH, Wang J, Knuth MW, Reeves WH. Role of a major autoepitope in forming the DNA binding site of the p70 (Ku) antigen. J Exp Med 1992; 175;1677–1684.
106. Asherson RA, Higenbottam TW, Dihn Xuan AT, et al. Pulmonary hypertension in a lupus clinic: experience with twenty-four patients. J Rheumatol 1990; 17:1292–1298.
107. Roncoroni AJ, Alvarez C, Molinas F. Plexogenic arteriopathy associated with pulmonary vasculitis in systemic lupus erythematosus. Respiration 1992; 59:52–56.
108. Simonson JE, Schiller NB, Petri M, et al. Pulmonary hypertension and systemic lupus erythematosis. J Rheumatol 1989; 16:918–925.
109. Schwartzberg M, Lieberman DH, Getzoff B, Ehrlich GE. Systemic lupus erythematosus and pulmonary vascular hypertension. Arch Intern Med 1984; 144:605–607.
110. Quismorio FP, Sharma O, Koss M, Boylen T, Edmiston AW, Thornton PJ, Tatter D.

Immunopathologic and clinical studies in pulmonary hypertension associated with systemic lupus erythematosus. Semin Arthritis Rheum 1984; 13:349–359.
111. Cervera R, Khamashta MA, Font J, Sebastiani GD, Gil A, Lavilla P, Domenech I, Aydintug AO, Jedryka-Goral A, de Ramon E, Galeazzi M, Haga H, Mathieu A, Houssiau F, Ingelmo M, Hughes G. Systemic lupus erythematosus: clinical and immunologic patterns of disease expression in a cohort of 1,000 patients. Medicine 1993; 72:113–124.
112. Desnoyers MR, Bernstein S, Cooper AG, Kopelman RI. Pulmonary hemorrhage in lupus erythematosus without evidence of an immunologic cause. Arch Intern Med 1984, 144:1398–1400.
113. Myers JL, Katzenstein AA. Micro angiitis in lupus-induced pulmonary hemorrhage. Am J Clin Pathol 1986; 85:552–556.
114. Bunch T, Tancredi R, Lie J. Pulmonary hypertension in polymyositis. Chest 1991; 79:105–107.
115. Rawson AJ, Woske HM. A study of etiologic factors in so called primary pulmonary hypertension. Arch Intern Med 1960; 105:81.
116. Badesch DB, Wynne KM, Bonvallet S, Voelkel NF, Ridgeway C, Groves BM. Hypothyroidism and primary pulmonary hypertension. Ann Intern Med 1993; 119: 44–46.
117. Martas VJ. Primary pulmonary hypertension associated with hyperthyroidism. Aten Primaria 1992; 9:163–4.
118. Speich R, Jenni R, Opravil M, Pfab M, Russi EW. Primary pulmonary hypertension in HIV infection. Chest 1991; 100:1268–71.
119. Jacques C, Richmond G, Tierney L, et al. Primary pulmonary hypertension and human immunodeficiency virus infection in a non-hemophiliac man. Pathologe 1992; 23:191–194.
120. Kim KK, Factor SM. Membraneoproliferative glomerulonephritis and plexogenic pulmonary arteriopathy in a homosexual man with acquired immunodeficiency syndrome. Pathologe 1987; 18:1293–1296.
121. Mette SA, Palevsky HI, Pietra GG, Williams TM, Bruder E, Prestipino, AJ, Patrick AM, Wirth JA. Primary pulmonary hypertension in association with human immunodeficiency virus infection. Am Rev Respir Dis 1992; 145:1196–1200.
122. Tuder RM, Weinberg A, Bates T, Hoeper M, Li Z, Voelkel N. *Tat*-protein of HIV enhances inflammatory cell binding and PDGF levels in CMV-infected endothelial cells. Circulation 1994; 90:2237.
123. Kaner RJ, Ursea R, Ursea B, Emanuel D, Hajjar DP. Cytomegalovirus-induced release of mitogenic stimulators and inhibitors from vascular cells in vitro. Am Rev Respir Dis 1993; 147:A490.
124. Louis M, Thorens FB, Chevrolet JC. Calcium channel blockers testing for primary pulmonary hypertension associated with HIV infection. Am Rev Respir Dis 1993; 147:A536.
125. Ruchelli ED, Nojadera G, Rutstein R, Rudy B. Pulmonary veno-occlusive disease. Arch Pathol Lab Med 1994; 118:664–666.
126. Gahl K, Fabel E, Greiser E, Harmjanz D, Ostertag H, Stender HS, Primary vascular pulmonary hypertension. Report on 21 patients. Z. Kreislaufforsch 1970; 59: 868–883.

127. Frank H, Miczoch J, Lang I, Kneussl M, Baur HR, Gurtner HP. Influence of warfarin therapy in primary pulmonary hypertension. In: Widimsky J, Hengett F, eds. Progress in Respiration Research, Basel: S. Karger, 1987:119–124.
128. Gurtner HP. Chronische pulmonale Hypertonie vaskulären Ursprungs, plexogene pulmonale Arteriopathie und der Appetitzügler Aminorex: Nachlese zu einer Epidemie. Schweiz Med Wochenschr 1985; 115:782–789.
129. Douglas JG, Munro JF, Kitchin AH, Muir AL, Proudfoot AT. Pulmonary hypertension and fenfluramine. Br Med J 1981; 283:881–883.
130. McMurray J, Bloomfield P, Miller HC. Br Med J 1986; 292:239–240.
131. Rubin LJ, et al. Primary pulmonary hypertension. Chest 1993; 104:236–250.
132. Swift GL, Gibbs A, Campbell CA, Wagenvoort CA, Tuthill D. Pulmonary veno-occlusive disease and Hodgkin's lymphoma. Eur Respir J 1993; 6:596–598.
133. McCarthy JT, Staats BA. Pulmonary hypertension, hemolytic anemia, and renal failure. A mitomycin C-associated syndrome. Chest 1986; 89:608–611.
134. Reindel JF, Ganey PE, Wagner JG, Clocombe RF, Roth RA. Development of morphologic, hemodynamic, and biochemical changes in lungs of rats given monocrotaline pyrrole. Toxicol Appl Pharmacol 1990; 106:179–200.
135. Wagner JG, Petry TW, Roth RA. Characterization of monocrotaline pyrrole-induced DNA cross-linking in pulmonary artery endothelium. Am J Physiol 1993; 264: L517–L522.
136. Furie B, Furie BC. Molecular and cellular biology of blood coagulation. N Engl J Med 1992; 366:800–806.
137. Powell JS, Clozel JP, Muller RKM, Kuhn H, Heti F, Hosang M, Baumgartner HR. Inhibitors of angiotensin-converting enzyme prevent myointimal proliferation after vascular injury. Science 1989; 245:186–188.
138. Bell L, Luthringer DJ, Madri JA, Warren SL. Autocrine angiotensin system regulation of bovine aortic endothelial cell migration and plasminogen activator involves modulation of proto-oncogene pp60$^{c\text{-}src}$ expression. J Clin Invest 1992; 89:315–320.
139. Nelken NA, Soifer SJ, O'Keefe J, Vu TH, Charo IF, Coughlin SR. Thrombin receptor expression in normal and atherosclerotic human arteries. J Clin Invest 1992; 90:1614–1621.
140. Fink LM, Eidt JF, Johnson K, Cook JM, Cook CD, Morser J, Marlar R, Collins CL, Schaefer R, Xie S, Hsu S, Hsu P. Thrombomodulin activity and localization. Int J Dev Biol 1993; 37:221–226.
141. Wagenvoort CA, Mulder PGH. Thrombotic lesions in primary plexogenic arteriopathy. Chest 1993; 103:844–49.
142. Ingelsby TV, Singer JW, Gordon DS. Abnormal fibrinolysis in familial pulmonary hypertension. Am J Med 1973; 55:5–14.
143. Tubbs RR, Levin RD, Shirey EK, Hoffman GC. Fibrinolysis in familial pulmonary hypertension. Am J Clin Pathol 1979; 71:384–387.
144. Kentera D, Susic D, Veljkovic V, Tucakovic G, Koko V. Pulmonary artery pressure in rats with hereditary platelet function defect. Respiration 1988; 54:110–114.
145. Bobik A, Campbell JH. Vascular derived growth factors: cell biology, pathophysiology, and pharmacology. Pharmacol Rev 1993; 45:1–41.
146. Mantovani A, Bussolino F, Dejana E. Cytokine regulation of endothelial cell function. FASEB J 1992; 6:2591–2599.

147. Voelkel NF, Tuder RM, Bridges J, Arend WP. Interleukin-1 receptor antagonist treatment reduces pulmonary hypertension generated in rats by monocrotaline. Am J Respir Cell Mol Biol 1994; 11:664–675.
148. Colotta F, Lampugnanii MG, Polentaretti N, Dejana E, Montovani A. Interleukin 1 induces c-*fos* protooncogene expression in cultured human endothelial cells. Biochem Biophys Res Commun 1988; 152:1104–1110.
149. Gerritsen ME, Bloor CM. Endothelial cell gene expression in response to injury. FASEB J 1993; 7:523–532.
150. Border WA, Ruoslahti E. Transforming growth factor-beta in disease: the dark side of tissue repair. J Clin Invest 1992; 90:1–7.
151. Perkett EA, Pelton RW, Gold LI, Meyrick B. Expression of transforming growth factor TGF-β_1, -β_2, and -β_3 in sheep lungs during the development of pulmonary hypertension secondary to air embolization: immunohistochemistry and in situ hybridization. Am Rev Respir Dis 1992; 145:A484.
152. Perkett EA, Pelton RW, Meyrick B, Gold LI, Miller DA. Expression of transforming growth factor-β mRNAs and proteins in pulmonary vascular remodeling in the sheep air embolization model of pulmonary hypertension. Am J Respir Cell Mol Biol 1994; 11:16–24.
153. Botney M, Parks WC, Crouch EC, Stenmark K, Mecham RP. TGF-β_1 is decreased in remodeling hypertensive bovine pulmonary arteries. J Clin Invest 1992; 89:1629–1635.
154. Border WA, Noble NA, Yamamoto T, et al. Natural inhibitor of transforming growth factor-β protects against scarring in experimental kidney disease. Nature 1992; 360:361–364.
155. Chen RH, Ebner R, Derynck R. Inactivation of the type II receptor reveals two receptor pathways for the diverse TGF-β activities. Science 1993; 260:1335–1338.
156. Giannini G, Clementi E, Ceci R, Marziali G, Sorrentino V. Expression of a ryanodine receptor-Ca^{2+} channel that is regulated by TGF-β. Science 1992; 257:91–94.
157. Nabel EG, Yang Z, Liptay S, San H, Gordon D, Haudenschild CC, Nabel GJ. Recombinant platelet-derived growth factor B gene expression in porcine arteries induces intimal hyperplasia in vivo. J Clin Invest 1993; 91:1822–1829.
158. Ferns GAA, Raines EW, Sprugel KH, Motani AS, Rediy MA, Ross R. Inhibition of neointimal smooth muscle accumulation after angioplasty by an antibody to PDGF. Science 1991; 253:1129–1131.
159. Voelkel NF. Role of platelet-derived growth factor and other growth factors in inflammation. In: Henson PM, Murphy RC, eds. Handbook of Inflammation, Vol 6: Mediators of the Inflammatory Process. Elsevier Science Publishers, 1989:269–299.
160. Dahlberg CGW, Spence CR, Quinn DA, Bonventre JV, Joseph PM, Thompson BT, Hales CA. Heparin interfers with PDGF-stimulated intracellular alkalinization of bovine pulmonary artery smooth muscle cells via inhibition of Na^+/H^+ exchange. Am Rev Respir Dis 1993; 147:A495.
161. Dvorak HF, Sioussat TM, Brown LF, Berse B, Nagy JA, Sotrel A, Manseau L, Van De Water L, Senger DR. Distribution of vascular permeability factor (vascular endothelial growth factor) in tumors: concentration in tumor blood vessels. J Exp Med 1991; 174:1275–1278.
162. Connolly DT, Heuvelman DM, Nelson R, Olander JV, Eppley BL, Delfino JJ, Siegel

NR, Leimgruber RM, Feder J. Tumor vascular permeability factor stimulates endothelial cell growth and angiogenesis. J Clin Invest 1989; 84:1470–1478.

163. Breier G, Albrecht U, Sterrer S, Risau W. Expression of vascular endothelial growth factor during embryonic angiogenesis and endothelial cell differentiation. Development 1992; 114:521–532.
164. Monacci WT, Merrill MJ, Oldfield EH. Expression of vascular permeability factor/vascular endothelial growth factor in normal rat tissues. Am J Physiol 1993; 264: C995–C1002.
165. Millauer B, Wizigmann-Voos S, Schnuerch H, Martinez R, Moller NPH, Risau W, Ullrich A. High affinity VEGF binding and developmental expression suggest Flk-1 as a major regulator of vasculogenesis and angiogenesis. Cell 1993; 72:835–846.
166. Houck KA, Leung DW, Rowland AM, Winer J, Ferrara N. Dual regulation of vascular endothelial growth factor bioavailability by genetic and proteolytic mechanisms. J Biol Chem 1992; 267:26031–26037.
167. Kim KJ, Li B, Winer J, Armanini M, Gillett N, Phillips HS, Ferrara N. Inhibition of vascular endothelial growth factor-induced angiogenesis suppresses tumour growth in vivo. Nature 1993; 362:841–843.
168. Gagliardi A, Hadd H, Collins DC. Inhibition of angiogenesis by suramin. Cancer Res 1992; 52:5073–5075.
169. Tuder RM. Plexiform lesions in primary pulmonary hypertension may represent an abnormal form of angiogenesis. Semin Respir Crit Care Med 1994; 15:207–214.
170. Voelkel NF, Tuder RM. Cellular and molecular mechanisms in the pathogenesis of severe pulmonary hypertension. Eur Respir J 1995; (in press).
171. Dempsey EC, Stenmark KR, McMurtry IF, O'Brien RF, Voelkel NF, Badesch DB. Insulin-like growth factor I and protein kinase C activation stimulate pulmonary artery smooth muscle cell proliferation through separate but synergistic pathways. J Cell Physiol 1990; 144:159–165.
172. Badesch DB, Lee PDK, Parks WC, Stenmark KR. Insulin-like growth factor I stimulates elastin synthesis by bovine pulmonary arterial smooth muscle cells. Biochem Biophys Res Commun 1989; 160:382–387.
173. Perkett EA, Badesch DB, Roessler MD, Stenmark KR, Meyrick B. Insulin-like growth factor I and pulmonary hypertension induced by continuous air embolization in sheep. Am J Respir Cell Mol Biol 1992; 6:82–87.
174. Cacoub P, Dorent R, Carayon A. Thromboxane and prostacyclin metabolites in pulmonary hypertension. N Engl J Med 1992; 327:1456–1457.
175. Zamora MR, Walchak SJ, Dempsey EC, Stelzner TJ. A selective endothelin-A receptor antagonist, inhibits endothelin-1 mediated proliferation of cultured human pulmonary artery smooth muscle cells (HPASMC). Am Rev Respir Dis 1993; 146: A493.
176. Bonvallet ST, Morris KG, Yano M, Zamora MR, McMurtry IF, Stelzner TJ. A selective ET_A receptor antagonist (BQ123) attenuates the development of hypoxic pulmonary hypertension in vivo. Am Rev Respir Dis 1993; 146:A493.

176a. Bonvallet ST, Oka M, Yano M, McMurtry IF, Selzner TJ. An endothelin receptor antagonist attenuates endothelin-1 (ET-1) induced vasoconstriction in the rat pulmonary circulation. Am Rev Respir Dis 1993; 146:A642.

177. Voelkel NF, Chang SW, McDonnell TJ, Westcott JW, Haynes J. Role of membrane lipids in the control of normal vascular tone. Am Rev Resp Dis 1987; 136: 214–217.
178. Voelkel NF. Regulation of pulmonary vascular tone. Eur Respir J 1993; 3:543–549
179. Meyrick B, Perkett EA, Brigham KL. Inflammation and models of chronic pulmonary hypertension. Am Rev Respir Dis 136:765–767.
180. O'Banion MK, Winn VD, Young DA. cDNA cloning and functional activity of a glucocortoid-regulated inflammatory cyclooxygenase. Proc Natl Acad Sci USA 1992; 89:4888–4892.
181. Badesch DB, Orton EC, Zapp LM, Westcott JY, Hester J, Voelkel NF, Stenmark KR. Decreased arterial wall prostaglandin production in neonatal calves with severe chronic pulmonary hypertension. Am J Respir Cell Mol Biol 1989; 1:489–498.
182. Voelkel NF, Badesch DB, Zapp LM, Stenmark KR. Impaired prostacyclin synthesis of endothelial cells derived from hypertensive calf pulmonary arteries. Prog Respir Res 1990; 26:63–69.
183. Wade ML, Voelkel NF, Fitzpatrick FA. Suicide inactivation of prostaglandin I_2 synthase. Arch Biochem 1995; 321:453–458.
184. Xu XM, Ohashi K, Sanduja SK, Ruan KH, Wang LH, Wu KK. Enhanced prostacyclin synthesis in endothelial cells by retrovirus-mediated transfer of prostaglandin H synthase cDNA. J Clin Invest 1993; 91:1843–1849.
185. Eliasen K, Mogensen T, Andersen JB, Hasselstrom L, Jensen NB, Brynjolf I, Godtfredsen J. Acute life threatening pulmonary hypertension treated with ibuprofen. Intensive Care Med 1983; 8:122.
186. Resnick N, Dewey CF, Atkinson W, Collins T, Gimbrone MA. Platelet-derived growth factor B chain promoter contains a cis-acting fluid shear-stress-responsive element. Proc Natl Acad Sci USA 1993; 90:4591–4595.
187. Levin DE, Errede B. A multitude of MAP kinase activation pathways. J NIH Res 1993; 5:49–52.
188. Dempsey EC. Hypoxia alone stimulates translocation of protein kinase C and when combined with PMA, can augment phorbol-ester-induced activation of the same pathway in bovine pulmonary artery smooth muscle cells. Am Rev Respir Dis 1992; 145:A568.
189. Dempsey EC, McMurtry IF, O'Brien RF. Protein kinase C activation allows pulmonary artery smooth muscle cells to proliferate to hypoxia. Am J Physiol 1991; 260: L136–L145.
190. Nishizuka Y. Intracellular signaling by hydrolysis of phospholipids and activation of protein kinase C. Science 1992; 258:607–614.
191. Dempsey EC, Das M, Frid M, Stenmark KR. Unique growth properties of neonatal pulmonary vascular cells: Importance of time- and site specific responses, cell-cell interaction and synergy. J Perinatol 1995 (in press).
192. Karin M. Signal transduction from cell surface to nucleus in development and disease. FASEB J 1992; 6:2581–2590.
193. Reichel RR, Jacob ST. Control of gene expression by lipophilic hormones. FASEB J 1993; 7:427–436.
194. Rittling SR, Coutinho L, Amram T, Kolbe M. AP-1/*jun* binding sites mediate serum inducibility of the human vimentin promoter. Nucleic Acids Res 1989; 17:1619–1633.

195. Voelkel NF, Reeves JT. Primary pulmonary hypertension. In: Moser K, ed. Pulmonary Vascular Diseases. Lung Biology in Health and Disease. Vol. 14, New York: Marcel Dekker, 1979.
196. Groves BM, Badesch DB, Turkevich D, et al. Correlation of acute prostacyclin response in primary (unexplained) pulmonary hypertension with efficacy of treatment with calcium channel blockers and survival. In: Weir EK, ed. Ion Flux in Pulmonary Vascular Control. New York: Plenum Press, 1993:317–330.
197. Eleftheriades EG, Durand J, Ferguson AG, Engelman GL, Jones SB, Samarel AM. Regulation of procollagen metabolism in the pressure-overloaded rat heart. J Clin Invest 1992; 91:1113–1122.
198. Tsutsui H, Ishihara K, Cooper G. Cytoskeletal role in contractile dysfunction of hypertrophied myocardium. Science 1993; 260:682–686.
199. Bristow MR, et al. β-Adrenergic neuroeffector abnormalities in the failing human heart are produced by local, rather than systemic mechanisms. J Clin Invest 1992; 89:803–815
200. Voelkel NF, Hegstrand L, Reeves JT, McMurty IF, Molincff PB. Effects of hypoxia on density of β-adrenergic receptors. Am Physiol Soc 1981; pp. 363–366.
201. Gibbs JSR, Cunningham AD, Shapiro LM, Park A, Poole-Wilson PA, Fox KM. Diurnal variation of pulmonary artery pressure in chronic heart failure. Br Heart J 1989; 62:30–35.
202. Somers VK, Dyken ME, Mark AL, Abboud FM. Sympathetic-nerve activity during sleep in normal subjects. N Engl J Med 1993; 328:303–7.
203. Niedenzu, Grasedyck C, Voelkel NF, Bittmann S, Lindner F. Proliferation of lung cells in chronically hypoxic rats, an autoradiographic and radiochemical study. Int Arch Occup Environ Health 1981; 48:185–193.
204. Olson JW, Altiere RJ, Gillespie MN. Prolonged activation of rat lung ornithine decarboxylase in monocrotaline-induced pulmonary hypertension. Biochem Pharmacol 1984; 33:3633–3637.
205. Haven CA, Olson JW, Arcot SS, Gillespie MN. Polyamine transport and ornithine decarboxylase activity in hypoxic pulmonary artery smooth muscle cells. Am J Respir Cell Mol Biol 1992; 7:286–292.
206. Eddahibi S, Adnot S, Carville C, Blouquit Y, Raffestin B. L-Arginine restores endothelium-dependent relaxation in pulmonary circulation of chronically hypoxic rats. Am J Physiol 1992; 263:L194–L200.
207. Dubois J-M, Rouzaire-Dubois B. Role of potassium channels in mitogenesis. Prog Biophys Molc Biol 1993; 59:1–24.
208. Fanburg, BL. Case Records of the Massachusetts General Hospital. N Engl J Med 1992; 327:1226–1233.

5

Risk Factors for Primary Pulmonary Hypertension

FRANÇOIS BRENOT[†] and GÉRALD SIMONNEAU

University of Paris XI School of Medicine
and Antoine Béclère Hospital
Clamart, France

I. Introduction

The clinical term "primary pulmonary hypertension" (PPH), sometimes referred to as "unexplained pulmonary hypertension" (1), is used to describe patients who had pulmonary hypertension in the absence of any of the known or supposed causes, outlined by the National Institutes of Health (NIH) Registry for the characterization of PPH (2), and listed in Table 1. When these potential etiologies have been excluded, patients with a mean pulmonary arterial pressure is excess of 25 mmHg at rest or 30 mmHg on exercise are considered to have PPH (2). However, from many case reports and some large case series of patients with PPH (2–6), there is no doubt that this definition may require amplification and raises the question as to how rigorously other conditions should be excluded. Indeed, there is increasing evidence that many patients with PPH often present with a medical history or life-style that may provide clues to an improved understanding of the pathogenesis of this disease.

†Deceased.

Table 1 Secondary Causes of Pulmonary Hypertension

Pulmonary hypertension within the first year of life
Congenital abnormalities of the lungs, thorax, and diaphragm
Congenital or acquired valvular or myocardial disease
Large-vessel chronic thromboembolic pulmonary disease
Sickle cell anemia
History of intravenous drug abuse
Obstructive lung disease (hypoxemia and reduced flow rates >2 SD)
Interstitial lung disease (reduced total lung capacity >2 SD and pulmonary infiltrates on chest roentgenogram)
Arterial hypoxemia associated with hypercapnia
Collagen vascular disease
Parasitic disease affecting the lungs
Pulmonary artery or valve stenosis
Pulmonary venous hypertension

SD, standard deviation from predicted values.
Source: From Ref. 2.

II. General Considerations

No single etiological factor has been identified in PPH, and it is possible that several different stimuli can give rise to a common final pathway of disease in the lung microvasculature, leading to smooth muscle cell proliferation and migration, intimal thickening, thrombosis, and ultimately chronic pulmonary hypertension (7). Our current knowledge of these potential risk factors is limited; since PPH is a very rare disease, its pathogenesis remains unknown and large case series are uncommon (1–6,8,9). Moreover, extensive epidemiological data are unavailable and should ideally be obtained from large-scale epidemiological investigations such as international case-control studies, which are currently not yet available (10). However, observations such as the increased incidence of the disease in young women, the familial predisposition, the association with autoimmune disorders, and recent immunogenetic studies (see below) favor the hypothesis that the development of PPH very likely depends on an *individual susceptibility* or predisposition, which is probably genetically determined. It is also hypothesized that the development of pulmonary hypertension in some predisposed individuals could be hastened or precipitated by various *expression factors*, such as ingestion of certain drugs or diets, hepatic cirrhosis and portal hypertension, or particular infectious disease states (Fig. 1).

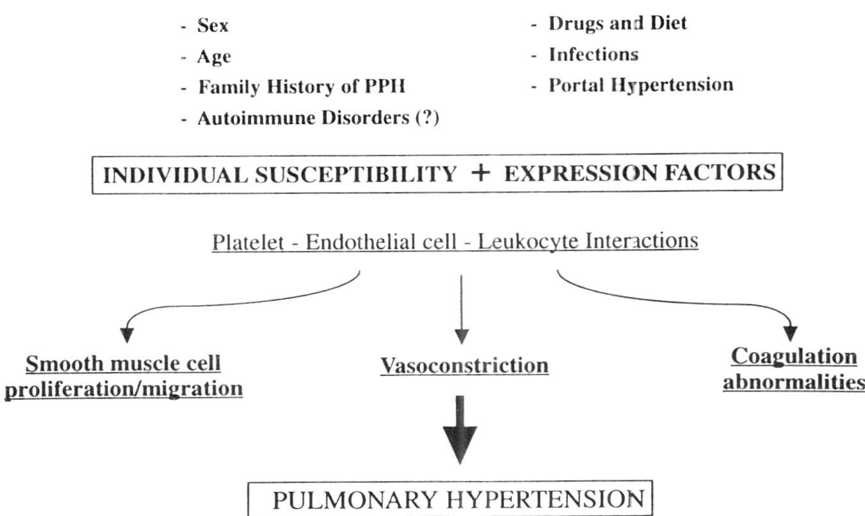

Figure 1 Possible pathways involved in the pathogenesis of primary pulmonary hypertension and associated conditions.

The risk factors that will be considered and discussed are derived both from previously published data and from a large retrospective single-center case series including 307 patients with PPH referred to our Center for Pulmonary Vascular Diseases between 1982 and February 1995 (5,6).

III. Age, Sex, and Race

PPH can present at any age, but occurs most commonly in young adults. The sex distribution is approximately equal in childhood, but shows a greater incidence in females and young adults (2,4–6) with a female-to-male (F:M) ratio of about 2:1, except in one large case series from Japan with an unexplained greater proportion of males in the third decade of life (11). As in the NIH Registry, our (F:M) ratio was 1.7:1 overall, but 2.4:1 in the third decade and 1.9:1 in the fourth decade of life. The mean age at the time of diagnosis is approximately 40 years in most large case series, with a peak of incidence in the third and fourth decades of life (2,5). PPH may also occur relatively late in life: 9% of the patients in the NIH Registry and 8% of the patients in our series had the diagnosis made at age 60 or later. No differences have ever been definitely documented in the geographical or racial incidence of the disease; however, both in the NIH Registry (2) and in our series, there was a greater incidence in black females with a (F:M) ratio of 4.3:1 in a 12.3% black population and a (F:M) ratio of 3:1 in a 5% black population, respectively. The reason for these findings is unclear, although black females are known to be more susceptible than white females to the development of autoimmune diseases, which is likely associated with PPH.

IV. Familial Pulmonary Hypertension

Familial cases were first described (12) as early as 1927 and since then have been commonly reported from Europe and North America (13–20). As first suggested in 1970 by Thompson and McRae (21), the inheritance of the disease has been established by Lloyd et al. in 1984 to be autosomal dominant, based on a review of 13 families with PPH in the North American literature (22). They also excluded an X linkage of the gene and showed that the transmission has incomplete penetrance, i.e., may skip generations and consequently may appear to be sporadic. It can thus be suspected that many cases of "nonfamilial" PPH will prove to be familial once careful family histories are taken. However, the number of reported cases of familial PPH from major case series is usually fairly low, with only 6.4% and 3% of the patient population analyzed in the American registry (2) and the French series (5), respectively. This strengthens the importance of expression factors for the development of the disease.

The genetic basis of familial PPH is still unknown (22), but the clinical presentation, pathological features, and disease evolution are the same as in sporadic PPH (23), except for a shorter time from symptom onset to diagnosis, as would be expected from earlier recognition of subsequent cases in families (0.61 year in the NIH Registry and 0.68 year in our series, compared with an average of 2 years in nonfamilial cases). Earlier studies had also found a tendency for the disease to develop at an earlier age in ensuing generations in affected families (15). This phenomenon, called genetic anticipation, has recently been confirmed as a characteristic of familial PPH, by analysis of 24 American families with 99 affected individuals (24). The molecular basis of genetic anticipation is the mechanism of trinucleotide repeat amplification, which is seen in other inherited disease states such as the fragile X syndrome, myotonic dystrophy, and Huntington's disease.

The link between PPH and autoimmune disorders (see below) has also recently prompted immunogenetic studies on familial pulmonary hypertension (25,26). An association was found with the major histocompatibility complex, with an increased frequency of HLA-DR 3, DR 52, and DQ 2 haplotypes in 17 children with primary pulmonary hypertension, whereas 13 other children with pulmonary hypertension and large congenital pulmonary-to-systemic communications had no HLA association. These findings led the authors to add juvenile

PPH to the "DR3+ group" of autoimmune diseases such as Sjögren's syndrome (27), systemic lupus erythematosus (28), one scleroderma subset (29), and immunoglobulin isotype deficiency (26).

There is no doubt that these recently discovered immunogenetic features are important clues providing direction for a search for the molecular basis of familial PPH.

V. Factors Related to Pregnancy and the Menstrual Cycle

The increased incidence of PPH in women of childbearing age (2–9) remains unexplained. There are several reports of onset of PPH during pregnancy (3,30,31); whether this indicates that the disease was present earlier and was exacerbated by the hemodynamic changes of pregnancy (30,32,33) or whether pregnancy and hormonal factors may be considered risk factors for PPH is unknown. The same limitations are true for the association of PPH with the use of oral contraceptives or progestational agents (34). The association with pregnancy is uncommon and was not supported by the NIH Registry data, which did not disclose an association with oral contraceptive use, either (2). Although many investigators share the notion that hormonal influences on the pulmonary circulation are important, conclusive findings are lacking (35–37).

VI. Autoimmune Disorders

Among the pulmonary complications that can occur in patients with known connective tissue diseases, pulmonary hypertension has been identified as one of the most common and life-threatening. It has been reported in association with scleroderma (38–40), particularly in its CREST variant (calcinosis, Raynaud's disease, esophageal dysmotility, sclerodactyly, and telangiectasis), with systemic lupus erythematosus (41–44), with mixed connective tissue disease (45–48), and to a lesser extent with rheumatoid arthritis (49,50), polymyositis (51), and dermatomyositis (52). These diseases also occur primarily in women. The strongest association with PPH seems to be with that part of the autoimmune spectrum represented by Raynaud's syndrome, which has been reported in 7–30% of patients with PPH. The NIH Registry reported a 10% frequency of Raynaud's syndrome (2) while we found it in 20% of our patients, almost exclusively in females and often preceding the appearance of PPH symptoms. Interestingly, in the familial cases, some family members not afflicted with PPH had Raynaud's syndrome (26).

The frequency of positive antinuclear antibodies (ANA) in PPH has been reported to be as high as 40% (53,54), but was 29% in the NIH Registry (range:

1:10–1:10,000) and only 12% of our 275 patients who were tested (ANA titers ⩾ 1:80 were considered significant, range 1:80–1:2650). Based on the data reviewed previously, it has been suggested that some patients with PPH might have a connective tissue disease confined to the lung with the features overlapping rheumatoid arthritis and scleroderma. In an attempt to define an autoantibody specific for PPH, Isern et al. proposed the anti-Ku because it was found in 23% of adults with the disease (55). However, anti-Ku, which is an autoantibody to a DNA-binding nuclear complex, has also been found in higher frequencies in a wide range of connective tissue diseases (56), making the specificity of the correlation with PPH uncertain. Whether these marker autoantibodies play a role in the pathogenesis of PPH, in addition to the pulmonary hypertension complicating connective tissue diseases, or whether they are merely nonspecific markers of vascular damage is unknown at the present time.

Recently, Badesch et al. suggested that there may be an association between PPH and autoimmune thyroid dysfunction, on the basis of four cases of women with severe pulmonary hypertension, low-titer positive ANA, and hypothyroidism (57). We retrospectively analyzed (unpublished data) the medical history of our first 219 patients with PPH who were seen prior to 1993, and we prospectively evaluated the next 88 consecutive patients with PPH for the presence of autoimmune thyroid disorders. In the retrospective study, only four of 219 (2%) had evidence of thyroid disease, which was due to Graves' disease in two patients and to chronic Hashimoto's thyroiditis in two. Among the 88 patients prospectively studied, 16 (18%) had positive antithyroid autoantibodies directed against either thyroglobulin (range: 110–20,000 U/ml; normal <130 U/ml), or peroxidase (range 130–23,340 U/ml; normal <130 U/ml), or both. Among these 16 patients, eight had evidence of hypothyroidism (Hashimoto's disease) and two had hyperthyroidism (Graves' disease). Whether thyroid dysfunction may have influenced the development and course of the pulmonary vascular disease, or whether it is a consequence of pulmonary hypertension, is unclear.

VII. Drugs and Diet

The possibility of a relationship between the ingestion of some drugs and the development of pulmonary hypertension was first suggested in the late sixties, when a 20-fold increased incidence of unexplained pulmonary hypertension was reported in Switzerland, Austria, and West Germany (58,59). This epidemic closely followed the introduction in these countries of the appetite depressant aminorex fumarate (2-amino-5-phenyl-2-oxazoline) and subsided shortly after the drug had been removed from the market. While only 2% of the population that had taken aminorex developed pulmonary hypertension (59), 61% of the 582 patients who were identified as new cases of PPH gave a history of aminorex intake (60).

The relative risk of developing pulmonary hypertension in aminorex users was estimated to be 52:1 compared with patients without any exposure to the drug (60). At that time, controversial conclusions were raised regarding the relationship between the total individual dose and the risk of developing the disease; however, there was no correlation between the disease severity and the number of tablets each individual patient had taken (59,60). During follow-up, some authors felt that after discontinuation of the drug, patients with a history of aminorex intake had a better long-term survival than "unexposed" patients with PPH (60), while other authors reported no differences in the survival rates (61,62). Aminorex resembles epinephrine and amphetamine, and a release of catecholamines from endogenous stores by this drug has been suggested as the mechanism (63); serotonin release may also be involved (64,65). However, all attempts to produce chronic pulmonary hypertension experimentally with chronic administration of aminorex in any species have failed (65–67). This has been explained by the low incidence of pulmonary hypertension in test animals as well as in humans, and by the fact that a prerequisite for the pulmonary circulation to constrict or proliferate when exposed to an offending agent is probably dependent on genetic susceptibility.

Since 1981, 10 cases of PPH associated with the use of the anorexic drug fenfluramine have been reported (68,75). Most of those cases were related to the use of DL-fenfluramine, whereas some cases were linked to the more recently marketed dexfenfluramine. We have recently reported 15 new cases of severe PPH in fenfluramine users, among 73 consecutive patients with PPH referred between 1988 and 1992 (76). Although this series was not quantitatively comparable to the aminorex-related outbreak, the question of a cause-and-effect relationship between fenfluramine exposure and PPH was raised. Indeed, the number of our patients with PPH possibly related to fenfluramine use had markedly increased in the early nineties, with a time course that appeared to parallel the increase in dexfenfluramine consumption in France. The proportion of fenfluramine users among our consecutive patients was fairly high, reaching 20% of the overall patient population and about one-third of all female patients, a rate that was probably higher than the proportion of fenfluramine users that could be estimated in the general female population of the same age in France. In about two-thirds of these fenfluramine users, there was a close temporal relationship between the period of use and the development and diagnosis of PPH. Right-side heart hemodynamic findings were those of severe pulmonary hypertension, as in previously reported cases related to fenfluramine use (68.75). We did not find any relationship between the total duration of appetite suppressant use and the level of pulmonary hypertension. Among the 10 cases of PPH associated with fenfluramine use in the literature, five showed spontaneous clinical and hemodynamic partial or complete remission, usually with 1–3 months after diagnosis and withdrawal of the drug (68,29,72,75). However, complete remission in pulmonary hypertension was not the rule with our patients, and occurred in only three. The notion of better prognosis commonly associated with "appetite suppressant–related" PPH was also not supported by the survival rate when compared to that of the group of fenfluramine "nonusers" who had been evaluated during the same time period. The mechanisms that may cause pulmonary hypertension in susceptible patients using fenfluramine or other amphetamine-related drugs are unclear. Most of them are structurally related and their anorectic activity is due to the phenylethylamine molecule (77). They all share various degrees of sympathomimetic and serotoninergic effects, the latter involving blocking of cellular uptake and metabolism of serotonin, inhibition of monoamine oxidase activity, and, more generally, a release of large amounts of serotonin from cellular stores (platelets, nerve endings). Serotonin has been shown to contract isolated pulmonary arteries in dogs and humans (78,79), and to have a synergistic effect with platelet-derived growth factor on vascular smooth muscle cell proliferation (80). It has also been recently demonstrated that patients with PPH have very high levels of free plasma serotonin, which are likely related to an increased serotonin release from platelets (81,82).

Biguanides have been widely used in the treatment of diabetes mellitus. In 1973, Fahlen et al. reported two patients who developed pulmonary hypertension during treatment with the antihyperglycemic biguanide phenformin, with pulmonary hypertension gradually subsiding on withdrawal of the drug (83). Phenformin has been withdrawn from the market in many countries because it can produce severe lactic acidosis, which, interestingly, induces pulmonary vasoconstriction in animal experiments.

Severe pulmonary hypertension has been reported as a complication of an epidemic disorder involving more than 20,000 patients that swept Spain in 1981 and was subsequently called "toxic oil syndrome" (TOS) (84,85). It was related to the ingestion of rapeseed oil intended for industrial use, which had been denatured with aniline and sold as cooking oil. The initial phase of the syndrome was characterized by an ill-defined lung disease with cough, fever, and dyspnea associated with radiographic findings of interstitial pneumonia; blood eosinophilia plus elevated levels of IgE were identified as early "markers" of the disease. Within the first 3 months after the onset of TOS, survivors developed neuropathy and myositis, Raynaud's phenomenon, and in 2–3% of patients, mostly women, severe pulmonary hypertension. In such cases, the histological findings included pulmonary artery medial thickening, a foamy intimal proliferation, polymorphonuclear neutrophils infiltrating the pulmonary blood vessels, but no plexiform lesions (86). Interestingly, some cases of pulmonary hypertension were reported in patients from the same families. A recent analysis of the morbidity data from the TOS patient registry (87) showed that the cumulative rate of pulmonary hypertension in a cohort of 914 affected patients was 8.2% from 1981 to 1992. The etiological role of the adulterated oil was certain, although the responsible compounds, suspected to be aniline or "aniline-oil complexes," were not definitely implicated (84). Whether such chemicals had caused a direct injury or an activation of the immune defense system of the patients, leading to platelet-endothelial damage and pulmonary arteriopathy, is still unknown.

More recently, chronic pulmonary hypertension has been described as a complication of the epidemic "eosinophilia-myalgia syndrome" (EMS), a disorder first recognized in 1989 in New Mexico (88). EMS was associated in almost all the cases with the ingestion of products containing L-tryptophan, taken as dietary supplements and publicized as useful for the treatment of insomnia, depression, and premenstrual symptoms (89–95). As of the beginning of 1990, the Centers for Disease Control had been notified of 1269 cases of EMS, with patients being predominantly non-Hispanic, previously healthy, white, middle-age women (96). Symptoms and signs typically progressed from an early and abrupt onset of incapacitating myalgia, fatigue, and intense blood eosinophilia to the later development of polyneuropathy, scleroderma-like skin changes, and pulmonary complications such as interstitial pneumonia or chronic pulmonary hypertension. The actual frequency of pulmonary hypertension in persons with EMS was estimated to be 5–7%, from the results of a few population-based case series (94,95). Clinically as well as etiologically, EMS shared striking similarities with TOS (91). Indeed, the leading possibility as a cause of the EMS epidemic was the contamination of tryptophan: One method of producing tryptophan is fermentation, during which the drug is synthesized by mutant bacteria from various nutrients and particularly anthranilic acid, which is similar to aniline, which was strongly implicated in the pathogenesis of TOS (97).

VIII. Hepatic Cirrhosis and Portal Hypertension

The association of portal hypertension and pulmonary hypertension was first described in 1951 (98) and later confirmed by several authors who demonstrated lung histological findings indistinguishable from those commonly found in PPH (99–101). Whether such a combination of conditions is relevant has been questioned for a long time, because of conflicting observations. From a large autopsy study (102), McDonnell et al. found that the prevalence of pulmonary hypertension in patients with proven hepatic cirrhosis was 0.73%, which was significantly higher than that in an unselected autopsy series (0.13%). Another autopsy study (103) in cirrhotic patients reported an incidence of 0.26%. In one clinical study, Lebrec et al. showed that this prevalence was also very low (0.25%) and suggested that this association may only be coincidental (104).

In 1985, Naeije et al. reported that among 100 patients with liver cirrhosis approximately 10% had significant pulmonary hypertension measured during right-side heart catheterization (105). More recently, Hadengue et al. prospectively evaluated 507 consecutive hospitalized patients with hepatic cirrhosis and portal hypertension (106). Regardless of respiratory symptoms and signs, each patient underwent right-side heart catheterization combined with splanchnic hemodynamic measurements. This study demonstrated that 10 patients (2%) had significant pulmonary hypertension. The proportion of patients with PPH and portal hypertension was 8% in the NIH Registry and 12% (37 patients) in our series (107). Portal hypertension had been diagnosed years before the onset of symptoms of pulmonary hypertension in about 80% of our patients. Hepatic cirrhosis, primarily alcoholic, was the leading cause of portal hypertension and was found in almost all the cases (91%), while Budd-Chiari syndrome was found in the remaining cases. Compared with a group of 235 consecutive patients with "isolated" PPH evaluated during the same time period, it appeared that patients with portal hypertension were diagnosed as having pulmonary hypertension at a more advanced age (49 ± 13 vs. 41 ± 15 years, $p < .05$), were significantly less severely disabled (NYHA functional class III or IV: 43% vs. 74%), had significantly lower levels of pulmonary hypertension, and had a better long-term survival with medical treatment than did their counterparts with "isolated" primary pulmonary hypertension (107).

The mechanism whereby portal hypertension facilitates the development of primary pulmonary hypertension remains unknown. Repeated pulmonary embolism from thrombus arising in the portal vein has been suggested (108), although lung pathological findings usually resemble typical plexogenic arteriopathy rather than the patchy changes of thromboembolism. In addition, thrombosis of the portal venous system is uncommon in these patients. Other etiological possibilities include unidentified endogenous or exogenous vasoconstrictor substances emanating from the splanchnic circulation, which bypass liver detoxification before reaching the lung vasculature. However, attempts to provoke pulmonary vascular alterations by the surgical production of portal hypertension in animals have failed so far (109,110).

IX. Infections

It has been postulated that viral infections might be at the origin of PPH in some patients in whom nonspecific infectious episodes preceded the diagnosis of the pulmonary vascular disease (7).

Since 1987, numerous cases of patients suffering from pulmonary hypertension associated with human immunodeficiency virus (HIV) infection have been reported in the literature (111–122). The first report concerned only patients with classic hemophilia, raising questions about a cause-and-effect relationship between PPH and the use of factor VIII concentrates of low purity, although these patients were all HIV-positive (112). It was subsequently shown that pulmonary hypertension may develop in HIV patients independent of immunosuppression and/or the risk factors for HIV infection, including a history of chronic intravenous heroin abuse. Intravenous drug abusers classically develop pulmonary hypertension due to foreign-particle embolism following injections of solutions derived from crushed tablets or pills containing insoluble microcrystals (123–126), and these patients are usually excluded from reports dealing with PPH (2). However, ordinary heroin does not contain sufficient crystalline debris to induce extensive pulmonary angiothrombosis, which is the main pathological finding in this condition (123). Furthermore, fewer than 5% of drug addicts frequently inject tablet derivatives (124,125), and pulmonary hypertension is rare in this group, as was shown in the late seventies before the HIV infection epidemic (127). Most of the cases of HIV-infected drug abusers with associated pulmonary hypertension reported so far included only patients with exclusive heroin addiction, and foreign body granulomas were usually absent in the lung pathological specimens (113,116,118). Thus, the etiological role of HIV infection in the development of pulmonary hypertension is more likely.

We have recently reported 20 new cases of HIV-infected patients with pulmonary hypertension (128). By comparing them with 93 non-HIV-infected patients with PPH referred during the same time period, we showed that HIV-infected patients were significantly younger and less severely disabled at the time of diagnosis of pulmonary hypertension. This finding, as well as the shorter time between symptom onset and diagnosis of pulmonary hypertension, was explained by the close medical attention usually devoted to HIV patients, although both conditions were simultaneously diagnosed in 25% of our patients. Survival in PPH is poor (129) and has been reported to be limited in HIV-infected patients with pulmonary hypertension as well. In our HIV patients, survival was not significantly different from that of non-HIV-infected patients with PPH who had been evaluated and treated in the same manner (128). However, considering that HIV patients had a shorter average duration of symptoms attributable to pulmonary hypertension prior to initial catheterization, a more rapid disease evolution in HIV-infected patients could not be ruled out.

The evidence for a cause-and-effect relationship between these two diseases would require a controlled epidemiological study, which is not currently available. However, in a recent retrospective study from a cohort of 1200 HIV-infected subjects (116), the incidence of pulmonary hypertension was estimated to be as high as 0.5%, which is probably higher than the estimated incidence of primary pulmonary hypertension in the general population (130).

The pathogenesis of the pulmonary arterial disease associated with HIV infection is unknown. The hypothesis of a direct involvement of the virus on the pulmonary vascular smooth muscle and/or endothelial cells has not been demonstrated (122). An indirect role of the HIV on the production of growth factors leading to abnormal endothelial and smooth muscle cell proliferation has also been discussed (117,131,132). Whatever the underlying mechanisms, this likely association obviously raises questions about a viral involvement in the pathogenesis of PPH in general (122).

With a better understanding of the influence of growth factors and cytokines on endothelial cell function in a variety of vascular diseases, it is plausible that the HIV infection leads to PPH by a generalized increase in cytokines or growth factors that affect the pulmonary vascular endothelium in susceptible individuals. Whether this involves the interleukins, endothelin, or other inducible growth factors is only now being explored. In this scenario, the pulmonary hypertension that develops would be expected to be very similar to PPH, which appears to be the case.

References

1. Fishman AP. Editorial: Unexplained pulmonary hypertension. Circulation 1982; 65:651.
2. Rich S, Dantzker DR, Ayres SM, Bergofsky EH, Brundage BH, Detre KH, Fishman AP, Goldring RM, Groves BM, Koener, SK, Levy PS, Reid LM, Vreim CE, Williams GW. Primary pulmonary hypertension: a national prospective study. Ann Intern Med 1987; 107:216–223.
3. Wagenvoort CA, Wagenvoort N. Primary pulmonary hypertension: a pathologic study of the lung vessels in 156 clinically diagnosed cases. Circulation 1970; 42: 1163–1184.
4. Fuster V, Steele PM, Edwards WD, Gersh BJ, Phil D, McGoon MD, Frye RL. Primary pulmonary hypertension: natural history and the importance of thrombosis. Circulation 1984; 70:580–587.
5. Brenot F. Primary pulmonary hypertension: case series from France. Chest 1994; 105:33S–36S.
6. Brenot F, Hervé P, Rain B, Simonneau G. Hypertension artérielle pulmonaire primitive: données de la littérature et expérience personnelle sur 125 cas en 10 ans. Rev Prat (Paris) 1991; 41:1560–1567.
7. Voelkel NF, Weir EK. Etiologic mechanisms in primary pulmonary hypertension. In: Weir EK, Reeves JT, eds. Pulmonary Vascular Physiology and Pathophysiology. New York: Marcel Dekker 1989:513–539.
8. Kanemoto N, Sasamoto H. Pulmonary hemodynamics in primary pulmonary hypertension. Jpn Heart J 1979; 20:395.
9. Kanemoto N. Natural history of pulmonary hemodynamics in primary pulmonary hypertension. Am Heart J 1987; 114:407–413.
10. Abenhaim L, Higenbottam TW, Rich S. International primary pulmonary hypertension study. Br Heart J 1994; 71:303 (letter).
11. Watanabe S, Ogata T. Clinical and experimental study upon primary pulmonary hypertension. Jpn Heart J 1976; 40:603.
12. Clarke RC, Coombes CF, Hadfield G. On certain abnormalities, congenital and acquired, of the pulmonary artery. Q J Med 1927; 21:51.

13. Lang F. Die essentielle Hypertonie der Lungenstrombahn und ihr familares Vorkommen. Deutsch Med Wochenschr 1948; 72:322.
14. Hood HB Jr. Primary pulmonary hypertension: familial occurrence. Br Heart J 1968; 30:336.
15. Kingdon HS, Cohen LS, Roberts WC, Braunwald E. Familial occurrence of primary pulmonary hypertension. Arch Intern Med 1966; 118:422–426.
16. Tubbs RR, Levin RD, Shirley EK, Hoffman GC. Fibrinolysis in familial pulmonary hypertension. Am J Clin Pathol 1979; 71:384–387.
17. Asmervik J. Familiaer primaer pulmonal hypertension. Tidsskr Nor Loegeforen nr 1985; 105:673–674.
18. Knaue M. Huffman W, Uhl J. Primary pulmonary hypertension in childhood. Med Welt 1982; 33:1238–1241.
19. Knight JA, Wilson JF. Primary pulmonary hypertension in childhood; a report on two brothers. Pediatr Pathol 1985; 4:13–23.
20. Massoud H, Puckett W, Auerbach SH. Primary pulmonary hypertension: a study of the disease in four young siblings. J Tenn Med Assoc 1970; 63:299–305.
21. Thompson P, McRae C. Familial pulmonary hypertension: evidence of autosomal dominant inheritance. Br Heart J 1970; 32:758–760.
22. Loyd JE, Primm RK, Newman JH. Familial primary pulmonary hypertension: clinical patterns. Am Rev Respir Dis 1984; 129:194–197.
23. Voelkel NF, Reeves JR. Primary pulmonary hypertension. In: Moser KM, ed. Pulmonary Vascular Diseases. New York: Marcel Dekker, 1979:573–649.
24. Loyd JE, Butler MG, Foroud TM, Conneally PM, Phillips JA, Newman JH. Genetic anticipation and abnormal gender ratio at birth in familial primary pulmonary hypertension. Am J Respir Crit Care Med 1995; 152:93–97.
25. Barst RJ, Flaster ER, Menon A, Fotino M, Morse JH. Evidence for the association of unexplained pulmonary hypertension in children with the major histocompatibility complex. Circulation 1992; 85:249–258.
26. Morse JH, Barst RJ, Fotino M. Familial pulmonary hypertension: immunogenetic findings in four caucasian kindreds. Am Rev Respir Dis 1992; 145:787–792.
27. Wilson RW, Provost TT, Bias WB, Alexander EL, Edlow DW, Hochberg MC, Stevens MB, Arnett FC. Sjögren's syndrome: influence of multiple HLA-D region alloantigens on clinical and serologic expression. Arthritis Rheum 1984; 7:1245–1253.
28. Hamilton RG, Harley JB, Bias WB, Roebber M, Reichlin M, Hochberg MC, Arnett FC. Two Ro (SSA) autoantibody responses in systemic lupus erythematosus. Arthritis Rheum 1988; 31:496–505.
29. Genth E, Mieran R, Genetzky P, von Muhlen CA, Kaufmann S, von Wilmowsky, Meurer M, Krieg T, Pollmann HJ, Hartl PW. Immunogenetic associations of scleroderma-related antinuclear antibodies. Arthritis Rheum 1990; 33:657–665.
30. Feijen HWH, Hein PR, van Lakwijk-Vondrovicova EL, Nijhuis GMM. Primary pulmonary hypertension and pregnancy. Eur J. Obstet Gynecol 1983; 15:159–164.
31. Dawkins KD, Burke CM, Billingham ME, Jamieson SW. Primary pulmonary hypertension and pregnancy. Chest 1986; 89:383–388.
32. Gatewood RP Jr, Yu PN. Primary pulmonary hypertension. In: Yu PN, Goodwin JG, eds. Progress in Cardiology. Philadelphia: Lea & Febiger, 1979:305–349.

33. Nelson DM, Main E, Crafford W, Ahumada GG. Peripartum heart failure due to primary pulmonary hypertension. Obstet Gynecol 1983; 62:58S–63S.
34. Kleiger RE, Boxer M, Ingham RE, Harrison DC. Pulmonary hypertension in patients using oral contraceptives. Chest 1976; 69:143–147.
35. McMurty IF, Frith CH, Will DH. Cardiopulmonary responses of male and female swine to simulated high altitude. J Appl Physiol 1973; 35:459–462.
36. Rabinovitch M, Gamble WJ, Miettinen OS, Reid L. Age and sex influence on pulmonary hypertension of chronic hypoxia and on recovery. Am J Physiol 1981; 240 (Heart Circ Physiol 9):H62–H72.
37. Moore LG, Reeves JT. Pregnancy blunts pulmonary vascular reactivity in dogs. Am J Physiol 1980; 239:H297.
38. Salerni R, Rodnan GP, Leon FL, Shaver JA. Pulmonary hypertension in the CREST syndrome variant of progressive systemic sclerosis (scleroderma). Ann Intern Med 1977; 86:394–399.
39. Ungerer RG, Tashkin DP, Furst D, Clements PG, Gong H Jr, Bein M, Smith JW, Roberts N, Cabeen W. Prevalence and clinical correlates of pulmonary arterial hypertension in progressive systemic sclerosis. Am J Med 1983; 75:65–74.
40. Stupi AM, Steen VD, Owens GR. Pulmonary hypertension in the CREST syndrome variant of systemic sclerosis. Arthritis Rheum 1986; 29:515–524.
41. Nair SS, Askari AD, Popelka CG, Kleinerman JF. Pulmonary hypertension and systemic lupus erythematosus. Arch Intern Med 1980; 140:109–111.
42. Simonson JS, Schiller NB, Petri M, Hellmann DB. Pulmonary hypertension in systemic lupus erythematosus. J Rheumatol 1989; 16:918–925.
43. Quismorio FP, Sharma O, Koss M, Boylen T, Edmiston AW, Thornton PJ, Tatter D. Immunopathologic and clinical studies in pulmonary hypertension associated with systemic lupus erythematosus. Semin Arthritis Rheum 1984; 13:349–359.
44. Asherson RA, Higenbottam TW, Dinh Xuan AT, Khamashta MA, Hughes GR. Pulmonary hypertension in a lupus clinic: experience with twenty-four patients. J Rheumatol 1990; 17:1292–1298.
45. Wiener-Kronish JP, Solinger A, Warnock ML, Churg A, Ordonez N, Golden JA. Severe pulmonary involvement in mixed connective tissue disease. Am Rev Respir Dis 1981; 124:499–503.
46. Alpert MA, Goldberg SH, Singsen BH, Durham JB, Sharp GC, Ahmad M, Madigan NP, Hurst DP, Sullivan WD. Cardiovascular manifestations of mixed connective tissue disease in adults. Circulation 1986; 68:1182–1193.
47. Sullivan WD, Hurst DJ, Harmon CE, Esther JH, Agia GA, Maltby JD, Lillard SB, Held CN, Wolfe JG, Sunderrajan EV, Maricq HR, Sharp GC. A prospective evaluation emphasizing pulmonary involvement in patients with mixed connective tissue disease. Medicine 1984; 63:92–107.
48. Hosoda Y, Suzuki Y, Takano M, Tojo T, Homma M. Mixed connective tissue disease with pulmonary hypertension: a clinical and pathological study. J Rheumatol 1987; 14:826–830.
49. Case Record of the Massachusetts General Hospital (Case 37-1992). N Engl J Med 1992; 327:873–880.

50. Baydur A, Mongan ES, Slager UT. Acute respiratory failure and pulmonary arteritis without parenchymal involvement: demonstration in a patient with rheumatoid arthritis. Chest 1979; 75:518–520.
51. Bunch TW, Tancredi RG, Lie JT. Pulmonary hypertension in polymyositis. Chest 1981; 79:105.
52. Caldwell IW, Aitchison JD. Pulmonary hypertension in dermatomyositis. Br Heart J 1956; 18:273.
53. Brundage BH, Rich S, Groves BM. Positive antinuclear antibody tests in primary pulmonary hypertension. J Am Coll Cardiol 1984; 3:596.
54. Rich S, Kieras K, Hart K, Groves BM, Stobo JD, Brundage BH. Antinuclear antibodies in primary pulmonary hypertension. J Am Coll Cardiol 1986; 8:1307–1311.
55. Isern RA, Yaneva M, Weiner E, Parke A, Rothfield N, Dantzker D, Rich S, Arnett FC. Autoantibodies in patients with primary pulmonary hypertension: association with anti-Ku. Am J Med 1992; 93:307–312.
56. Yaneva M, Arnett FC. Antibodies against Ku protein in sera from patients with autoimmune diseases. Clin Exp Immunol 1989; 76:366–372.
57. Badesch DB, Wynne KM, Bonvallet S, Voelkel NF, Ridgway C, Groves BM. Hypothyroidism and autoimmune primary pulmonary hypertension: an pathogenetic link? Am Intern Med 1993; 119:44–46.
58. Gurtner HP, Gertsch M, Salzmann C, et al. Haeufen sich die primaer vasculaeren formen des chronischen cor pulmonale? Schweiz Med Wochenschr 1968; 98:1579–1581, 1695–1707.
59. Gurtner HP. Pulmonary hypertension, plexogenic pulmonary arteriopathy and the appetite depressant drug aminorex: post or propter? Bull Eur Physiopathol Respir 1979; 15:897–923.
60. Greiser E. Epidemiologische untersuchungen zum zusammenhang zwischen appetitzueglere innahme und primaer vasculaer pulmonaler hypertonie. Internist 1973; 14:437–442.
61. Mlezoch J, Probst P, Szeless S, et al. Primary pulmonary hypertension: follow up of patients with and without anorectic drug intake. Cor Vasa 1980; 22:251–257.
62. Turina J, Wirz P, Krayenbuehl HP, Verlauf und prognose der primaeren pulmonalen hypertonie. Schweiz Med Wochenschr 1977; 107:1825–1828.
63. Kraupp O. Studies on the etiology of primary pulmonary hypertension in animal experiments. Wien Z Inn Med 1969; 50(10):493–496.
64. Lullmann H, Parwaresch MR, Sattler M, Seiler KU, Siegfriedt A. The effects of anorectic agents on the pulmonary pressure and morphology of rat lungs after chronic administration. Arzneimittelforsch 1972; 22:2096.
65. Mielke H, Seiler KU, Stumpf U, Wassermann O. Influence of aminorex (menocil) on pulmonary pressure and on the content of biogenic amines in the lungs of rats. Naunyn Schmiedeberg's Arch Pharmacol 1972; 274(s):R79.
66. Byrne-Quinn E, Grover RF. Aminorex (Menocil) and amphetamine: acute and chronic effects on pulmonary and systemic hemodynamics in the calf. Thorax 1972; 27:127.

67. Kay JM, Smith P, Heath D. Aminorex and the pulmonary circulation. Thorax 1971; 26:262–270.
68. Douglas JG, Munro JF, Kitchin AH, Muir AL, Proudfoot AT. Pulmonary hypertension and fenfluramine. Br Med J 1981; 283:881–883.
69. Gaul G, Blazek G, Deutsch E, Heeger H. Ein fall von chronischer pulmonaler hypertonie nach Fenfluramineinahme. Wien Klin Wochenschr 1982; 22:618–621.
70. Loogen F, Worth H, Schwan G, Goeckenjan, Lösse B, Horstkotte D. Long term follow-up of pulmonary hypertension in patients with and without anorectic drug intake. Cor Vasa 1985; 27(213):111–124.
71. McMurray J, Bloomfield P, Miller HC. Irreversible pulmonary hypertension after treatment with fenfluramine. Br Med J 1986; 292:239–240.
72. Pouwels HMM, Smeets JLRM, Cheriex EC, Wouters EFM. Pulmonary hypertension and fenfluramine. Eur Respir J 1990; 3:606–607.
73. Fotiadis I, Apostolou T, Koukoulas A, Michelacakis N, Kremastinos D. Fenfluramine-induced irreversible pulmonary hypertension. Postgrad Med J 1991; 67:776–777.
74. Atanassoff PG, Weiss BM, Schmid ER, Tornic M. Pulmonary hypertension and dexfenfluramine. Lancet 1992; 339:436 (letter).
75. Roche N, Labrune S, Braun JM, Huchon G. Pulmonary hypertension and dexfenfluramine. Lancet 1992; 339:436–437 (letter).
76. Brenot F, Hervé P, Petitpretz P, Parent F, Duroux P, Simonneau G. Primary pulmonary hypertension and fenfluramine use. Br Heart J 1993; 70:537–541.
77. Pinder RM, Brogden RN, Sauryer PR, Speight TM, Avery GS. Fenfluramine: a review of its pharmacological properties and therapeutic efficacy in obesity. Drugs 1975; 10:241–323.
78. McGoon MD, Vanhoutte PM. Aggregating platelets contract isolated canine pulmonary arteries by releasing 5-hydroxytryptamine. J Clin Invest 1984; 74:828–833.
79. Boe J, Somonsson BG, Stahl E. Effect of histamine, 5-hydroxytryptamine and prostaglandins on isolated pulmonary arteries. Eur J Respir Dis 1980; 61:12–19.
80. Nemecek GM, Coughlin SR, Handley DA, Moskowitz MA. Stimulation of aortic smooth muscle cell mitogenesis by serotonin. Proc Natl Acad Sci USA 1986; 83: 674–678.
81. Hervé P, Launay JM, Scrobohaci ML, Brenot F, Simonneau G, Petitpretz P, Poubeau P, Cerrina J, Duroux P, Drouet L. Increased plasma serotonin in primary pulmonary hypertension. Am J Med 1995; 99:249–254.
82. Hervé P, Drouet L, Bosquet C, Launay JM, Rain B, Simonneau G, Caen J, Duroux P. Primary pulmonary hypertension in a patient with a familial platelet storage pool disease. Role of serotonin. Am J Med 1990; 89:117–120.
83. Fahlen M, Bergman H, Helder G, et al. Phenformin and pulmonary hypertension. Br Heart J 1973; 35:824–828.
84. Kilbourne EM, Rigau-Perez JG, Heath CW Jr et al. Clinical epidemiology of toxic-oil syndrome: manifestations of a new illness. N Engl J Med 1983; 309:1408–1414.
85. Garcia-Dorado D, Miller DD, Garcia EJ, Delca J-L, Maroto E, Chaitman BR. An epidemic of pulmonary hypertension after toxic rapeseed oil ingestion in Spain. J Am Coll Cardiol 1983; 1:1216–1222.
86. Martinez-Tello FJ, Navas-Palacio JJ, Ricoy JR. Pathology of a new toxic syndrome

caused by ingestion of adulterated oil in Spain. Wirchows Arch Pathol Anat 1982; 327:261–285.

87. Philen RM, Hill RH. Pulmonary hypertension in patients with eosinophilia-myalgia syndrome or toxic oil syndrome. Mayo Clin Proc 1993; 68:823–824.
88. Eosinophilia-myalgia syndrome—New Mexico MMWR 1989; 38:765–767.
89. Hertzman PA, Blevins WL, Mayer J, Greenfield B, Ting M, Gleich GJ. Association of the eosinophilia-myalgia syndrome with the ingestion of tryptophan. N Engl J Med 1990; 322:869–873.
90. Silver RM, Heyes MP, Maize JC, Quearry B, Vionnet-Fuasset M, Sternberg EM. Scleroderma, fasciitis, and eosinophilia associated with the ingestion of tryptophan. N Engl J Med 1990; 322:874–881.
91. Medsger TA Jr. Tryptophan-induced eosinophilia-myalgia syndrome. N Engl J Med 1990; 322:926–928 (editorial).
92. Tazelaar HD, Myers JL, Drage CW, King TE Jr, Aguayo S, Colby TV. Pulmonary disease associated with L-tryptophan-induced eosinophilic myalgia syndrome: clinical and pathologic features. Chest 1990; 97:1032–1036.
93. Philen RM, Eidson M, Kilbourne EM, Sewell M, Voorhees R. Eosinophilia-myalgia syndrome: a clinical case series of 21 patients. Arch Intern Med 1991; 151:533–537.
94. Martin RW, Duffy J, Engel AG, Lie JT, Bowles CA, Moyer TP, Gleich GJ. The clinical spectrum of the eosinophilia-myalgia syndrome associated with L-tryptophan ingestion: clinical features in 20 patients and aspects of pathophysiology. Ann Intern Med 1990; 113:124–134.
95. Culpepper RC, Williams RG, Mease PJ, Koepsell TD, Kobayashi JM. Natural history of the eosinophilia-myalgia syndrome. Ann Intern Med 1991; 115:437–442.
96. Clinical spectrum of eosinophilia-myalgia syndrome—California. MMWR 1990; 112:85–87.
97. Kilbourne EM, Bernert JT, Posada de la Paz, Hill RH Jr, Abaitua Borda I, Kilbourne BW et al. Chemical correlates of pathogenicity of oils related to the toxic oil syndrome epidemic in Spain. Am J Epidemiol 1988; 127:1210–1227.
98. Mantz FA, Craige E. Portal axis thrombosis with spontaneous portocaval shunt and resulting cor pulmonale. Arch Pathol 1951; 52:91–97.
99. Segel N, Kay JM, Bayley TJ, Paton A. Pulmonary hypertension with hepatic cirrhosis. Br Heart J 1968; 30:575–578.
100. Senior RM, Britton RL, Turino GM, Wood JA, Langer GA, Fishman AP. Pulmonary hypertension associated with cirrhosis and with portocaval shunts. Circulation 1968; 37:88–96.
101. Edwards BS, Weir EK, Edwards WD, Ludwig J, Dykoski RK, Edwards JE. Coexistent pulmonary and portal hypertension: morphologic and clinical features. J Am Coll Cardiol 1987; 10:123–138.
102. McDonnell PJ, Toye PA, Hutchins GM. Primary pulmonary hypertension: are they related? Am Rev Respir Dis 1983; 127:437–441.
103. Ruttner JR, Bartschi JP, Niedermann R, Schneider J. Plexogenic pulmonary arteriopathy and liver cirrhosis. Thorax 1980; 35:133–136.
104. Lebrec D, Capron JP, Dhumeaux D, Benhamou JP. Pulmonary hypertension complicating portal hypertension. Am Rev Respir Dis 1979; 120:849–856.

105. Naeije RL, Mélot C, Hallemans R, Mols P, Lejeune P. Pulmonary hemodynamics in liver cirrhosis. Semin Respir Med 1985; 7:164–170.
106. Hadengue A, Benhayoun MK, Lebrec D, Benhamou JP. Pulmonary hypertension complicating portal hypertension: prevalence and relation to splanchnic hemodynamics. Gastroenterology 1991; 100:520–528.
107. Sitbon O, Brenot F, Hervé P, Parent F, Azarian R, Taravella O, Simonneau G. Pulmonary hypertension associated with portal hypertension. Comparison with primary pulmonary hypertension. Am J Respir Crit Care Med 1995; 151:A723 (abstract).
108. Naeije RL. "Primary" pulmonary hypertension with coexisting portal hypertension: a retrospective study of six cases. Circulation 1960; 22:376–384.
109. Khaliq SU, Kay Jm, Heath D. Porto-pulmonary venous anastomoses in experimental cirrhosis of the liver in rats. J Pathol 1972; 107:167–174.
110. Chang S, Ohara N. Pulmonary circulatory dysfunctions in rat biliary cirrhosis. Am Rev Respir Dis 1992; 145:798–805.
111. Kim KK, Factor SM. Membrano-proliferative glomerulonephritis and plexogenic pulmonary arteriopathy in a homosexual man with acquired immunodeficiency syndrome. Hum Pathol 1987; 18:1293–1296.
112. Goldsmith GH, Baily RG, Brettler DB, Davidson WR, Ballard JO, Driscoll TE, Greenberg JM, Kasper CK, Levine PH, Ratnoff OD. Primary pulmonary hypertension in patients with classic hemophilia. Ann Intern Med 1988; 108:797–799.
113. Rouveix E, Job D, Delorme G, Jouin H, Franc B, Saveuse H, Dorra M. Hypertension arterielle pulmonaire mortelle chez un toxicomane à l'héroïne et aux amphétamines. Presse Med 1989; 140:153.
114. Bray GL, Martin GR, Chandra R. Idiopathic pulmonary hypertension, hemophilia A and infection with human immunodeficiency virus. Ann Intern Med 1989; 111:689–690.
115. Himelman RB, Dohrmann M, Goodman P, Schiller NB, Straksen NF, Warnock M, Cheitlin MD. Severe pulmonary hypertension and cor pulmonale in the acquired immunodeficiency syndrome. Am J Cardiol 1989; 64:1396–1399.
116. Speich R, Jenni R, Opravil M, Pfab M, Russi EW. Primary pulmonary hypertension in HIV infection. Chest 1991; 100:1268–1271.
117. Coplan NL, Shimony RY, Ioachim HL, Wilentz JR, Posner DH, Lipschitz A, Ruden RA, Bruno MS, Sherrid MV, Gaetz H, Englard A, Kukin M, Packer M. Primary pulmonary hypertension associated with human immunodeficiency viral infection. Am J Med 1990; 89:96–99.
118. Polos PG, Wolfe D, Harley RA, Strange C, Sahn SA. Pulmonary hypertension and human immunodeficiency virus infection: two reports and a review of the literature. Chest 1992; 101:474–478.
119. Piette AM, Legoux B, Gepner P, Chapman A. Hypertension artérielle pulmonaire "primitive" associée à l'infection par le VIH: deux observations. Presses Med 1992; 21:616–618.
120. Jacques C, Richmond G, Tierney L, Curtis JL, McKerron J, Warnock ML. Primary pulmonary hypertension and human immunodeficiency virus infection in a non hemophiliac man. Hum Pathol 1992; 23:191–194.

121. Aarons EJ, Nye FJ. Primary pulmonary hypertension and HIV infection. AIDS 1991; 5:1276–1277.
122. Mette SA, Palevsky HI, Peitra GG, Williams TM, Bruder E, Prestipino AJ, Patrick AM, Wirth JA. Primary pulmonary hypertension in association with human immunodeficiency virus infection: a possible viral etiology for some forms of hypertensive pulmonary arteriopathy. Am Rev Respir Dis 1992; 145:1196–1200.
123. Tomashefski JF, Hirsch CS. The pulmonary vascular lesions of intravenous drug abuse. Hum Pathol 1980; 11:133–145.
124. Arnett EN, Battle WE, Russo JV, Roberts WC. Intravenous injection of talc-containing drugs intended for oral use: a cause of pulmonary granulomatosis and pulmonary hypertension. Am J Med 1976; 60:711–718.
125. Robertson CH, Reynolds RC, Wilson JE. Pulmonary hypertension and foreign body granulomas in intravenous drug abusers: documentation by cardiac catheterization and lung biopsy. Am J Med 1976; 61:657–664.
126. Hind CRK. Pulmonary complications of intravenous drug misuse: epidemiology and non infective complications. Thorax 1990; 45:891–898.
127. Overland ES, Nolan AJ, Hopewell PC. Alteration of pulmonary function in intravenous drug abusers: prevalence, severity and characterization of gas exchange abnormalities. Am J Med 1980; 68:231–237.
128. Petitpretz P, Brenot F, Azarian R, Parent F, Rain B, Hervé P, Simonneau G. Pulmonary hypertension in patients with human immunodeficiency virus infection: comparison with primary pulmonary hypertension. Circulation 1994; 89:2722–2727.
129. D'Alonzo GE, Barst RJ, Ayres SM, Bergofsky EH, Brundage BH, Detre KM, Fishman AP, Goldring RM, Groves BM, Kernis JT, Levy PS, Pietra GG, Reid LM, Reeves JT, Rich S, Vreim CE, Williams GW, Wu M. Survival in patients with primary pulmonary hypertension: results from a national prospective study. Ann Intern Med 1991; 115:343–349.
130. Hughes JD, Rubin L. Primary pulmonary hypertension: an analysis of 28 cases and a review of the literature. Medicine 1986; 65:56–72.
131. Humbert M, Monti G, Petitpretz P, Brenot F, Rain B, Magnan A, Galanaud P, Duroux P, Simonneau G. Pulmonary hypertension in HIV-1 infected patients is associated with an increased intrapulmonary PDGF production. Am J Respir Crit Car Med 1994; 149:A824 (abstract).
132. Tuder RM, Hoeper MM, Bates T, Voelkel NF. TAT-protein of HIV enhances vascular growth factor production by endothelial cells and monocytes. Am J Respir Crit Care Med 1995; 151:A735 (abstract).

6

Familial Primary Pulmonary Hypertension

JAMES E. LOYD and JOHN H. NEWMAN

Vanderbilt University School of Medicine
Nashville, Tennessee

I. Historical Perspective

Within 3 years of Dresdale's original clinical description of primary pulmonary hypertension (PPH) in 1951 (1), the same author was the first to record the occurrence of PPH in several members of one family (2). Although much has been learned about PPH in the subsequent four decades, this initial report was astonishing for the depth and accuracy of its clinical commentary. The authors noted that "primary pulmonary hypertension is not limited to any age group, having been described in patients as young as twenty months and found in the eighth decade. The majority of cases, however, fall in the age group of twenty to forty years. There appears to be a slightly greater incidence in the female sex."

The first reported PPH family (2) suffered deaths in four patients, including a mother and son, in whom disease was documented by right heart catheterization, and two maternal siblings, in whom PPH was suspected on clinical grounds. Pulmonary artery pressure was 122/52 mmHg in the mother, who died of right ventricular failure at age 43 and was 78/33 in the son, who died at age 21. A sister of the mother had radiographic and electrocardiographic documentation of right ventricular hypertrophy (RVH), and PPH was diagnosed clinically; she died at age 31. A brother of the mother died of heart disease in his youth. Later efforts to identify and locate PPH families from early reports have often been successful, but this first reported family has not been identified.

This informative manuscript (2) was prescient, both for the description of the first-reported PPH family, but also in the reporting of hemodynamic responsiveness to vasodilating agents, as reflected in its title, *Recent Studies in Primary Pulmonary Hypertension, Including Pharmacodynamic Observations on Pulmonary Vascular Resistance*.

Subsequently, reports of PPH in families were infrequent. During the three decades after the first report in 1954, there were reports of only 13 PPH families in the United States (3).

II. Incidence and Distribution of Familial Primary Pulmonary Hypertension

Estimates of the incidence of familial PPH derive from the National Institutes of Health (NIH) registry for PPH (4), a natural history study that enrolled 187 PPH patients between 1981 and 1985 from 32 U. S. centers. Twelve of the registry patients (6%) had a first-order relative with PPH. An analysis to determine whether the clinical presentation or outcome in familial PPH was different from those of sporadic PPH showed no differences in the ages, hemodynamics, or other clinical findings. The 12 familial PPH patients in the registry included seven males and five females; this small sample of familial PPH does not accurately reflect the preponderance of females in larger studies.

Patients who had a positive family history were diagnosed sooner after the onset of symptoms than were the other registry patients (0.68 vs. 2.56 years; $p = 0.0002$). Familial PPH appears to be identical with sporadic PPH in every other respect. The long time (2.5 years) to diagnosis in sporadic PPH suggests that, for most physicians, the index of suspicion is not very high for this disorder. In families with PPH, a heightened index of suspicion is often present in both the families and their physicians. Aside from more rapid diagnosis in familial than in sporadic PPH, no clinical or pathological difference has ever been demonstrated. The remarkable variability that occurs in some aspects of PPH, such as the age of onset varying from 1 to 60 years, is a feature of both familial and sporadic PPH alike.

Scant data are available on the prevalence of familial PPH. The best estimate derives from the 6% of the total cases in the PPH registry that were recognized to be familial. We suspect that there may be substantial variation in the geographic distribution of familial PPH. It is a further impediment that there are no reported data on the geographic distribution of sporadic PPH patients.

We have direct knowledge of 35 families in the United States who have two or more members who had PPH, and we have indirect knowledge of 15 other families in the United States who are known to several colleagues, so there appears to be at least 50 total. Conclusive information is not available on the total number of PPH families in the United States, but the 50 proved families seems to be a larger number than one might expect from the low incidence (6%) of familial disease in the PPH registry data.

Review of the geographic distribution suggests that there appears to be clustering in Tennessee, because we have direct knowledge of 13 PPH families in this state. This number is also a minimum, because there may be other families unknown to us. In the absence of data describing the prevalence of familial PPH in other states or regions, it cannot be ascertained whether this is true clustering or not. Tennessee contains 1⁄50 of the United States population. If the prevalence of PPH families in Tennessee is not a cluster, but instead is representative of the distribution of disease throughout the United States, there may be 650 or more PPH families.

Other reports confirm that familial PPH is distributed worldwide. Three PPH families have been reported from England, and others originate from France, Germany, Sweden, Italy, Poland, India, and Australia.

III. Clinical Features

The symptoms of familial PPH are identical with those of patients with sporadic PPH (4). The most common symptoms are dyspnea, fatigue, chest pain, syncope, near syncope, edema, and palpitations. In the PPH registry (4), dyspnea was nearly universal, occurring in 98% of patients by the time of entry in the registry. Fatigue was also present in most patients, whereas the other symptoms were less common.

As noted earlier, familial PPH patients were diagnosed sooner after the onset of symptoms than were the other registry patients (0.68 vs. 2.56 years), but even in familial PPH, the time to diagnosis appears slow (0.68 years). Many possible explanations for delayed diagnosis may exist, but both the patient and physician may be deceived in the early course of PPH. The symptoms noted are nonspecific, and their onset may be insidious. Many patients initially believe that their exertional symptoms are due to deconditioning or advancing age. The condition may also deceive the physician, who sees the patient only at rest. In the original clinical description of PPH (1), Dresdale noted astutely that "An impressive feature ... was the contrast between the appearance of good health when at rest and the striking discomfort evoked by even mild exertion."

The gender ratio of PPH demonstrates excess disease in females in both sporadic and familial PPH. The female/male ratio in the PPH registry (4) was 1.7 females for each male. Familial PPH has a similar predisposition for females, with a 2:1 ratio (3,21). Of interest, other causes of pulmonary hypertension also disproportionately affect females, including individuals born with atrial septal

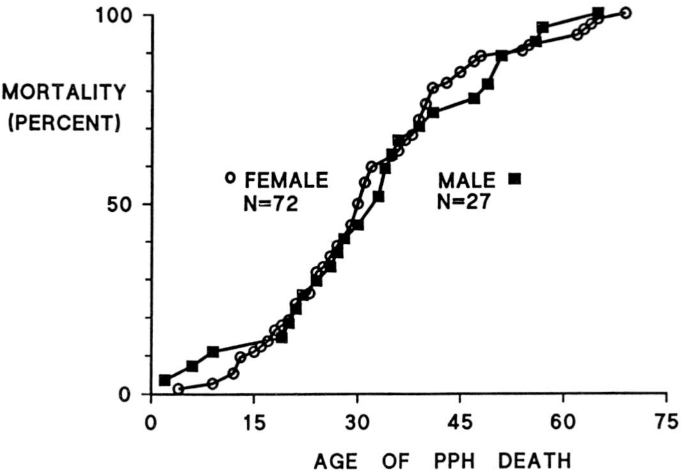

Figure 1 Cumulative mortality curves for males and females who died of familial PPH.

defect (5), and individuals who smoke crack cocaine (6). Although incidence of disease is greater in females, the severity of disease and outcome are similar between sexes. Cumulative mortality curves (Fig. 1) for males and females dying of familial PPH are very similar.

Survival does not differ between sporadic and familial PPH. This is best shown in an analysis (3) of 36 familial PPH patients, compared with 41 sporadic patients, for whom survival did not differ. The median survival of all patients in the PPH registry was 2.8 years (7), and the survival of the 12 familial PPH patients was no different.

IV. Associated Abnormalities in Families with Primary Pulmonary Hypertension

A. Fibrinolytic Defect

Investigations of the fibrinolytic system in two families with pulmonary hypertension have been reported that examined the hypothesis that its pathogenesis may be related to impaired ability to lyse recurrent microthrombi or emboli.

In 1973, Inglesby et al. (8) reported a family who demonstrated pulmonary hypertension in five members; the authors found abnormal elevations of antiplasmin in seven members. In contrast, Tubbs et al. (9) studied another family who had three members with pulmonary hypertension; plasminogen, antiplasmin, and fibrinolytic titers of antiurokinase did not differ significantly from those of the control group. Thus, defective fibrinolysis is not the universal cause of primary pulmonary hypertension, at least in this family.

B. Human Leukocyte Antigen Association

Indirect evidence demonstrates that pulmonary hypertension may be associated with autoimmune disease. Low-titer antinuclear antibodies occur commonly in PPH (4). The human leukocyte antigen (HLA) alleles and neighboring genes are involved in antigen presentation and lymphocyte interactions. Increased risk of autoimmune disease has been associated with genes closely linked to HLA.

Barst et al. (10) recently reported an association of PPH with the major histocompatibility complex (MHC). They studied 17 children with PPH and 13 children with shunt-related pulmonary hypertension. The PPH patients had increased frequencies of HLA-DR3 ($p = 0.01$), DRw52 ($p = 0.04$), and DQw2 ($p = 0.01$), and decreased DR5 ($p = 0.045$). The children with shunt-related pulmonary hypertension had no statistically significant alterations in any *DR* or *DQ* allele.

More recently the same investigators reported an HLA association of familial PPH in 15 members from four families with PPH (11). Eight FPPH patients were HLA-DRw52, and seven were HLA-DR3,DRw52,DQw2. The authors concluded that there is a susceptibility factor for FPPH located within or near the major histocompatibility locus on chromosome 6p21.3.

C. Platelet or Serotonin Abnormality

Platelet abnormalities could be pathogenetically related to pulmonary hypertension through the release of vasoactive substances or substances that stimulate cellular proliferation. Herve et al. (12) described a 46-year-old man who developed pulmonary hypertension in the setting of an inherited bleeding disorder, platelet delta storage pool disease, associated with a high level of 5-hydroxytryptamine (5-HT) in plasma. Therapy with ketanserin and prostacyclin was initially successful, but he died 2 years after the diagnosis of pulmonary hypertension. Postmortem examination revealed plexiform lesions and intimal proliferation and fibrosis.

D. Abnormal Hemoglobin

Rich et al. (13) recently reported a mother and three sons with familial pulmonary hypertension in association with an abnormal hemoglobin. The hemoglobin has an abnormality of the β-chain containing a phenylalanine to valine substitution at position β-42, which is associated with a lower than normal oxygen affinity, sufficient to cause cyanosis. In this family the hemoglobinopathy was transmitted as an autosomal dominant trait and was present in those family members who had PPH. Many hemoglobin variants with decreased oxygen affinity have been identified previously, but they are generally without important clinical manifestations such as pulmonary hypertension.

V. Pathology

Clinically, PPH is a diagnosis of exclusion. The presence of pulmonary hypertension is confirmed by catheterization, and secondary causes are excluded by clinical testing. This disorder can be the presenting clinical syndrome of several different diseases. Disorders that selectively cause disease in the small vessels of the lungs (such as pulmonary veno-occlusive disease [PVOD] and pulmonary capillary hemangiomatosis [PCH]) may be clinically indistinguishable from classic plexogenic PPH. In series of PPH patients selected by clinical criteria alone, a few patients are eventually found to even have other types of lung disease, such as interstitial lung disease (14) or, rarely, even normal lung vessels (15). Although a clinical definition of PPH is not universally correct, it remains as the standard of clinical care for PPH because the risk/benefit ratio of surgical lung biopsy is generally less favorable, unless discordant clinical data suggests that another treatable diagnosis might be present. In families with classic PPH, when a family member develops the onset of symptoms compatible with PPH, and noninvasive testing supports the diagnosis, the prior occurrence of PPH in the family is further support to the clinical diagnosis, and the need for biopsy confirmation is lower still, as compared with sporadic PPH.

In addition, the pathological changes alone are not specific for PPH. Although the pathological changes for classic PPH are typical, they are not pathognomonic; plexogenic arteriopathy is typical of many secondary causes of pulmonary hypertension, including congenital heart disease, toxic oil syndrome, portal hypertension, and others. The individual vessels in the lungs of patients with primary pulmonary hypertension exhibit a variety of types of pathological changes, which have been used to categorize patients into subsets. Whether the different pathological subsets represent different basic disease processes, or whether they are simply different manifestations of the same underlying mechanism is not known.

We sought to determine the nature and variety of pathological lesions in PPH families, and to discover whether the pattern of pathological lesions would provide support for the existence of more than one type of disease. The two pathological subsets of PPH reported to be most common are plexogenic PPH, defined by concentric intimal fibrosis and plexogenic lesions, and thromboembolic PPH, defined by vessels with eccentic intimal fibrosis. Families with PPH offer a unique opportunity to investigate the distribution of pathological lesion types, because there should be a single pathogenetic basis within each family. Thus, the breadth of pathological lesions should reflect only that underlying mechanism. We recovered and analyzed lung specimens from 23 affected members of 13 PPH families (16). Four patients were from 1 family, 3 patients from each of 2 families, 2 patients from each of 3 families, and 1 patient from each of the others. Every lung vessel was assessed and categorized. We analyzed 2516 vessels, with a mean of 109 vessels per patient (range 38–264).

The results suggest that these most common pathological subsets—plexogenic and thromboembolic PPH—are different pathological manifestations of the same process, and not different disease processes. We found marked heterogeneity of the types of vascular lesions within and among families, including frequent coexistence of thrombotic and plexiform lesions.

In one PPH family the most common lesion type was different in each of the three patients. The predominant lesion type was concentric intimal fibrosis (the defining lesion of plexogenic PPH) in a father who died of PPH at age 51; eccentric intimal fibrosis (the defining lesion of thromboembolic PPH) in his niece, who died of PPH at age 40; and isolated medial hypertrophy in his daughter with PPH, who died at age 25. Different PPH pathological subsets would not be expected to occur among members of the same family unless they had the same basic pathogenesis.

Most importantly the pathological analysis suggested that all of the families had a single disease process. There was a broad spectrum of lesions within and among families, but there were no features that distinguished a different disease process among or between them. It is our experience that, although the categorization of patients by pathological subsets may be crisply distinguished in a narrative classification schema, the designation of a specific pathological subset for an individual patient is more interpretive than is recognized by most clinicians.

The occurrence of familial PPH has been reported for each of the pathological subsets of PPH, even the extremely rare ones, except for thromboembolic PPH. Familial occurrence has been described in two families with pulmonary veno-occlusive disease (18,19), a subset identified in pathological specimens of only seven patients in the NIH registry. Pulmonary capillary hemangiomatosis appears to be extremely rare, so much so that there were no patients with that subset in the PPH registry; however, there is at least one family with pulmonary capillary hemangiomatosis (20). The observation that all of the PPH subsets, except thromboembolic PPH, have been reported in families, even the rare subsets, might further suggest that thromboembolic PPH is not a truly different basic disease process. The future identification of molecular mechanisms of PPH will surely hold the answer to the true number of different disease processes that give rise to the clinical syndrome of PPH.

VI. Genetics

Transmission of PPH in families (Fig. 2) is unpredictable, and the mode of transmission has not been proved. Incomplete penetrance, in which the gene is

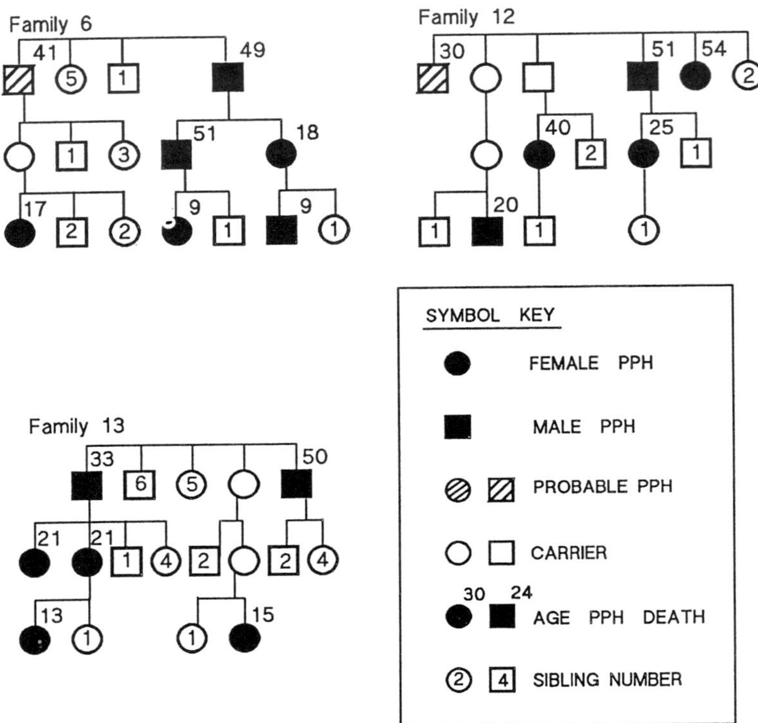

Figure 2 Pedigrees of three families with familial PPH.

transmitted to affected progeny by persons who manifest no evidence of disease, is a major confounding feature to genetic analysis (3). Because there is no marker for the gene, its presence can be documented only by the development of disease in an individual or in their progeny.

Vertical transmission affecting four generations in some PPH families strongly suggests the action of a single dominant gene. Father to son transmission of familial PPH (see Fig. 2, family 6) has been shown in many families, which excludes X-linked disease. It appears that the PPH gene is autosomal dominant, but the complex features of its transmission have prevented confirmation by formal segregation analysis to date.

A. Genetic Anticipation

Genetic anticipation is a phenomenon in which there is worsening of familial disease in subsequent generations, which can be manifested by earlier age of onset, or by greater severity of disease. In the past, genetic anticipation was attributed to artifact and ascertainment bias, but it has recently been shown with certainty to have a biological basis in several unrelated neurological diseases. This new molecular mechanism also explains incomplete penetrance and variability in clinical severity. Genetic anticipation is dramatic in familial PPH (Fig. 3) and manifests as younger age of death in subsequent generations. It was originally noted in early reports of individual PPH families, as shown in Figure 2, and we confirmed it in our initial analysis of 14 families with PPH (3) and again more recently (21). Genetic anticipation in familial PPH has also been further supported recently by other investigators (11). The presence of genetic anticipation in FPPH implicates a molecular mechanism similar to that recently discovered in other diseases that manifest this phenomenon.

A molecular basis for genetic anticipation was first elucidated for the fragile X syndrome, in 1991 (22,23). A trinucleotide (CGG) in the 5′-region of the *FMR-1* gene is repeated 6–54 times in tandem in normal individuals, but it occurs more than 200 times in patients with fragile X syndrome. The triplet repeat becomes unstable, particularly during female meiosis, once the repeat number exceeds about 52. The transcript that contains the massively expanded repeat sequence is not expressed in patients who have the fragile X syndrome. Currently, there is a virtual explosion of investigations into triplet-repeat expansion as a mechanism of human disease (24,25). A recent review summarizes the impor-

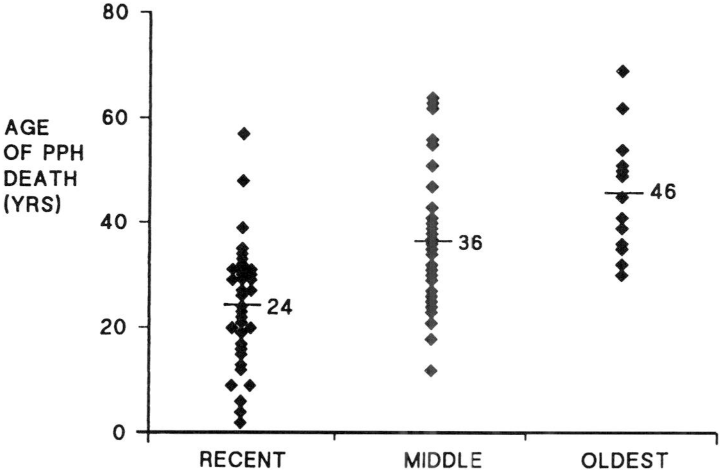

Figure 3 Genetic anticipation in familial PPH, indicating the younger ages at death in subsequent generations.

tance of this mechanism in the statement "Finding a mutagenesis mechanism in humans that hadn't been described years ago in *Drosophila* or some other organism is unprecedented.... These mutations have quickly gone from being an anomaly to being one of the hottest topics in human genetics (25)."

A new molecular method (26), repeat expansion detection (RED) has been developed to detect single copies of large trinucleotide repeats. It uses genomic DNA as a template for the annealing and ligation of repeat-specific oligonucleotides. It does not require flanking sequence information, or single-copy probes. The fact that this method can identify the presence of pathological repeat expansions without prior knowledge of chromosomal location, is precisely the capability needed to study diseases such as FPPH, for which anticipation suggests a trinucleotide-repeat expansion, but the gene or its location is unknown. The presence of genetic anticipation in FPPH clearly implicates such a molecular mechanism (triplet-repeat expansion) similar to that recently discovered in the other diseases with genetic anticipation (27).

In summary, familial PPH is clinically and pathologically identical with the sporadic form. There is little data on geographic distribution of sporadic or familial PPH, but 13 of 35 PPH families known to us reside in Tennessee, which has 1/50 of the U. S. population; either familial PPH clusters in this state, or if not, an estimate for total PPH families in the United States would approach 650 families. Pathological studies of familial PPH, especially those examining different patients in the same family, have important implications for the number of different diseases causing the clinical syndrome of PPH. Vertical transmission in families suggests a single dominant gene. The mode of gene transmission appears to be autosomal dominant, but confirmation by formal segregation analysis has not yet been achieved. An uncommon genetic phenomenon, genetic anticipation, suggests that the molecular basis of familial PPH may be trinucleotide-repeat expansion, which has recently been discovered to be the molecular basis of several unrelated neurological diseases that manifest this phenomenon.

Acknowledgment

Supported by NIH Grants HL 48164, 41952, and 45107, National Heart, Lung, and Blood Institute.

References

1. Dresdale DT, Schultz M, RJ Michtom. Primary pulmonary hypertension. I. Clinical and hemodynamic study. Am J Med 1951; 11:686–701.
2. Dresdale DT, Michtom RJ, Schultz M. Recent studies in primary pulmonary hypertension, including pharmacodynamic observations on pulmonary vascular resistance. Bull NY Acad Med 1954; 30:195.

3. Loyd JE, Primm RK, Newman JH. Transmission of familial primary pulmonary hypertension. Am Rev Respir Dis 1984; 129:194–197.
4. Rich S, Dantzker DR, Ayres SM, et al. Primary pulmonary hypertension: a national prospective study. Ann Intern Med 1987; 107:216–223.
5. Steele PM, Fuster V, Cohen M, Ritter DG, McGoon DC. Isolated atrial septal defect with pulmonary vascular obstructive disease—long-term follow-up and prediction of outcome after surgical correction. Circulation 1987; 76:1037–1042.
6. Russell LA, Spehlmann JC, Clarke M, Lillington GA. Pulmonary hypertension in female crack users (abstr). Am Rev Respir Dis 1992; A717.
7. D'Alonzo GE, Barst RJ, Ayres SM, et al. Survival in primary pulmonary hypertension. Ann Intern Med 1991; 115:343–349.
8. Inglesby TV, Singer JW, Gordon DS. Abnormal fibrinolysis in familial pulmonary hypertension. Am J Med 1973; 55:5–14.
9. Tubbs RR, Levin RD, Shirey EK, Hoffman GC. Fibrinolysis in familial pulmonary hypertension. Am J Clin Pathol 1979; 71:384–387.
10. Barst RJ, Flaster ER, Menon A, Fotino M, Morse JH. Evidence for the association of unexplained pulmonary hypertension in children with the major histocompatibility complex. Circulation 1992; 85:249–258.
11. Morse JH, Barst RJ, Fotino M. Familial pulmonary hypertension: immunogenetic findings in four Caucasian kindreds. Am Rev Respir Dis 1992; 145:787–792.
12. Herve P, Drouet L, Dosquet C, Launay JM, Rain B, Simonneau G, Caen J, Duroux P. Primary pulmonary hypertension in a patient with a familial platelet storage pool disease: role of serotonin. Am J Med 1990; 89:117–120.
13. Rich S, Hart K. Familial pulmonary hypertension in association with an abnormal hemoglobin. Chest 1991; 99:1208–1210.
14. Palevsky HI, Schloo BL, Pietra GG, Wever KT, Janicki JS, Rubin E, Fishman AP. Primary pulmonary hypertension: vascular structure, morphometry, and responsiveness to vasodilator agents. Circulation 1989; 80:1207–1221.
15. Pietra GG, Edwards WD, Kay JM, et al. Histopathology of primary pulmonary hypertension: a qualitative and quantitative study of pulmonary blood vessels from 58 patients in the National Heart, Lung, and Blood Institute, primary pulmonary hypertension registry. Circulation 1989; 80:1198–1206.
16. Loyd JE, Atkinson JB, Virmani R, Pietra GG, Newman JH. Heterogeneity of pathologic lesions in familial PPH. Am Rev Respir Dis 1988; 138:952–957.
17. Wagenvoort CA, Mulder PGH. Thrombotic lesions in primary plexogenic arteriopathy. Chest 1993; 103:844–849.
18. Davies P, Reid L. Pulmonary veno-occlusive disease in siblings: case report and morphometric study. Hum Pathol 1982; 13:911–915.
19. Voordes CG, Kuipers JRG, Elema JD. Familial pulmonary veno-occlusive disease: a case report. Thorax 1977; 32:763–766.
20. Langleben D, Heneghan JM, Batten AP, Wang NS, Fitch N, Schlesinger RD, Guerraty A, Rouleau JL. Familial pulmonary capillary hemangiomatosis resulting in primary pulmonary hypertension. Ann Intern Med 1988; 109:106–109.
21. Loyd JE, Butler MG, Foround TM, Conneally PM, Phillips JA, Newman JH. Genetic anticipation and abnormal gender ratio at birth in familial primary pulmonary hypertension. Am J Respir Crit Care Med 1995; 152:93–97.

22. Fu YH, Kuhl DPA, Pizzuti A, Pieretti M, Sutcliffe JS, Richards S, Verkerk AJMH, Holden JJA, Fenwick RG, Warren ST, Oostra BA, Nelson DL, Caskey CT. Variation of the CGG repeat at the fragile X site results in genetic instability: resolution of the Sherman paradox. Cell 1991; 67:1047–1058.
23. Verkerk AJMH, Pieretti M, Sutcliffe JS, Fu YH, Kuhl DPA, Pizzuti A, Reiner O, Richards S, Victoria MF, Zhang F, Eussen BE, van Ommen GJB, Blonden LAJ, Riggins GJ, Chastain JL, Kunst CB, Galjaard H. Identification of a gene (*FMR-1*) containing a CGG repeat coincident with a breakpoint cluster region exhibiting length variation in fragile X syndrome. Cell 1991; 65:905–914.
24. Morell V. The puzzle of the triplet repeats. Science 1993; 260:1422–1423.
25. Mandel, J-L. Questions of expansion. Nature Genet 1993; 14:8–9.
26. Schalling M, Hudson TJ, Buetow KH, Housman DE. Direct detection of novel expanded trinucleotide repeats in the human genome. Nature Genet 1993; 4:135–139.
27. Slovis BS, Loyd JE, Newman JH, Krishnamani MRS, Phillips JA. Investigation of trinucleotide repeat expansion as the genetic basis of familial primary pulmonary hypertension (FPPH). Am J Respir Crit Care Med 1995; 151:A724.

7

Epidemiology of Primary Pulmonary Hypertension

YOLA MORIDE
and LUCIEN ABENHAIM

McGill University
and Sir Mortimer B. Davis Jewish General Hospital
Montreal, Quebec, Canada

JIWEI XU

McGill University
Montreal, Quebec, Canada

I. The Nature of Primary Pulmonary Hypertension

Primary pulmonary hypertension (PPH) is used to define a subcategory of pulmonary hypertension. In the medical community, it is agreed that the diagnosis of PPH first requires the exclusion of secondary causes of pulmonary hypertension. However, the criteria to define the secondary causes vary from those proposed by the World Health Organization (WHO), following a meeting on PPH in 1973 (1), to those of a recent American College of Chest Physicians (ACCP) consensus statement in 1993 (2). The operational definition of PPH used in the scarce observational studies stems from the United States national prospective study of PPH (3). Although the terminology to define pathological changes is highly heterogeneous, classified into plexogenic pulmonary arteriopathy, thrombotic pulmonary arteriopathy, and pulmonary venous occlusive disease by the WHO, or pulmonary capillary hemangiomatosis and pulmonary veno-occlusive by the ACCP, the clinical presentation of PPH appears to be typical. The epidemiological knowledge about PPH is very limited.

II. Primary Pulmonary Hypertension in the Population

Validated indices commonly used to quantify the occurrence of PPH in the population, such as incidence, prevalence, and mortality, are not available in the literature. Nevertheless, the incidence (number of new cases per year in a well-defined population) has been estimated to vary from approximately 1 per million to 2 per million inhabitants in countries such as France or the United States (4).

Pulmonary hypertension, as a whole, l[illegible]ggested to account for approximately 20% of all hospital admissions [illegible] cardiology unit, from which fewer than 5% could be classified as primary (5). So far in the literature, the only available data on the frequency of PPH are based on the proportion of PPH cases obtained from autopsy data (6), or from those found in a population of cardiopulmonary patients (7). In 1954, Goodale et al. reported only 2 cases of PPH in a series of 10,000 autopsies (6). Wood identified 17 cases of PPH in a consecutive series of 10,000 patients seen in a cardiovascular clinic, of which 14 were females and 3 were males (7). Given these figures, PPH may account for less than 1% of the total number of patients who undergo catherization in the United States.

Under a public health perspective, the effect of PPH, in terms of absolute number of cases, is not expected to be huge. However, the burden is extremely high, considering the poor survival and prohibitive cost of treatment. Epidemiological studies, therefore, should be oriented toward an etiological perspective; that is, they should attempt to identify promoting or predisposing factors for the onset of the disease, to ultimately identify high-risk groups and apply preventive measures.

III. Survival

Survival analyses are useful to assess prognostic factors and to evaluate the effectiveness of therapy. Most often, clinical traits, hemodynamic characteristics, and drug responsiveness are important factors that influence survival. Such analyses can be useful only if uniform diagnostic procedures are applied to a large and representative sample of patients. Survivorship must be assessed from the onset of symptoms or from diagnosis (most likely the date of cardiac catheterization) (4) to endpoint events. Also, there should be a sufficient time of follow-up and sensible outcome assessment intervals. Accurate measurements and definitions of prognostic factors, as well as appropriate control of confounding factors, are absolutely necessary. Unfortunately, studies on PPH are not consistent in meeting all these criteria.

A. Survival Rates

Rich and Levy documented 12 patients with PPH in one hospital setting and found that among the 7 patients who survived at least 2 years after diagnosis (4 males and

3 females) the average survival time was 5.2 ± 2 years and among 5 nonsurvivors, those who survived less than 6 months after diagnosis (all females), the average survival time was 0.3 ± 0.2 year (3). The duration between the onset of symptoms to diagnosis was about 1.3 ± 0.8 years for survivors and 0.7 ± 0.5 year for nonsurvivors. A national survey on PPH was conducted in all hospitals of Japan between 1975 and 1978 (8). A total of 87 cases were identified, with a female to male ratio of 3.6:1. The age of patients ranged from 14 to 69 years old (average 33). The diagnostic exclusion criteria did not consider drug-related human immunodeficiency virus (HIV) infection, and portal hypertension as secondary causes. The average survival rate was 2.5 years, with a follow-up time of up to 100 months. In a series of 137 cases from the Untied Kingdom, the median survival time was 3.4 years, and the range from onset of symptoms to death varied between 2 months and 42 years (9). In another case series of 137, "moderate" and "severe" PPH patients who underwent transplantation had a similar survival time (75% at 1 year, and 60% at 2 years) (10). Both groups were better than patients with "severe" PPH who received medical treatment only. These findings are concordant with those by Gilbert et al. in a series of 90 cases referred for heart–lung transplantation, who had a median survival from diagnosis of 3.6 years (11). The survival advantage of these patients may be due to a highly selected candidate pool for heart–lung transplantation, which excluded patients either too young or too old, or with other clinical conditions not meeting the requirements for heart–lung transplantation.

B. Prognostic Factors

Studies found in the literature differ relative to factors that predict best survival. The stroke volume index and right atrial pressure were good predictors of clinical course in one study (8), whereas, in another, cardiac index (CI; L $min^{-1}m^{-2}$) was considered to be the best prognostic factor (9). However, the best understanding of survivorship probably came from the Patient Registry for the Characterization of Primary Pulmonary Hypertension, established by the U.S. National Heart, Lung, and Blood Institute of the National Institutes of Health (3,12). A total of 32 clinical centers were involved nationwide, and 194 cases were registered between 1981 and 1985, and followed through 1988. The estimated median survival of those patients was 2.8 years. The best predictors of mortality were mean pulmonary artery pressure, mean right atrial pressure, and cardiac index. Survival was not affected by age, age at onset of symptoms, symptom duration, sex, smoking history, the presence or absence of a serum antinuclear antibody titer, family history of PPH, history of oral contraceptive use, or pregnancy.

C. Survival in Children and the Elderly

Survival in a group of eight children with PPH included in an acute vasodilator trial (average age 7.4 years) was much shorter: 37% at 1 year, and 12% at 2.5 years

(13). These figures are lower than those reported in the National Prospective Registry, 64% at 1 year and 48% at 3 years (3). Another study found that the mean survival in children whose ages were younger than 1 year to 15 years, was 8.7 years (17). In eight PPH patients aged 65 and over, survival was 2.5 years (range: 0.25–6.7) (14,15). Relatively little information is available in the elderly population, despite the fact that 8% of the cases included in the National Registry for PPH, were over 60 years old.

IV. Risk Factors for Primary Pulmonary Hypertension

Most researchers agree that PPH is an expression of multiple causes. A set of minimal conditions and events can be defined as a sufficient cause, but all those components are as yet unknown (16). Some individuals may be predisposed to develop the disease. To be considered a causal factor for a disease, a suspected variable must covary with the disease statistically, not by chance; its presence must precede the occurrence of the disease, and the association between the suspected variable and the disease must not be entirely due to biases, such as those from study subject, measurement of suspected factor, and disease condition (17).

When dealing with a disease of unknown etiology, such as PPH, an epidemiological approach usually has to take a wider range of factors into consideration. Most often suspected factors fall into the following domains: hereditary or genetic trait, which may be represented by family cluster; tobacco smoking, alcohol consumption, and substance abuse; occupational exposure, such as mechanical, chemical, and infectious agents; environmental characteristics, such as air, water, and food quality; hazardous materials; dietary and nutritional pattern; deficiencies and excess; prenatal exposure; nosocomial or iatrogenic exposure, particularly medications; abnormal metabolic or physiological status; and comorbidity. Among this plethora of possible risk factors, very few have been addressed, and even fewer have been shown to be associated with the risk of PPH. The following summarizes findings available for each of the domains.

A. Hereditary or Genetic Taint

Since the first report of familial PPH, confirmed by catheterization, published research has suggested that the pattern of inheritance may be autosomal dominant with a 2:1 female to male ratio (18,19). Heterogeneity of pathological changes within and among the families existed, and the survival after the onset of symptoms was the same as in nonfamilial PPH. This disease may be initiated by abnormalities of the pulmonary vascular bed that may predispose to in situ thrombosis (20,21). Interested readers may refer to Chapter 6 of this volume for details.

B. Personal Characteristics and Lifestyle

Age and Gender

Primary pulmonary hypertension can affect individuals of all age groups, from newborns to the elderly over 80. A national study in the United States showed that the mean age was 36 years old, with a range of 1–81 (3). In females the highest percentage was in the 21–30 age group, whereas males tended to be older, in the 31–40 age group. A preponderance of females among PPH patients was noted in several large case series, and the female to male ratio varied from 1.7:1 to 3.5:1. The highest ratio was found among black people (4:1). In a large case series from India, a male preponderance was noted. It was suggested that this ratio may be influenced by local economic conditions, for which women of the poorer social classes may not be able to afford medical attention. Childhood PPH includes equal proportions of boys and girls. Overall, age, gender, and race have not been quantitatively demonstrated to be risk factors for PPH. To our knowledge, no study has been conducted to assess the risk associated with smoking, alcohol consumption, or socioeconomic status.

Substance Abuse

An association between PPH and substance abuse has been reported in children, young women, and men. So far, evidence was obtained from case series, which usually include selected populations and do not allow for an account of the baseline risk in the population. Among 18 boys, with a history of chronic glue (toluene) abuse, pulmonary hypertension was found in some of them (22). A man with a 10-year history of "crack" and "peanut butter methamphetamine" inhalation also was seen with marked pulmonary hypertension (23). Four young women, with a history of smoking crack cocaine, were reported to develop clinical pulmonary hypertension. Cocaine abuse by a mother also produced signs of persistent pulmonary hypertension in a newborn (24,25).

Altitude

Residents of highland areas usually show some signs of pulmonary vascular reaction to chronic alveolar hypoxia. Among 160 natives living in the Himalayas, at altitudes of 3000–5000 meters (m), 5% presented with right ventricular hypertrophy, as assessed by electrocardiogram, whereas 27% of those living between 4500 and 5000 m had clinical evidence of pulmonary hypertension (26). Another study reported that pulmonary arterial pressure and pulmonary vascular resistance were normal in five men who were lifelong residents at $\geq$ 3600 m (27). It was suggested that immigrants from lowlands to high altitude may be more likely to react to chronic hypoxia than lifelong residents. High altitude has not yet been explored as a potential risk factor for PPH.

C. Pregnancy and Primary Pulmonary Hypertension

Pregnancy and labor increase the demand on the heart–pulmonary system. Cardiac output and blood values increase by approximately 40% by the 20th–24th week of pregnancy, and oxygen consumption increases by 20% during pregnancy (28). To adapt to those changes, pregnant women develop a low pulmonary vascular resistance and less pulmonary vasoconstriction in response to hypoxia. Although serial and sporadic cases have been reported on a coexistence between PPH and pregnancy, the association is unclear. Pregnancy has not been identified as a risk factor for PPH, nor as a promoting factor that would make asymptomatic PPH become symptomatic. Dawkins et al. observed that in 6 of 73 women patients with PPH who were of childbearing age and who were waiting for heart–lung transplants, the disorder appeared to be associated with their pregnancies (29). The time of onset was heterogeneous: a few days before delivery (4 cases), to the second trimester of pregnancy (1 case), and 3 months after birth (1 case). Because of the insidious nature and clinical presentation of PPH, it is not known with certainty that the temporal sequence between pregnancy and the onset of PPH is consistent. Other causes of pulmonary hypertension may also be associated with pregnancy, such as trophoblastic embolism, thromboembolic pulmonary hypertension, and Eisenmeger's syndrome, which could be misdiagnosed as PPH. The role of pregnancy, if any, is expected to be very small, since only 5–8% of PPH cases were combined with pregnancy (30).

D. Comorbidity

Human Immunodeficiency Virus Infection and AIDS-Related Pulmonary Hypertension

More than 30 cases of HIV or acquired immunodeficiency syndrome (AIDS) patients with PPH have now been reported worldwide (31–39). In a series of 33 cases of PPH with AIDS or HIV infection, almost all were men; fewer than one-third were intravenous drug users; and half had a plexogenic lesion (32). The probability of noninfectious cardiopulmonary manifestations, such as cardiomyopathy, pericardial and pleural effusion, pulmonary thromboembolism, and cor pulmonale, as well as other conditions believed to be associated with PPH (cirrhosis and portal hypertension), were ruled out in all reported cases. The causal association between HIV infection or AIDS with PPH is not well established. Although Rudolf et al. reported that, among 1200 HIV-positive subjects, 0.5% of them had PPH diagnosed (39), very few studies have clearly documented the HIV infection really preceded the occurrence of PPH. Although direct damage to the vascular endothelium by the virus was not demonstrated, HIV-induced immunological response was suggested to be responsible for PPH (33). It has also been suggested that intravenous drug users, who have been reported to constitute a great part of the HIV-infected population, had an increased chance of having an embolism in the small pulmonary arteries caused by a foreign body (39). The hypotheses of direct or indirect HIV infection are worth further investigation. In one study, five patients, with classic hemophilia who had more than a 10-year history of self-administered lyophilized concentrates of factor VIII, had PPH diagnosed. It was suggested that exposure to factor VIII might be used as an alternative explanation for PPH (40).

Portal Hypertension

The association between portal hypertension and PPH has been postulated and debated for more than 40 years since it was first proposed in 1951 (41). McDonnell et al. reviewed 17,901 autopsy records between 1944 and 1981 in one hospital setting (42). Among them, 24 cases of PPH (0.13%) were identified. Also, 1241 cases of cirrhosis were examined and 9 PPH cases (0.73%) were pathologically diagnosed. The difference in prevalence of PPH between the autopsy and cirrhosis population was considered statistically significant. To reduce the possibility that PPH may make the patient predisposed to cirrhosis, patients with cardiac cirrhosis were excluded from the case series, leaving only alcoholic cirrhosis, postnecrotic cirrhosis, and chronic active hepatitis with cirrhosis. Of the 2459 cases of cirrhosis diagnosed by biopsy during a 20-year period, 15 cases of PPH were diagnosed (0.61%), which was very close to the proportion in an autopsy population. Despite the high prevalence of cirrhosis in males of all age groups, a preponderance of females with PPH did exist, with a female to male ratio of 2:1. Thus, the co-existence of cirrhosis and PPH was considered not likely to be due to chance. Robalino and Moodie (43) reviewed 78 cases of PPH combined with portal hypertension and found that the time interval between the onset of portal and pulmonary hypertension in 52 patients was 5.7 years (± 4.8). The mean survival time was only about 1 year, much shorter than patients with PPH only, which was about 2–3 years. No gender preponderance was noted in this study. Hadengue et al. (44) reported 10 cases of PPH among 507 patients hospitalized with portal hypertension. In their study, patients with PPH who had clinical signs of portacaval shunt showed a significantly shorter interval between the diagnosis of portal and pulmonary hypertension than did patients without the shunt (12.3 years versus 3.7 years). Although many hypotheses were put forward to explain the association between portal hypertension and PPH, such as thromboembolism or pulmonary vasoconstriction caused by vasoactive substances (43–46), there is no evidence of a causal association because the autopsy population and case series are highly selected populations.

Antinuclear Antibodies and Primary Pulmonary Hypertension

It has been suggested that autoimmune connective tissue disease could be associated with PPH because Raynaud's phenomenon and serum antinuclear antibodies (ANA) were frequently seen in PPH patients. The pulmonary vascular lesions were similar to those observed in certain connective tissue diseases, especially scleroderma. Isern et al. (47) reported that anti-Ku titers were significantly elevated in 31 cases of PPH, compared with 24 cases of secondary pulmonary hypertension. Rich et al. reported that 40% of PPH patients had positive ANA titers, compared with only 6% in secondary pulmonary hypertension patients, the latter figure representing that of the normal population (48).

E. Drugs

The identification of drug-related risk poses a great challenge to both the physician and the epidemiologist. The temporality between exposure to a given drug and the onset of the disease must be demonstrated (49). In a disease such as PPH, for which there may be a long period between the onset of the first symptoms and the diagnosis, it is very difficult to ascertain that exposure to suspected drugs occurred before the onset of the symptoms (4,50). Furthermore, because the diagnosis of PPH is one of exclusion and there are no objective criteria, it is possible that a patient may be classified as secondary pulmonary hypertension because of exposure to a suspected drug.

Anorectic Agents

Aminorex

A dramatic increase in the number of diagnoses of PPH was first noted in a Swiss medical clinic in 1967, which rose from 0.87% to 13.5% of adults who underwent cardiac catherization. There were no apparent changes in either size or composition of the population, nor of diagnostic procedures. About half of the patients were more or less overweight, with a female preponderance. Afterward, 582 cases were identified in a study conducted in Germany, Switzerland, and Austria, among which 68% had claimed they had used the drug aminorex, either alone or in combination with other anorectic agents. The overall incidence of developing PPH in patients who used aminorex was estimated to be about 1–2% (51–53). In a cohort of 731 patients known to have taken aminorex and who were covered by a single health insurance company, 3% developed PPH (54). The number of cases varied geographically, consistent with the marketing, and temporally with the intake of aminorex. The clinical manifestations, hemodynamic measures, and pathological changes were reported to be indistinguishable from those of PPH. Survival rate at 5 years was 75%, and at 10 years it was 44%, which is much better than figures obtained in the NIH registry (34% at 5 years) (3). Despite that a dose–response effect between aminorex intake and severity of pulmonary hypertension has not been established, and that the evidence has not been substantiated by an animal model, it is widely accepted that the epidemic of pulmonary hypertension was due to aminorex.

Chlorphetermine and Phenmetrazine

Chlorphentermine and phenmetrazine were suggested to contribute to the development of pulmonary hypertension, but no report has been issued on humans since 1972 (55).

Fenfluramine

Fenfluramine (DL-fenfluramine, dexfenfluramine), a phenylethylamine derivative, has been widely prescribed as an anorectic drug since the early 1960s. Until now, all reported cases of PPH with a history of fenfluramine intake were women, from 20 to 58 years old. The length of time between exposure to fenfluramine or its derivatives until the presentation of early symptoms of pulmonary hypertension, such as dyspnea on exertion, or to hospital admission, varied from 3 months to 8 years (56–59). For some patients, the condition resolved completely after withdrawal of the drug (57), although reversibility is debatable (58,60). Brenot et al. (59) followed a group of 73 PPH patients and found that about 25% of them had been exposed to fenfluramine. The relation between fenfluramine and PPH is still unclear, as it has been documented only in case reports. Further investigations are required to confirm temporality between drug intake and disease occurrence, as well as the control of potential biases (4).

Nonsteroidal Anti-inflammatory Drugs

Indomethacin

Indomethacin is used to treat premature labor and polyhydramnios. It has been reported that the risk of PPH in the newborn may be increased after prolonged therapy (61). In a randomized clinical trial, Besigner et al. found three cases of PPH in newborns whose mothers received indomethacin treatment for intact membranes in preterm labor (62). Subsequently, Dalens et al. found that five premature newborns, whose mothers had received indomethacin, had clinical and biological symptoms similar to those of pulmonary hypertension (63). In two of the cases, autopsy showed an important reduction of the lumen of pulmonary artery owing to a thickening of the tunica media. Findings found in the literature are inconsistent (64–66). These results should be interpreted with caution, as the diagnosis of PPH in the newborn is difficult to make because anatomical abnormalities have to be considered.

Naproxen

Naproxen can be used to delay parturition by inhibiting prostaglandin synthesis. Persistent pulmonary hypertension has been noted in three newborns whose mothers had a history of exposure to naproxen, which was associated with very low plasma concentration of prostaglandin (67).

Chemotherapy-Related Drugs

Mitomycin-C

Mitomycin-C is used in chemotherapy for malignant tumors. Pulmonary veno-occlusive disease, which involves about 8% of the PPH cases in the NIH registry, occurred in patients with metastatic cervical carcinoma, or with metastatic gastric adenocarcinoma after treatment with mitomycin-C (68,69).

Carmustine, Etoposide, and Cyclophosphamide

Pulmonary veno-occlusive disease was reported in two children suffering from acute lymphoblastic leukemia treated with marrow allograft transplant, followed by high doses of carmustine [*N*,*N*-bis(2-chloroethyl)−*N*-nitrosourea; BCNU], etoposide, and cyclophosphamide. Open-lung biopsy demonstrated pulmonary veno-occlusive disease (70).

Phenformin

Phenformin has been used to treat diabetes mellitus and was reported to be associated with severe lactic acidosis, which could induce pulmonary vasoconstriction in animal experiments. Two cases of pulmonary hypertension, believed to be associated with treatment with phenformin, have been reported (71). These two patients, without any sign of pulmonary hypertension at treatment initiation, came to medical attention after 1 and 3 years administration of phenformin, respectively. Improvement of right-sided heart failure was observed after the withdrawal of phenformin, and proliferative changes, consistent with PPH, were found in the lung vessels at necropsy.

Oral Contraceptives

Kleiger et al. (72) reported six cases of pulmonary hypertension in women with a history of oral contraceptive use. In three of them PPH was diagnosed after they had been exposed to oral contraceptives for about 5 years. There was no evidence of thromboembolism in the lungs or the veins of the leg. However, because oral contraceptives are used frequently in the population, further research is needed to rule out a coincidental association. On the other hand, the high proportion of females among PPH cases is worth further consideration to assess the potential role of oral contraceptives in the development of PPH (73).

F. Herb Toxins

In rats, monocrotaline, a pyrolizidine alkaloid found in a plant called *Crotalaria*, and fulvine found in *Crotalaria fulva*, have induced pulmonary hypertension and right-sided heart failure (74). Bush tea is made with extracts from seeds and leaves from these plants. The occurrence of pulmonary hypertension, originating from pulmonary venous occlusion after the ingestion of bush tea, has been implicated in the pathogenesis of PPH (75).

G. L-Tryptophan

L-Tryptophan is a food supplement used for ailments such as premenstrual syndrome, insomnia, depression, and drug detoxification. Since 1989, it has been etiologically linked with a newly recognized disease, eosinophilia-myalgia syndrome (EMS). More than 1500 cases of EMS have been reported in the United States, and the number of cases has been estimated to be as high as 5000. Of the reported cases, 83% were women, and 94% were non-Hispanic whites, with a median age of 48 years, which data are believed to reflect the pattern of L-tryptophan users, rather than potential risk factors. In its serious, multisystemic, and progressive course, many cases of EMS presented with cough and dyspnea, interstitial infiltrates, and pleural effusion. Pulmonary involvements consisted of eosinophilic and vasculitis syndromes, interstitial lung disease, and pulmonary hypertension (76,77,80). Few cases have been reported with pulmonary hypertension (77,78). Biopsy specimens showed vasculitis and perivasculitis to be associated with a mild chronic interstitial pneumonitis and eosinophilia (79,80). Considering multisystemic manifestations of EMS and its linkage with L-tryptophan consumption, pulmonary hypertension related to the intake of L-tryptophan should be considered as a separate item in the definition criteria of pulmonary hypertension.

H. Contaminated Rapeseed Oil

Although not recognized as primary pulmonary hypertension per se, the "toxic oil syndrome" is an interesting example of the relations between exposure to chemicals and pulmonary hypertension. The occurrence of a multisystemic disease, first recognized as a typical pneumonia, according to pulmonary symptoms and interstitial infiltrates on chest roentgenograms, suddenly increased in Spain in early 1981. The failure of patients to respond to antibiotic therapy, the clustering of the disease within families, without any evidence of a pathogenic agent, and the lack of cases among infants, were factors that favored the suggestion of a potential exposure to a toxic agent. These findings were evidence that the consumption of rapeseed oil was the responsible agent or the vehicle for the epidemic (81–83). Hypotheses were made that the oil was contaminated. A World Health Organization Expert Committee (81) defined the condition as the toxic oil syndrome (TOS). A total of 20,688 cases were officially registered; among them, 835 have died. Exposure to toxic oil was loosely defined as the consumption of oil, presumed to be toxic, before the onset of the disease or the occurrence of the disease within the nuclear family, or an epidemic outbreak in the community. Pulmonary hypertension was found in about 20% of hospitalized patients at the second to fourth month since the onset of the disease (85). Alonso-Ruiz et al. (86) followed 332 cases of TOS for up to 8 years and found that 8.1% of them developed pulmonary hypertension; the condition regressed in 74% of them, and only 2% developed a malignant form of pulmonary hypertension at the end of a follow-up period of 8 years. It was estimated that pulmonary hypertension accounted for about 1.6% of all deaths caused by toxic oil. In a group of 40 cases of severe pulmonary hypertension due to TOS, aged from 8 to 58 years old and a female to male ratio of 4:1, 83% died within 6 years of follow-up (84). Pathological changes in pulmonary arteries were characterized by medial hypertrophy, intimal fibrosis, and plexiform lesions.

V. Conclusion

In the literature, several factors have been suggested to be associated with PPH. These can be divided into etiologic factors and risk factors. So far, strong evidence supports the etiologic role of only aminorex. The toxic oil syndrome is considered as a different entity. Other risk factors, such as HIV infection and portal hypertension, are documented, and most evidence comes from case series. The preponderance of young females among reported cases may reflect a physiological predisposition of this group to develop PPH, or a higher exposure to an initiation or promoting factor. Other risk factors, such as pregnancy and anorectic agents, remain to be established. In view of the lack of evidence about the role of these suspected factors there is a strong demand for epidemiological investigations.

References

1. Hatano S, Strasser T, eds. Primary pulmonary hypertension: Report on a WHO meeting. Geneva: World Health Organization, 1973.
2. Rubin LJ. ACCP consensus statement: primary pulmonary hypertension. Chest 1993; 104:236–250.
3. Rich S, et al. Primary pulmonary hypertension: a national prospective study. Ann Intern Med 1987; 107:216–223.
4. The International Primary Pulmonary Hypertension Study Group. The international primary pulmonary hypertension study (IPPHS). Chest 1994; 105(suppl):37S–41S.
5. Olivari MT. Southwestern internal medicine conference: Primary Pulmonary Hypertension. Am J Med Sci 1991; 302:185–198
6. Goodale F, Thomas WA. Primary pulmonary arterial disease, observations with special reference to medical thickening of small arteries and arterioles. Arch Pathol 1954; 58:568.
7. Wood P. Pulmonary hypertension. In: Wood P, ed. Diseases of the Heart and Circulation. 3rd ed. London: Eyre & Spottiswoode, 1968:976.

8. Kanemoto N. Natural history of pulmonary hemodynamics in primary pulmonary hypertension. Am Heart J 1987; 114:407–413.
9. Oakley CW. Primary pulmonary hypertension: case series from the United Kingdom. Chest 1994; 105(suppl):29S–32S.
10. Brenot F. Primary pulmonary hypertension: case series from France. Chest 1994; 105(suppl):33S–36S.
11. Gilbert E, et al. Survival in patients with primary pulmonary hypertension: results from a national prospective registry. Ann Intern Med; 1991:343–349.
12. David RD. Primary pulmonary hypertension: the American experience. Chest 1994; 105(suppl):26S–28S.
13. Houde C, et al. Profile of pediatric patients with pulmonary hypertension judged by responsiveness to vasodilator. Br Heart J 1993; 70:461–468.
14. Rozkovec A, et al. Factors that influence the outcome of primary pulmonary hypertension. Br Heart J 1986; 55:449–458.
15. Sidney S, et al. Primary pulmonary hypertension in the elderly. Arch Intern Med 1991; 151:2433–2438.
16. Rothman KJ. Modern Epidemiology. Boston: Little Brown & Company, 1986.
17. Kleinbaum DG, Kupper LL, Morgenstern H. Epidemiologic Research: Principles and Quantitative Methods. New York: Van Nostrand Reinhold, 1982.
18. Langleben D. Familial primary pulmonary hypertension. Chest 1994; 105(suppl): 13S–16S.
19. Loyd JE, Primm RK, Newman JH. Familial primary pulmonary hypertension: clinical patterns. Am Rev Respir Dis 1984; 129:194–197.
20. Langleben D, et al. Familial pulmonary capillary hemangiomatosis resulting in primary pulmonary hypertension. Ann Intern Med 1988; 109:106–109.
21. Rich S, Hart K. Familial pulmonary hypertension associated with an abnormal hemoglobin: insights into the pathogenesis of primary pulmonary hypertension. Chest 1991; 99:1208–1210.
22. Devathasan G, et al. Complications of chronic glue (toluene) abuse in adolescents. Aust NZ J Med 1984; 14:39–43.
23. Schaiberger PH, et al. Pulmonary hypertension associated with long-term inhalation of "crank" methamphetamine. Chest 1993; 104:614–616.
24. Russell LA, et al. Pulmonary hypertension in female crack users. Am Rev Respir Dis 1992; 145:A717.
25. Collins E, Hardwick H, Jeffery H. Perinatal cocaine intoxication. Med J Aust 1989; 150:331–332.
26. Sharma S. Clinical, biochemical, electrocardiographic and noninvasive hemodynamic assessment of cardiovascular status in natives at high to extreme altitudes (3000 m–5000 m) of the Himalaya region. Indian Heart J 1990 42:375–379.
27. Groves BM, et al. Minimal hypoxic pulmonary hypertension in normal Tibetans at 3,658 m. J Appl Physiol 1993; 74:312–318.
28. Roberts NV, Keast PJ. Pulmonary hypertension and pregnancy—a lethal combination. Anaesth Intensive Care 1990; 18:366–374.
29. Dawkins KD, Burke CM, Billingham ME, et al. Primary pulmonary hypertension and pregnancy. Chest 1986; 89:383–388.

30. Wagenwoort CA, Wagenvoort N. Primary pulmonary hypertension: a pathologic study of lung vessels in 156 clinically diagnosed cases. Circulation 1970; 42:1163–1184.
31. Mani S, Smith W. HIV and pulmonary hypertension: a review. South Med J 1994; 87:357–362.
32. Martos A, Carratala J, Cabellow C, et al. AIDS and primary pulmonary hypertension (letter). Am Heart J 1993; 125:1819.
33. Diaz PT, Clanton TL. Marker pulmonary function abnormalities in a case of HIV-associated pulmonary hypertension. Chest 1993; 104:313–315.
34. Legoux B, Piette AM, Bouchet PE, et al. Pulmonary hypertension and HIV infection. Am J Med 1990; 89:122.
35. Polos PG, Wolfe D, Harley RA, et al. Pulmonary hypertension and human immunodeficiency virus infection: two reports and a review of the literature. Chest 1992; 101: 474–478.
36. Wright EJ, et al. Review of 33 HIV positive patients referred to cardiac assessment. Int Conf AIDS 1992; 8:85.
37. Rafi I, et al. Factor associated with death in a cohort of HIV positive women in Washington DC. Int Conf AIDS 1992; 8:182.
38. Schulman S, Johnson H. Beneficial effect of an ultrapure factor VIII concentrate on hypergammaglobulinemia in HIV-positive hemophiliacs. Int Conf AIDS 1989; 5:416.
39. Rudolf S, Jenni R, Opracil M, et al. Primary pulmonary hypertension in HIV infection. Chest 1991; 100:1265–1271.
40. Goldsmith GH, Baily RG, Brettler DB, et al. Primary pulmonary hypertension in patients with classic hemophilia. Ann Intern Med 1988; 108:797–799.
41. Mantz FA Jr, Craige E. Portal axis thrombosis with spontaneous portacaval shunt and resultant cor pulmonale. Arch Pathol 1951; 52:91–97.
42. McDonnell PJ, Toye PA, Hutchins GM. Primary pulmonary hypertension and cirrhosis: are they related? Am Rev Respir Dis 1983; 127:437–441.
43. Robalino BR, Moodie DO. Associated between primary pulmonary hypertension and portal hypertension: analysis of its pathophysiology and clinical, laboratory and hemodynamic manifestations. J Am Coll Cardiol 1991; 17:492–498.
44. Hadengue A, Benhayoun MK, Lebrec D, et al. Pulmonary hypertension complicating portal hypertension: prevalence and relation to splanchnic hemodynamics. Gastroenterology 1991; 100:520–528.
45. Levine OR, Newark NJ, Harris RC, et al. Progressive hypertension in children with portal hypertension. J Pediatr 1973; 83:964–972.
46. Haworth SG, Hislop A, Reid L. Progressive pulmonary hypertension in children with portal hypertension. J Pediatr 1974; 84:783–785.
47. Isern RA, Yaneva M, Weiner E, et al. Autoantibodies in patients with primary pulmonary hypertension: association with anti-Ku. Am J Med 1992; 93:307–312.
48. Rich S, Kieras K, Hart K. Antinuclear antibodies in primary pulmonary hypertension. J Am Coll Cardiol 1986; 8:1307–11.
49. Sackett DL. The diagnosis of causation. In: Gent M, Shigematsu, eds. Epidemiological Issues in Reported Drug-Induced Illnesses—S.M.O.N. and Other Examples. Hamilton, Ontario; McMaster University Library Press, 1976:106–113.
50. Miettinen O, Slone D, Shapiro S. Current problems in drug-related epidemiologic

research. In: Colombo F, Shapiro S, Slone D, et al., eds. Epidemiological Evaluation of Drugs. Littleton, MA: PSG Publishing, 1977:295–307.
51. Gurtner HP. Aminorex and pulmonary hypertension. Cor Vasa 1985; 27:160–171.
52. Follath F, Burrart F, Schweizer W. Drug-induced pulmonary hypertension? Br Med J 1971; 1:265–266.
53. Kay JM, Smith P, Heath D. Aminorex and the pulmonary circulation. Thorax 1971; 26:262–269.
54. Loogen F, Worth H, Schwan G, et al. Long-term follow-up of pulmonary hypertension in patients with and without anorectic drug intake. Cor Vasa 1985; 27:111–124.
55. Mlczoch J. Drug and dietary induced pulmonary hypertension In: Weir KE, Reeves JT, eds. Pulmonary Hypertension. Mount Kisco, NY: Futura Publishing, 1981: 341–359.
56. Douglas JG, Munro JF, Kitchin AH, et al. Pulmonary hypertension and fenfluramine. Br Med J 1981; 283:881–883.
57. Pouwels HM, Smeets JL, Cheriex EC, et al. Pulmonary hypertension and fenfluramine. Eur Respir J 1990; 3:606–607.
58. McMurray J, Bloomfield P, Miller HC. Irreversible pulmonary hypertension after treatment with fenfluramine (letter). Br Med J 1986; 293:51–52.
59. Brenot F, Herve P, Petitpretz P, et al. Primary pulmonary hypertension and fenfluramine use. Br Heart J 1993; 70:537–541.
60. Watters K, Le Ridant A. Irreversible pulmonary hypertension after treatment with fenfluramine (letter). Br Med J 1986; 292:1137.
61. Niebyl JR. Drug therapy during pregnancy. Curr Opin Obstet Gynecol 1992; 4:43–47.
62. Besinger RE, Niebyl JR, Keyes WG, et al. Randomized comparative trial of indomethacin and ritodrine for the long-term treatment of preterm labor. Am J Obstet Gynecol 1991; 164:981–986.
63. Dalens B, Dechelotte P, Gaulme J, et al. Maternal treatment with indomethacin and severe neonatal pulmonary hypertension. Arch Fr Pediatr 1981; 38:261–265.
64. Niebyl JR, Blake DA, White RD, et al. The inhibition of premature labor with indomethacin. Am J Obstet Gynecol 1980; 136:1014–1091.
65. Zuckerman H, Shalev E, Gilad G. Further study of the inhibition of premature labor by indomethacin. J Perinat Med 1984; 12:25–29.
66. Morales WJ, Smith SG, Angel JL, et al. Efficacy and safety of indomethacin versus ritodrine in the management of preterm labor: a randomized study. Obstet Gynecol 1989; 74:567–572.
67. Wilkinson AR, Aynsley-Green A, Mitchell MD. Persistent pulmonary hypertension and abnormal prostaglandin E levels in preterm infants after maternal treatment with naproxen. Arch Dis Child 1979; 54:942–945.
68. Joselson R, Warnock M. Pulmonary veno-occlusive disease after chemotherapy. Hum Pathol 1983; 14:88–91.
69. Waldhorn RE, Tsou E, Smith FP, et al. Pulmonary veno-occlusive disease associated with microangiopathic hemolytic anemia and chemotherapy of gastric adenocarcinoma. Med Pediatr Oncol 1984; 12:394–396.
70. Hackman RC, Madtes OK, Petersen FB, et al. Pulmonary venoocclusive disease following bone marrow transplantation. Transplantation 1989; 47:989–992.

71. Fahlen M, Bergman H, Helder G, et al. Phenformin and pulmonary hypertension. Br Heart J 1973; 35:824–828.
72. Kleiger RE, Boxer M, Ingham RE, et al. Pulmonary hypertension in patients using oral contraceptives: a report of six cases. Chest 1976; 69:143–147.
73. Masi AT. Pulmonary hypertension and oral contraceptive usage. Chest 1976; 69: 451–453.
74. Fishman AP. Dietary pulmonary hypertension. Circ Res 1974; 35:657–660.
75. Olivari MT. Southwestern internal medicine conference: Primary pulmonary hypertension. Am J Med Sci 1991; 302:185–198.
76. Philen RM, Posada M. Toxic oil syndrome and eosinophilia-myalgia syndrome: May 8–10, 1991, World Health Organization Meeting Report. Semin Arthritis Rheum 1993; 23:104–124.
77. Tazelaar HD, Myerd JL, Drage CW, et al. Pulmonary disease associated with L-tryptophan-induced eosinophilic myalgia syndrome: clinical and pathologic features. Chest 1990; 97:1032–1036.
78. Campagna AC, Blanc PD, Criswell LA, et al. Pulmonary manifestations of the eosinophilia-myalgia syndrome associated with tryptophan ingestion. Chest 1992; 101:1274–1281.
79. Sack KE, Criswell LA. Eosinophilia-myalgia syndrome: the aftermath. South Med J 1992; 85:878–882.
80. Criswell LA, Sack KE. Tryptophan-induced eosinophilia-myalgia syndrome. West J Med 1990; 153:269–274.
81. Philen RM, Posada M. Toxic oil syndrome and eosinophilia-myalgia syndrome: May 8–10, 1991, World Health Organization Meeting Report. Semin Arthritis Rheum 1993; 23:104–124.
82. Diaz de Rojas F, Castro Garcia M, Abaitus Bordal, et al. The association of oil ingestion with toxic-oil syndrome in two convents. Am J Epidemiol 1987; 125:907–911.
83. Rigau-Perez JG, Perez-Alvarez L, Duenas-Castro S, et al. Epidemiologic investigation of an oil-associated pneumonic paralytic eosinophilic syndrome in Spain. Am J Epidemiol 1984; 119:250–260.
84. Gomez-Sanchez MA, Mestre de Juan MJ, Gomez-Pajuelo C, et al. Pulmonary hypertension due to toxic oil syndrome: a clinicopathologic study. Chest 1989; 95:325–331.
85. Castro Garcia M, Posada de la Paz F, Diaz de Rojas F, et al. Pulmonary hypertension after toxic rapeseed oil ingestion. J Am Coll Cardiol 1984; 4:443.
86. Alonso-Ruiz A, Calabozo M, Perez-Ruiz F, et al. Toxic oil syndrome: a long-term follow-up of a cohort of 332 patients. Medicine 1993; 72:285–295.

8

Primary Pulmonary Hypertension in Children

ROBYN J. BARST

Columbia University
College of Physicians and Surgeons
New York, New York

I. Introduction

Primary pulmonary hypertension is characterized by progressive elevation of pulmonary artery pressure, which eventually leads to right ventricular failure and death. Although the histopathology in children with primary pulmonary hypertension is often the same as that seen with adult patients, the clinical presentation, natural history, and factors influencing survival may differ. These differences appear to be most apparent in the youngest children. Before the era of vasodilator treatment, most children died within 1 year of diagnosis (1), as opposed to a 2- to 3-year median survival in adult primary pulmonary hypertension patients (2).

Adults with primary pulmonary hypertension often have severe plexiform lesions and fixed pulmonary vascular changes. On the other hand, pathological studies show greater pulmonary vascular medial hypertrophy and less intimal fibrosis and fewer plexiform lesions in younger patients with primary pulmonary hypertension (3). In the classic studies by Wagenvoort and Wagenvoort in 1970, medial hypertrophy was severe in patients younger than 15 years of age, and it was usually the only change in young infants. Among the 11 patients younger than 1 year of age, all with severe medial hypertrophy, 2 had only minimal and a third had moderate intimal fibrosis. With increasing age, intimal fibrosis and plexiform lesions were seen more frequently. These postmortem studies suggest that pulmonary vasoconstriction, leading to medial hypertrophy, occurs early in the course of the disease and precedes the development of plexiform lesions and fixed pulmonary vascular changes. These observations by Wagenvoort and Wagenvoort may offer clues to the observed differences in the natural history and factors influencing survival in children with primary pulmonary hypertension compared with adult patients. In general, younger children appear to have a more reactive pulmonary vascular bed relative to both active vasodilatation and vasoconstriction, with severe acute pulmonary hypertensive crises occurring in response to pulmonary vasoconstrictor triggers more often than in older children or adults.

II. Definition

Primary pulmonary hypertension (PPH), in children, as in adults, continues to be referred to as unexplained or idiopathic pulmonary hypertension, as the disease was first described by Romberg in 1891. The definition for primary pulmonary hypertension in children is the same as for adult patients: the presence of pulmonary hypertension (mean pulmonary artery pressure greater than 25 mmHg at rest, or greater than 30 mmHg during exercise), with a normal pulmonary artery wedge pressure and the absence of secondary causes. The inclusion of exercise hemodynamic abnormalities in the definition of PPH is important, since children with PPH often have an exaggerated response of the pulmonary vascular bed to exercise, compared with their adult counterparts. We have seen children with a history of recurrent exertional syncope who have a resting mean pulmonary artery pressure of approximately 25 mmHg, but demonstrate marked increases in their pulmonary artery pressure with exercise.

The workup in children to exclude secondary causes of pulmonary hypertension is similar to adult patients, although there are several differences (Table 1). There appears to be age dependency in the degree of the vascular response to hypoxia, with hypoxic pulmonary vasoconstriction more profound in infants than in adults (4,5). Variability in pulmonary vascular reactivity among individuals of the same age in response to hypoxia appears similar to the variability seen in response to various other pulmonary vasoconstrictor triggers (6–8).

Although the physiology of persistent fetal circulation resembles primary pulmonary hypertension (9), differences between the two entities suggest that primary pulmonary hypertension and persistent fetal circulation are two separate disorders. Persistent fetal circulation is almost always transient (10), with infants either recovering completely without chronic vasodilator therapy or dying during the neonatal period, despite maximal cardiopulmonary therapeutic interventions. In contrast, patients with primary pulmonary hypertension who respond to vasodilator therapy appear to need treatment indefinitely to maintain improved pulmonary hemodynamics (11). Persistent fetal circulation occurs when there is

Table 1 Causes of Pulmonary Hypertension

- Heart disease
  - Hyperkinetic pulmonary arterial hypertension—systemic to pulmonary communications with increased pulmonary blood flow
  - Pulmonary venous hypertension—disease of left heart obstruction or dysfunction
- Lung disease—hypoxia
  - Parenchymal lung disease
    - —Obstructive, i.e., cystic fibrosis
    - —Restrictive, i.e., interstitial pneumonitis
  - Upper airway obstruction
  - Diminished ventilatory drive, i.e., Ondine's curse
  - Congenital anomalies
  - Hypoxia-induced, i.e., high-altitude
  - Disorders of the chest wall, i.e., kyphoscoliosis
- Thromboembolic disease—pulmonary vascular obstruction
  - Pulmonary thromboembolism
  - Hemoglobinopathies, i.e., sickle cell disease
  - Mediastinal tumors or fibrosis
  - Ova emboli, i.e., schistosomiasis
  - Foreign bodies, i.e., talc
  - Ventriculovenous shunts for hydrocephalus
  - Tumor emboli
  - Sepsis and/or dehydration
  - Right-sided endocarditis
  - Right atrial myxoma
- Collagen vascular and granulomatous diseases
  - Scleroderma
  - Systemic lupus erythematosus
  - Mixed connective tissue disease
  - Rheumatoid arthritis
  - Sarcoidosis
- Exogenous substances
  - Anorexic agents
  - Toxic rapeseed oil
  - Psychotropic drugs, i.e., L-tryptophan, crack cocaine
- HIV infection
- Portal hypertension
  - Portal vein thrombosis
  - Liver disease
- Primary pulmonary hypertension
  - Pulmonary arteriopathy
  - Pulmonary veno-occlusive disease

hypoplasia of the lung and pulmonary vascular bed, maladaptation of the pulmonary vascular bed postnatally as a result of perinatal stress, and maladaptation of the pulmonary vascular bed in utero from unknown causes. Some infants with persistent fetal circulation may have a genetic predisposition to hyperreact to pulmonary vasoconstrictive triggers, such as alveolar hypoxia. It is possible that the pulmonary vascular resistance may not fall normally after birth in some infants, who never had a diagnosis of persistent fetal circulation, but subsequently, primary pulmonary hypertension was diagnosed as progressive pulmonary vascular disease developed. Pathological studies examining the elastic pattern of the main pulmonary artery (12,13) also suggest that primary pulmonary hypertension is present from birth in some patients, but is acquired later in life in others. Despite the questions that remain about the similarities and differences between persistent fetal circulation and PPH in children, this chapter will focus on primary pulmonary hypertension diagnosed after the neonatal period, since the natural history of these two disorders is quite different.

By definition, neither congenital heart disease nor acquired disease of the left side of the heart can be the initiating mechanism for the vasculopathy in primary pulmonary hypertension. On occasion, one may find small anatomical congenital heart defects, such as a small patent ductus arteriosus or ventricular septal defect, associated with severe pulmonary hypertension (apparently out of proportion to the congenital heart defect), or severe pulmonary hypertension in infancy associated with a congenital heart defect that is not known to cause pulmonary vascular obstructive disease until much later in life, such as an atrial septal defect. Whether these represent two distinct phenomena, or a genetic predisposition to the development of pulmonary hypertension with a hemodynamically insignificant congenital heart defect, remains uncertain (14–16). The pulmonary vascular disease from congenital heart disease usually follows a period of decreased pulmonary resistance and high pulmonary flow, but may occur in patients who never manifested a large left-to-right shunt, suggesting that the pulmonary hypertension in these children may be primary, rather than secondary, to congenital heart disease. Support for this comes from the observation of severe pulmonary hypertension in an eight-year-old child, following repair of partial anomalous pulmonary venous return and a sinus venosus atrial septal defect at 6 years of age, whose mother had primary pulmonary hypertension (17), and in another child following repair of a small secundum atrial septal defect at 4 years of age, with severe pulmonary hypertension at 10 years, whose mother also had primary pulmonary hypertension (personal communication).

III. Epidemiology

The frequency of primary pulmonary hypertension in children as well as in adults remains unknown. Although the disease certainly is rare, increasingly frequent

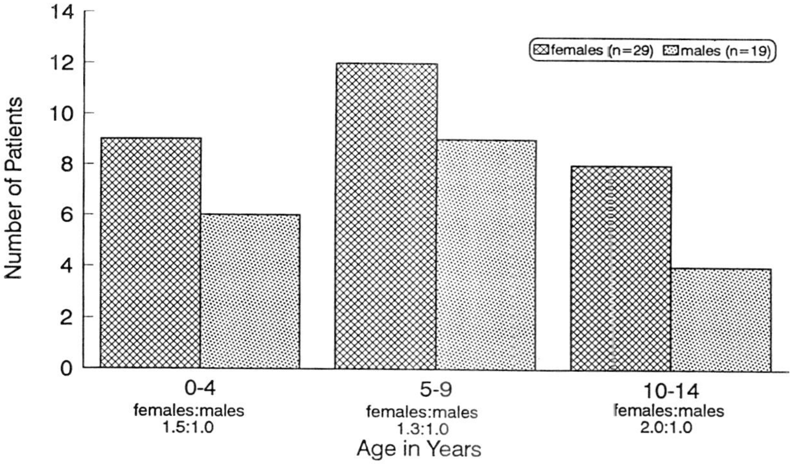

Figure 1 Distribution of children with primary pulmonary hypertension by age at the onset of symptoms. Similar to the sex incidence in adult patients, girls are affected more frequently throughout childhood.

reports of confirmed cases suggest that more patients (children and adults) have primary pulmonary hypertension than has previously been recognized. On occasion, dead infants have had the diagnosis of sudden infant death syndrome, when postmortem examination confirms a diagnosis of primary pulmonary hypertension. The sex incidence in adult patients with primary pulmonary hypertension is 1.7:1 women to men. In children, the sex incidence has been reported to vary between equal frequency before adolescence, to an increased frequency in girls to boys of approximately 1.5:1. In our experience with 48 children in whom primary pulmonary hypertension diagnosed before 15 years of age, we found a 1.5:1 female to male ratio, with no significant difference in the ratio in the younger children, compared with the older children (Fig. 1). The incidence of familial primary pulmonary hypertension is approximately 6% (18). The mode of genetic transmission appears to be autosomal dominant, with incomplete penetrance (19,20). With familial primary pulmonary hypertension, the disease presents in subsequent generations at younger ages (genetic anticipation; 19,20).

IV. Pathogenesis and Pathophysiology

A. Endothelial Dysfunction

The pathogenesis of primary pulmonary hypertension in children remains speculative (Fig. 2). The most widely proposed mechanism for PPH, pulmonary vasoconstriction, is based on histopathological studies and clinical responses to

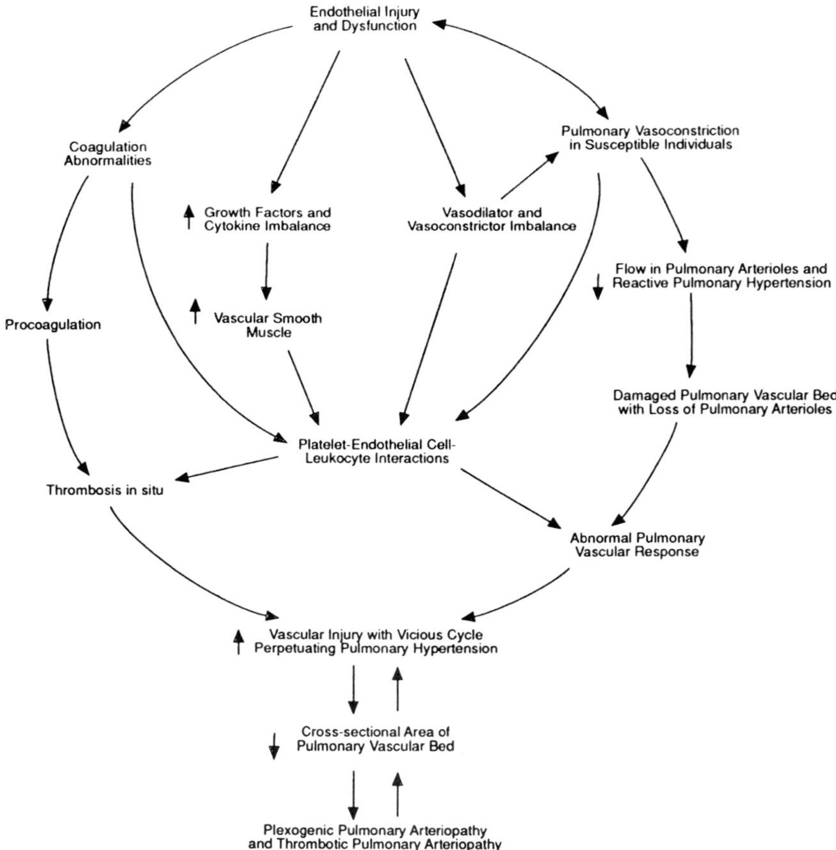

Figure 2 Possible pathogenesis of primary pulmonary hypertension.

vasodilator therapy (3,21–25). These studies suggest that PPH is a disease of predisposed individuals, in whom various stimuli may initiate the development of the characteristic vascular lesions. Whether or not vasoconstriction is the *primary* event in the pathogenesis of PPH, it is an important component in the pathophysiology of the disease. Possible triggers of pulmonary vasoconstriction in susceptible individuals include normobaric or hypobaric (high-altitude) hypoxia, autoimmune disorders, drugs and toxins, increased pulmonary blood flow (with or without increased pressure and shear stress), lung injury, and increased sympathetic tone, resulting in catecholamine-induced injury (26–32). Many of these vasoconstrictor stimuli can damage the pulmonary endothelium, resulting in alterations in the balance between vasoactive mediators. Several studies have looked at the possible role of an imbalance favoring vasoconstrictor mediators, including thromboxane and prostacyclin (33–35), as well as other endothelial-derived factors (36,37). Coagulation abnormalities may occur, initiating or further exacerbating the pulmonary vascular disease (38,39). For example, elevated levels of thromboxane promote not only pulmonary vasoconstriction, but also activate platelet aggregation. The interactions between the humoral and cellular elements of the blood on an injured endothelial cell surface result in remodeling of the pulmonary vascular bed and contribute to the process of vascular injury (40,41).

Migration of smooth-muscle cells in the pulmonary arterioles occurs with release of an unidentified chemotactic agent from injured pulmonary endothelial cells (42). Endothelial cell damage can also produce thrombosis in situ, transforming the pulmonary vascular bed from its usual anticoagulant state (owing to release of prostacyclin and plasminogen activator inhibitors) to a procoagulant state (43). Fibrinopeptide A levels are elevated in primary pulmonary hypertension patients, suggesting that in situ thrombosis is occurring (44). Further support for the role of coagulation abnormalities at the endothelial cell surface in the pathogenesis of primary pulmonary hypertension comes from the demonstration that treatment with anticoagulation therapy increases survival (25).

Although the pathogenesis for pulmonary hypertension secondary to sickle hemoglobinopathies is most often thought to be due to pulmonary thromboembolism, pulmonary vascular remodeling is also known to occur, further supporting the role of endothelial dysfunction in the pathogenesis of primary pulmonary hypertension (45).

Several studies have emphasized the importance of the pulmonary endothelial cell in the metabolism of vasoactive mediators known to modulate pulmonary vascular tone, and have implicated the local release of vasoactive agents, producing modification of smooth-muscle tone (46–50). We have looked at the role of an imbalance in arachidonic acid metabolites, specifically excess thromboxane, a potent vasoconstrictor, and decreased prostacyclin, a potent vasodilator (33), in children with primary pulmonary hypertension before and during attempts at pharmacological vasodilatation (51). In 4 out of 16 patients, thromboxane levels were increased, and in 3 of the 4 the concentrations of thromboxane were greater in the aorta than in the pulmonary artery, suggesting pulmonary release of thromboxane. These studies suggest that altered endothelial cell function may modify arachidonate metabolism and exacerbate or perpetuate pulmonary hypertension in some patients. Recent findings of increased endothelin levels in children and adults with pulmonary hypertension (52,53) is further support for the theory of an imbalance between pulmonary vasoconstrictors (e.g., endothelin) and pulmonary vasodilators (e.g., endothelial-derived relaxing factor—nitric oxide) in the pathogenesis of primary pulmonary hypertension.

Several studies (54,55) suggest that arachidonate metabolism in pulmonary endothelial cells is altered by changes in flow dynamics, and that endothelial cell deformation in response to shear stress can increase the release of arachidonate and prostacyclin. These studies support the hypothesis offered by Rodbard (56) that vascular shear stress controls vessel diameter. Since an increase in shear stress (caused by high flow and a large pressure drop across the vascular bed) can damage the endothelium (57,58), and injured endothelial cells may fail to release prostacyclin, the arachidonate released by shear stress may be diverted into the thromboxane synthetase pathway. This may lead to a vicious cycle of vasoconstriction, increased shear force, and progressive damage, with perpetuation of the pulmonary hypertension.

Celermajer et al. recently reported impairment of endothelial-dependent pulmonary artery relaxation in vivo in children with pulmonary vascular disease and congenital heart disease (59). Their study supports the potential role for endothelial dysfunction as an early event in the pathophysiology of pulmonary vascular disease, preceding morphological changes.

α-Adrenergic stimulation increases pulmonary vascular tone with the release of norepinephrine from the lung (60), and β-adrenergic agonists can induce vasodilatation when pulmonary vascular tone is increased (61). Several studies suggest a defect in the endothelial uptake and degradation of norepinephrine in pulmonary hypertension. The normal lung endothelium extracts 17–30% of the norepinephrine that passes through its circulation (46,47,62), whereas the loss of the lung's ability to extract circulating norepinephrine in patients with pulmonary hypertension has been described (63–65). In addition, increased circulating levels of norepinephrine have been measured in some patients with pulmonary hypertension (64–66).

It is possible that the sympathetic nervous system contributes toward the maintenance or exacerbation of pulmonary hypertension in some patients. We have observed that, in patients with increased sympathetic tone and pulmonary hypertension, crying or agitation may further increase norepinephrine levels and pulmonary pressures. It is possible that elevated norepinephrine concentrations may identify patients in whom enhanced sympathetic tone contributes to pulmonary vasoconstriction. Some patients may respond to α-adrenergic blocking agents with a decrease in pulmonary artery pressure (21,67).

The known association between PPH and portal hypertension is consistent with the role of an imbalance in vasoactive substances, favoring vasoconstriction in the pathogenesis of primary pulmonary hypertension (68). It is proposed that, in portal hypertension, the pulmonary vasculature is exposed to vasoactive substances normally metabolized by the liver that lead to pulmonary hypertension by inducing vasoconstriction or injury to the pulmonary endothelium.

Identification of the contribution to pulmonary vasoconstriction made by changes in the endothelial metabolism of vasoactive substances may lead to a more fundamental understanding of the control of the pulmonary circulation and, hence, lead to more specific modes of therapy for pulmonary hypertension. Pharmacological attempts at antagonizing these vasoconstrictors (e.g., norepinephrine or thromboxane) has resulted in prolonged survival and decreased pulmonary hypertension in some patients (21,69).

B. Autoimmunity

Pulmonary hypertension occurs in the setting of several autoimmune disorders, such as systemic lupus erythematosus, scleroderma, rheumatoid arthritis, polydermatomyositis, or mixed connective tissue disease (70–74). Pulmonary hypertension is also associated with immune dysregulation seen with drug therapy, pregnancy, and human immunodeficiency virus (HIV) infection. Although an increased frequency of positive antinuclear antibodies has been reported in adult patients with primary pulmonary hypertension (27), this finding has not been demonstrated in children. Interestingly, we found a significantly increased incidence of positive antinuclear antibodies (ANA) in the mothers of children with PPH (4/16; 25%) (28) in the absence of clinical findings of autoimmune disease. In addition, 3 of 17 (18%) children, who were initially ANA-negative, seroconverted during follow-up over several years. We also found an increased incidence of antibodies in the families of children with familial primary pulmonary hypertension (17). These data suggest that primary pulmonary hypertension may be a forme fruste of an autoimmune disease in some patients. Interestingly, we also found an increased incidence of antinuclear antibodies in mothers of children with pulmonary hypertension associated with anatomically trivial congenital pulmonary-to-systemic communications (i.e. a small PDA, VSD, or ASD; 5/13; 39%).

Most autoimmune diseases are associated with increased frequencies of certain HLA-DR, DQ, or DP (class II) alleles. We found an increased frequency of HLA-DR3, DR52, and DQ2 in children with primary pulmonary hypertension (28). This finding of an HLA class II association for childhood PPH suggests that it is an autoimmune disease in some children. We also found immunoglobulin isotype deficiencies and autoimmunity in distinct immunogenetically defined subsets of familial PPH, susceptibility to which is determined in part by gene(s) within or near the HLA region on chromosome 6 (17). The increase in DR3, DR52, and DQ2 in primary pulmonary hypertension and familial pulmonary hypertension was interesting, because these linked alleles are usually part of a haplotype frequently observed in systemic lupus erythematosus, common variable immunodeficiency, and IgA deficiency. To study if there is an increased incidence of shared HLA-DR, DQ alleles in the parents of children with primary pulmonary hypertension, we performed serological HLA-DR, DQ, and sequence-specific oligonucleotide (DNA) typing of DRB1,3,4,5 and DQB1. Preliminary data suggest that the inheritance of shared parental HLA-DR, DQ (class II) alleles is increased in children with PPH (75), further supporting the role of autoimmunity in the pathogenesis of this disorder in a subset of children.

C. Pathophysiology

Children with primary pulmonary hypertension appear to have differences in hemodynamic parameters measured at the time of diagnosis compared with adult patients (Table 2; 76). The increased cardiac index in children may reflect an earlier diagnosis and may partly explain why children tend to respond more favorably to vasodilator therapy than adults. The finding of higher heart rates and lower systemic artery pressures in children is expected.

Syncopal episodes in children with PPH are usually effort-related and are due to a limitation in cardiac output. Other mechanisms, including sympathetic and parasympathetic alterations, may also play a role.

From the pathogenesis and pathophysiology of primary pulmonary hypertension, the two most frequent mechanisms of death are progressive right ventricular failure and sudden death, with the former occurring far more often (2). With progressive right ventricular failure, the scenario, as described in the foregoing, leads to dyspnea, hypoxemia, and a progressive decrease in cardiac output. Pneumonia may be fatal owing to alveolar hypoxia, causing further pulmonary vasoconstriction, resulting in an inability to maintain adequate cardiac output, cardiogenic shock, and death. When arterial hypoxemia and acidosis occur, life-threatening arrhythmias may also occur. Postulated mechanisms for sudden death with primary pulmonary hypertension include brady- and tachyarrhythmias, acute pulmonary embolism, massive pulmonary hemorrhage, and sudden right ventricular ischemia.

Table 2 Baseline Hemodynamics in Children Versus Adults with Primary Pulmonary Hypertension

	Children (n = 24)	Adults (n = 77)
Mean pulmonary artery pressure (mmHg)	70 ± 15*	55 ± 16
Mean systemic artery pressure (mmHg)	75 ± 15*	91 ± 12
Cardiac index (L/min/M^2)	4.3 ± 3.9*	2.1 ± 0.7
Pulmonary vascular resistance (units/M^2)	28.1 ± 18.1*	15.4 ± 8.2
Systemic vascular resistance (units/M^2)	27.7 ± 17.9	25.2 ± 9.8
Heart rate (bpm)	121 ± 29*	83 ± 13

*$p < 0.05$ children vs. adults.
Source: Adapted with permission from Ref. 76.

V. Diagnosis

Although the diagnosis of primary pulmonary hypertension is one of exclusion, it can be made with a high degree of accuracy if care is taken to exclude all likely secondary causes. A thorough and detailed history and physical examination, as well as appropriate tests, must be performed to uncover potential causative or contributing factors, many of which may not be readily apparent. Questions should be asked about family history—pulmonary hypertension, connective tissue disorders, congenital heart disease, and other congenital anomalies, and early unexplained deaths. If the family history suggests familial PPH, careful screening of all siblings is recommended, including consideration of cardiac catheterization. Early therapy in "asymptomatic" siblings with familial primary pulmonary hypertension may improve outcome (personal experience). Additional issues to address include a careful, detailed birth and neonatal history, detailed drug history, prolonged medications [i.e., methylphenidate (Ritalin), appetite suppressants, psychotropics], exposure to high altitude or to toxic cooking oil (77,78), travel history, and a history of frequent respiratory tract infections. Problems with coagulation should also be queried. The answers to these questions frequently offer clues to a possible trigger for the development of the pulmonary vascular disease. For example, we have seen a 6-year-old boy with a diagnosis of primary pulmonary hypertension who had moved to New York from Spain at 1 year of age after having been exposed to rapeseed cooking oil during infancy. Another example is an 11-year-old boy, with suspected PPH, who had evidence of severe pulmonary schistosomiasis at autopsy. The child was from Brazil and had not been treated for schistosomiasis.

The diagnostic evaluation in children with primary pulmonary hypertension is similar to that of adult patients (Table 3).

A. Symptoms

The presenting symptoms in children with primary pulmonary hypertension may differ when compared with adult patients. Infants with primary pulmonary hypertension may present with signs of low cardiac output (i.e., poor appetite, failure to thrive, lethargy, diaphoresis, tachypnea, and tachycardia). In addition, infants and older children with primary pulmonary hypertension may be cyanotic with exertion, owing to right-to-left shunting through a patent foramen ovale. Children without adequate shunting through a patent foramen ovale can present with syncope, which is more often effort-related in children than in adult patients. After early childhood, children with primary pulmonary hypertension present with the same symptoms as adults. In the older children, the most common symptoms are exertional dyspnea and, occasionally, chest pain. Clinical right ventricular failure is rare in the younger children, occurring most often in children older than 10 years

Table 3 Primary Pulmonary Hypertension: Workup and Evaluation

- Chest X-ray
- Electrocardiogram—telemetry
- 2-Dimensional echocardiogram with cavitation study
- Pulmonary function tests—DLCO, KCO
- Progressive exercise test
- Continuous O_2 saturation monitoring overnight
- Holter (24-hr ECG) monitor
- CBC, urinalysis, SMAC-LFTs, GGTP
- Coagulation studies
  - Coagulation profile
  - Bleeding time
  - Platelet aggregation studies
  - Coagulation factors
    - Factor VIII
    - von Willebrand Ag
    - von Willebrand ristocetin cofactor
    - von Willebrand multimers
    - Antithrombin III
    - Protein C
    - Protein S
    - Factor VII
    - Factor II
    - Factor V
  - Serum viscosity
  - Serum protein electrophoresis
  - Hgb electrophoresis
  - Quantitative immunoglobulins
- Fractionated plasma catecholamines
- Fasting lipid profile
- HIV test
- Thyroid function tests
- Collagen vascular workup
  - Lupus anticoagulant
  - ESR
  - ANA
  - Anti-DNA
  - Anticardiolipin antibodies
  - CH_{50} complement and components
  - Special ANAs
  - Anticentromere
  - Rheumatoid factor
  - Latex fixation
  - HLA typing
- Magnetic resonance imaging
- Radionuclide angiocardiography (MUGA)
- Quantitative ventilation-perfusion Lung scan
- Cardiac catheterization with acute vasodilator drug testing and pulmonary angiography
- Lung biopsy
- Transplantation evaluation

of age with severe, long-standing primary pulmonary hypertension. The interval between onset of symptoms and time of diagnosis is usually shorter in children than in adults, particularly in those children who present with syncope. Some infants with PPH have crying spells, presumably as a result of chest pains that cannot be otherwise verbalized. Children of all ages also commonly complain of nausea and vomiting.

B. Physical Examination

Many of the physical findings in children are typical of any patient, child or adult, with pulmonary hypertension. An increased pulmonic component of the second heart sound is usually audible; however, a right-sided fourth heart sound is not heard as often in children. Children may have distortion of their chest wall, secondary to severe right ventricular hypertrophy. Tricuspid regurgitation is very common, whereas pulmonary insufficiency is heard less often. Clinical signs of right-sided heart failure (e.g., hepatomegaly, peripheral edema, and acrocyanosis) are rare in young children, particularly in those who present with syncope. Clubbing is not a typical feature of primary pulmonary hypertension, although it has been observed in patients who have had long-standing primary pulmonary hypertension who develop chronic hypoxemia secondary to right-to-left shunting through a patent foramen ovale.

C. Diagnostic Evaluation

The workup for children with suspected primary pulmonary hypertension is similar to the workup for adults (see Table 3).

The Electrocardiogram

The electrocardiogram (ECG) characteristically shows increased right-sided forces in the chest leads and right axis deviation.

The Chest Radiograph

A chest radiograph usually shows an enlarged right ventricle and dilated proximal pulmonary arteries. The attenuated ("pruned") distal pulmonary vasculature, which is a common finding in adult patients, is rarely seen.

Ventilation–Perfusion Scintigraphy

Although we perform ventilation–perfusion scintigraphy in children with suspected primary pulmonary hypertension, we are not as concerned about ruling out chronic thromboembolic disease as a cause of the elevated pulmonary pressure in this population. Chronic thromboembolic disease can be found in children with hemoglobinopathies or schistosomiasis. Because we have seen children with presumed primary pulmonary hypertension who had sickle cell disease first documented at autopsy, we perform hemoglobin electrophoresis on all children with unexplained pulmonary hypertension. A complete coagulation profile is performed to rule out hereditary or acquired hypercoagulable states that could be etiologic or potentiating factors.

Pulmonary Angiography

Pulmonary angiography should be performed if the perfusion lung scan shows more than a single segmental or multiple subsegmental defects, to rule out thromboembolic disease, since chronic thromboembolic pulmonary hypertension may be amenable to thromboendarterectomy (79). Quantitative pulmonary wedge angiography, using the balloon occlusion technique, may give additional information on the severity of pulmonary vascular disease. Rabinovitch et al. have reported the usefulness of the rate of taper, the background filling of peripheral vessels, and the pulmonary circulation time, as additional tools in evaluating disease progression (80).

Echocardiography

Echocardiography is extremely important in the pediatric patient to exclude associated congenital or acquired heart disease. The typical echocardiographic appearance in children with primary pulmonary hypertension is similar to adult patients: right ventricular and right atrial enlargement, with a normal or decreased left ventricular cavity dimension. Tricuspid and pulmonary insufficiency are detected with Doppler interrogation, and the size of the tricuspid and pulmonary regurgitant jets are useful in estimating pulmonary systolic and diastolic pressures. Posterior bowing of the interventricular septum occurs with significant pulmonary hypertension, and posterior bowing of the interatrial septum is seen with elevation of the right atrial pressure. Although transesophageal echocardiography is often helpful with adult patients, it is rarely necessary with children. A contrast study during two-dimensional echocardiography can be performed to determine the presence and size of an anatomical interatrial communication. The rate of disappearance of the bubbles is useful as a qualitative assessment of right heart function and resting cardiac output.

Continuous Oxygen Saturation Measurements

We recommend that all patients have a sleep evaluation, including continuous oxygen saturation monitoring performed to rule out airway obstruction or hypoventilation. Even modest decreases in systemic arterial oxygen saturation can significantly increase pulmonary artery pressures in children with a reactive pulmonary vascular bed. If nocturnal systemic arterial oxygen desaturation is observed, the patient is restudied with supplemental oxygen to determine the appropriate concentration of oxygen necessary for correction.

Holter Monitor

Patients with primary pulmonary hypertension rarely have significant arrhythmias, although an occasional patient may have complex ventricular or supraventricular arrhythmias that require treatment. Although syncope is rarely due to a conduction abnormality in primary pulmonary hypertension, we have occasionally seen various degrees of heart block in a child with unexplained pulmonary hypertension and a history of syncope. Accordingly, our patients undergo baseline Holter (24-h ECG) monitoring, with repeat studies as clinically indicated. Ambulatory monitoring is also useful before initiating medical therapy, particularly if treatment with drugs such as diltiazam, which affect AV node conduction, will be used.

Radionuclide Angiocardiography and Magnetic Resonance Imaging

These are noninvasive studies that can be used to assess right and left ventricular function in children with PPH before initiating therapy. Additionally, these imaging studies can be used to monitor the effects of therapy (81,82).

Pulmonary Function Testing

Adults with primary pulmonary hypertension have mild restrictive abnormalities, low-diffusing capacity and oxygen desaturation at rest, on pulmonary function testing (18). In 31 children and young adults with PPH, small-airway obstruction was the most frequent abnormality in pulmonary function test (83). Reductions in the FEF_{25-75} correlated with clinical disability and hemodynamic abnormalities. These studies suggest that pulmonary function testing may provide a noninvasive method for following the progression of the disease.

Cardiopulmonary Exercise Tests

Although limitations in exercise capacity are seen in most patients, the pattern of response to exercise in PPH is nonspecific. Rhodes et al. reported that exercise capacity correlated with right atrial pressure, pulmonary artery pressure, and cardiac index, and was useful in predicting prognosis and survival (84). Mean right atrial pressure, a variable found to be one of the best predictors of survival in patients with PPH (2), correlated best with exercise capacity (Fig. 3).

Patients with severely limited exercise capacity ($<$ 10% of the predicted value) are at high risk for complications during cardiac catheterization (84). Progressive cycle ergometry is a safe procedure that can identify these patients: We do not routinely perform acute vasodilator drug testing during cardiac catheterization in patients who cannot exceed 10% of the predicted workload. Conversely, an exercise capacity of more than 75% of the predicted value may identify the subgroup of patients capable of active pulmonary vasodilatation (84). Serial exercise studies may identify disease progression and influence timing of more aggressive medical or surgical treatment.

Laboratory Testing

We perform a battery of studies to assess multiorgan dysfunction secondary to pulmonary hypertension, to exclude underlying causes for secondary pulmonary hypertension and to further elucidate our understanding of the pathogenesis and pathophysiology of the disease in children. An HIV test is performed to rule out the association of HIV infection with pulmonary hypertension (85). Assays for a

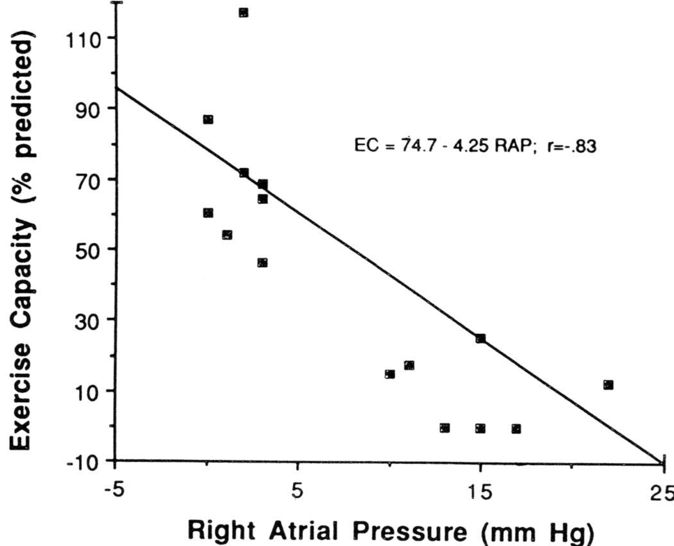

Figure 3 Regression plot of exercise capacity versus mean right atrial pressure in 16 patients with primary pulmonary hypertension. (Two patients had right atrial pressures of 13 mmHg and exercise capacities of 0% predicted.) (From Ref. 84.)

lupus anticoagulant and anticardiolipin antibody are performed to determine whether or not a patient has the antiphospholipid syndrome, which predisposes to secondary thromboembolic events (86,87). Liver function tests are done to assess liver function, with additional studies performed to rule out portal hypertension (88). A liver biopsy may be useful in selected patients to differentiate between hepatic cirrhosis, with secondary pulmonary hypertension, versus primary pulmonary hypertension, with passive hepatic congestion. Quantitative immunoglobulins are obtained, since immunoglobulin deficiencies are seen with children and adults with PPH. Additionally, patients with a deficiency could be predisposed to an acute pulmonary hypertensive crisis during the administration of blood products, such as fresh-frozen plasma (89). Low levels of antithrombin III, protein C, or protein S can be due to a genetic defect, or may be the result of ongoing consumption (90). Serial determinations of coagulation studies may be useful in evaluating the effect of therapy on endothelial dysfunction. Serum protein electrophoresis is obtained to rule out plasma cell dyscrasias, which have been associated with unexplained pulmonary hypertension (91). Thyroid function testing is performed, since in addition to the recently described association between thyroid disease and primary pulmonary hypertension reported in adults (92), we have seen children with thyroid abnormalities as well. Iron concentration studies are useful to identify children who need supplemental iron therapy to prevent iron deficiency, which results in less distensible red blood cells and increased thrombosis in situ.

Fractionated Plasma Catecholamines

Some children and adults with primary pulmonary hypertension have elevated resting levels of circulating catecholamines and exaggerated increases in catecholamines during exertion or agitation (51). In these patients, consideration of α-adrenergic blockade therapy may be appropriate.

Lung Biopsy

Lung biopsy, either open or thorascopic, is not routinely performed in patients suspected of having PPH, owing to the risks associated with performing a lung biopsy in patients with this disorder and the limited value of the information gained. Lung biopsy is reserved for the rare case for whom there is uncertainty concerning the etiology.

The necessity for performing a lung biopsy to diagnose pulmonary veno-occlusive disease remains controversial, since a careful and complete noninvasive evaluation, in most circumstances, will allow diagnosis of pulmonary veno-occlusive disease without the need for histopathological confirmation. Noninvasive findings suggestive of pulmonary veno-occlusive disease include (1) increased interstitial markings on chest radiography, with or without clinical signs of increased interstitial water on physical examination; and (2) pulmonary function tests demonstrating marked reductions in diffusion capacity and K_{CO} (diffusion capacity corrected for lung volume). Since the natural history of pulmonary veno-occlusive disease is significantly worse than primary pulmonary hypertension (93) and the response to vasodilator therapy may be extremely unpredictable (94), early recognition of the disease may be important in making therapeutic decisions.

Cardiac Catheterization

Cardiac catheterization is recommended for confirmation of the diagnosis of PPH. In adults, hemodynamic values obtained at catheterization can also be used to predict survival, although this has not been validated in children. Cardiac output can be accurately measured by the thermodilution technique in patients without significant pulmonary or tricuspid regurgitation or shunting through a patent foramen ovale, but the Fick method should be used when the latter conditions are present. Because of the increased risk of cardiac catheterization in patients with severe pulmonary hypertension, special precautions should be taken during cardiac catheterization: adequate sedation to minimize anxiety without depressing respiration, and prevention of hypovolemia and hypoxemia are important issues that should be addressed.

VI. Therapy

Treatment for this disease has improved significantly over the past 15 years, with sustained clinical improvement and increased long-term survival in children with PPH (21,98). Noninvasive studies obtained before starting therapy, and periodically thereafter, can be useful in guiding changes in the therapeutic regimen. Repeated cardiac catheterization may not be necessary if these noninvasive studies indicate stability or remission.

A. General Measures

The pediatrician plays an invaluable role in the care of children with primary pulmonary hypertension. Since children often have a more reactive pulmonary vascular bed than adult patients, any respiratory tract infection that results in ventilation–perfusion mismatching and subsequent alveolar hypoxia can result in a catastrophic event if not aggressively treated. Annual influenza vaccination is recommended, unless there is a specific contraindication. Children with pneumonia should be hospitalized for the initiation of antibiotic therapy, and antipyretics should be administered for temperature elevations higher than 101°F (38°C) to minimize the consequences of increased metabolic demands. Diet or medical therapy should be prescribed to prevent constipation, since Valsalva maneuvers transiently decrease venous return to the right side of the heart and can precipitate syncope.

Children may require aggressive therapy for acute pulmonary hypertension crises occurring with episodes of pneumonia or other infectious illnesses. We have seen adult respiratory distress syndrome occur in a child with PPH following viral gastroenteritis, requiring intravenous prostacyclin for several weeks, in addition to conventional maximal cardiopulmonary support.

B. Anticoagulation

The role for chronic anticoagulation in children is based on studies in adult primary pulmonary hypertension patients (25,96). Low-dose anticoagulation may be effective in preventing thrombosis in situ, which can exacerbate the underlying pulmonary vascular obstructive disease. Unfortunately, antiplatelet therapy with aspirin or dipyridamole does not appear to be effective in areas of low flow in the lung, where thrombosis in situ is known to occur. Warfarin is used in doses that increase the international normalized ratio (INR) to 2.3–3.0. Parents should be advised to avoid administering other medications that could interact with the warfarin. Frequent adjustments in warfarin dosage may be needed when right-sided heart failure is present.

C. Vasodilator Therapy

The rationale for the use of vasodilator drugs to treat pulmonary hypertension is based on histopathological studies that demonstrated an apparent progression in vascular remodeling from medial hypertrophy to plexiform arteriopathy (97). Medial hypertrophy is presumably associated with vessel constriction, whereas plexiform lesions are associated with fixed pulmonary vascular obstructive disease. Given these studies, Wagenvoort and Wagenvoort hypothesized, in 1977, that primary pulmonary hypertension is a disease of individuals with hyperreactive lung vessels, in whom various stimuli may initiate vasoconstriction, with subsequent development of the characteristic vascular lesions. It is believed that, early in the course of the disease, most pulmonary vessels are affected by vasoconstriction, with an increased proportion affected with fixed obstruction as the disease progresses. This is schematically shown in Figure 4. In the 1970s, the advent of vasodilator drugs to treat systemic hypertension led to vasodilator therapy for PPH beginning in the late 1970s to early 1980s.

Because one does not know exactly at which point a given patient is in the natural history of the disease, acute vasodilator drug testing is *necessary* to safely assess vasodilator therapy. Acute vasodilator trials using short-acting agents in the cardiac catheterization laboratory are performed to evaluate pulmonary vasoreac-

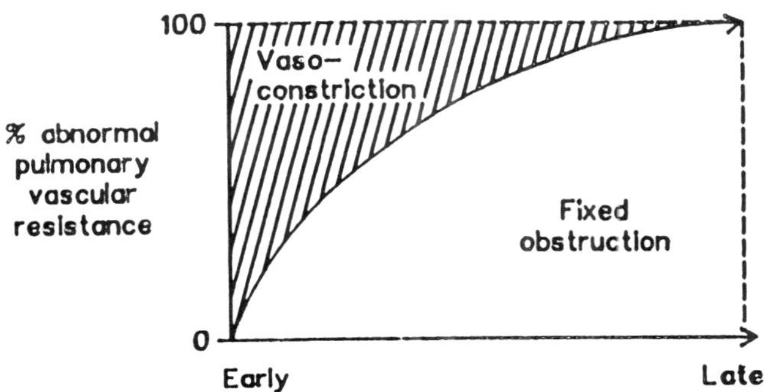

Figure 4 Hypothetical scheme illustrating that, with the passage of time in primary pulmonary hypertension, the hypertensive component caused by vasoconstriction decreases, whereas that caused by fixed obstruction increases. (The alternative hypothesis is that the vasoconstrictive and the obstructive components represent different diseases.) (From Ref. 11.)

tivity. Because passive distention or recruitment of pulmonary vessels can reduce pulmonary vascular resistance, without necessarily indicating a decrease in pulmonary vascular tone (99,100), and because spontaneous variability in pulmonary artery pressure and pulmonary resistance is observed in some patients with PPH (101), the following criteria are used to indicate acute drug-induced active pulmonary vasodilatation: (1) 20% or greater decrease in mean pulmonary artery pressure and (2) no change or an increase in cardiac index. In our laboratory, patients are considered responders to acute prostacyclin testing if they demonstrate both criteria. On the basis of the acute drug testing, long-term vasodilator drug treatment may be initiated. We have previously shown that children who have a reactive pulmonary vascular bed, defined by their response to acute prostacyclin testing, also respond to calcium channel blockers (Fig. 5; 21). In addition, acute pulmonary vasodilatation appears to be age-related, with the

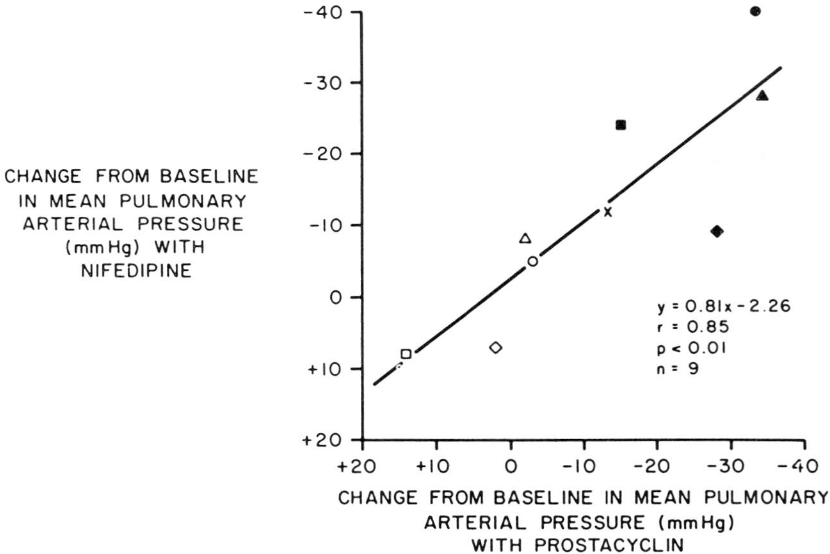

Figure 5 Correlation between the absolute change from baseline in mean pulmonary arterial pressure (mmHg) with prostacyclin infusion and the absolute change from baseline in mean pulmonary arterial pressure (mmHg) with sublingual nifedipine administration. Significant correlation ($r = 0.85$; $p < 0.01$) indicates that prostacyclin and nifedipine produce similar pulmonary vasodilator responses in patients with primary pulmonary hypertension. A similar correlation was observed between the percentage of change in pulmonary arterial pressure with prostacyclin and the percentage of change in pulmonary arterial pressure with nifedipine ($r = 0.89$, $p < 0.01$). (From Ref. 21.)

youngest patients demonstrating the greatest degree of reversible pulmonary hypertension (Fig. 6). In 41 children tested acutely with prostacyclin, the frequency of a positive response was greatest in the youngest children (86% in infants younger than 1 year of age, 47% in children 1–7 years of age, and 27% in children older than 7 years of age at the time of diagnosis; Fig. 7; 21).

Our early studies suggested that short-term survival could be enhanced by chronic vasodilator treatment (21,95). We recently reported improved long-term survival in children with PPH treated with long-term vasodilator therapy, compared with historical controls who never received vasodilator therapy (5-year survival 55% vs. 9%, respectively, $p < 0.005$; Fig. 8; 98). Age at the time of diagnosis was the most important predictor of survival, with an 88% 5-year survival for children younger than 6 years of age, compared with 25% for older patients ($p < 0.02$). In addition to age at diagnosis, children with a positive response to acute prostacyclin testing had a trend toward prolonged survival, compared with nonresponders: the 5-year survival for the responders was 86%, compared with 33% 5-year survival for the nonresponders ($p = 0.06$; Fig. 9). Five of the seven responders to acute prostacyclin testing had follow-up cardiac cathe-

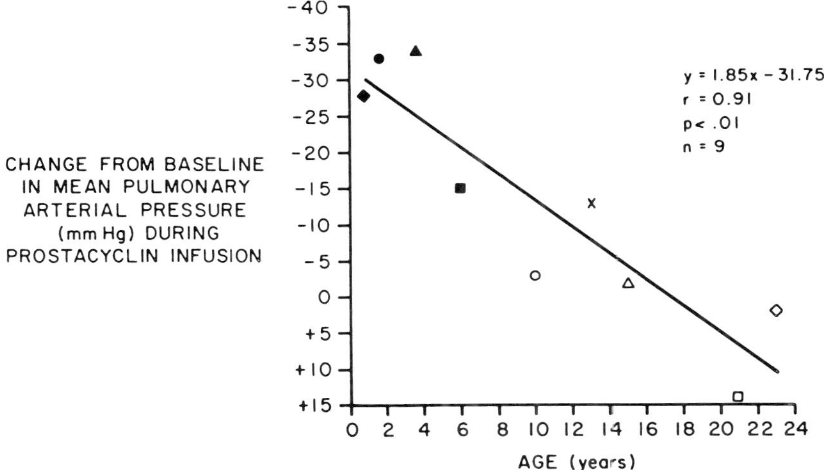

Figure 6 Relation between the age of the patient and the change from baseline in mean pulmonary arterial pressure with prostacyclin infusion. Significant inverse correlation ($r = 0.91$, $p < 0.01$) indicates that prostacyclin produces a greater fall in pulmonary arterial pressure in younger patients with primary pulmonary hypertension than in the older ones. A similar inverse correlation ($r = 0.82$, $p < 0.01$) was observed between the age of the patient and the change from baseline in mean pulmonary arterial pressure with sublingual nifedipine administration. (From Ref. 21.)

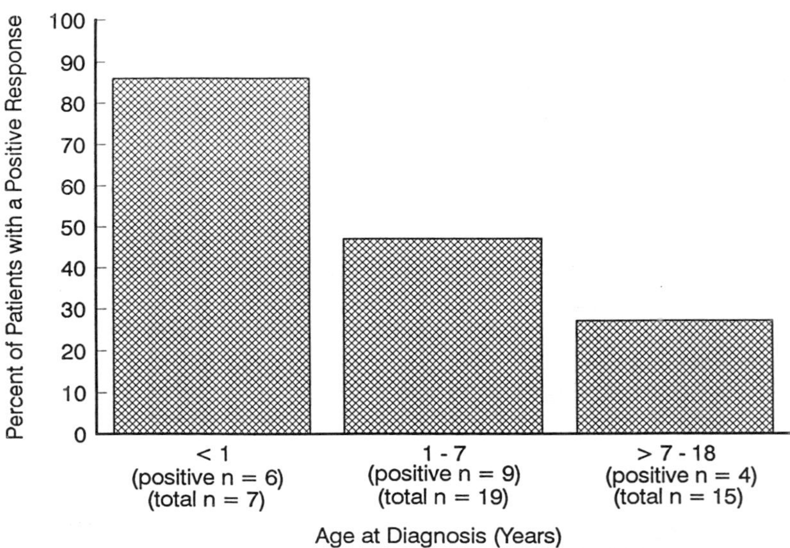

Figure 7 Positive response to acute prostacyclin testing in 41 children with primary pulmonary hypertension. The younger the child is at the time of initial evaluation, the greater is the likelihood of a positive response (86% in infants younger than 1 year of age, 47% in children 1–7 years of age, and 27% in children older than 7 years of age, at the time of diagnosis).

terizations while receiving chronic vasodilator therapy (2.6–11 years, mean ± SD, 7.0 ± 3.8 years; 89). Mean pulmonary artery pressure decreased from 74 ± 33 mmHg at baseline, to 36 ± 21 mmHg on long-term vasodilator therapy (p <0.04). Pulmonary vascular resistance index decreased from 22 ± 20 U·m^2 to 9 ± 8 U·m^2 (p <0.08; Fig. 10).

The recommended approach for children is similar to that used in adult patients with PPH: use of a potent, short-acting, titratable vasodilator, such as prostacyclin, during cardiac catheterization to determine the potential and magnitude of pulmonary vasoreactivity. The advantages of prostacyclin are its potency as a pulmonary vasodilator, its titratability, and its short half-life in circulation (3–5 min; 103). In general, acute prostacyclin testing is done with incremental doses from 2 to 12 ng/kg per minute; most adult patients cannot tolerate doses higher than 8–10 ng/kg per minute. In contrast, children tolerate short-term doses of 20–40 ng/kg minute, and it is not unusual to observe pulmonary vasodilatation only when the dose is increased to greater than 20 ng/kg minute. Prostacyclin is now commercially available in the United States; however, it is expensive. Alter-

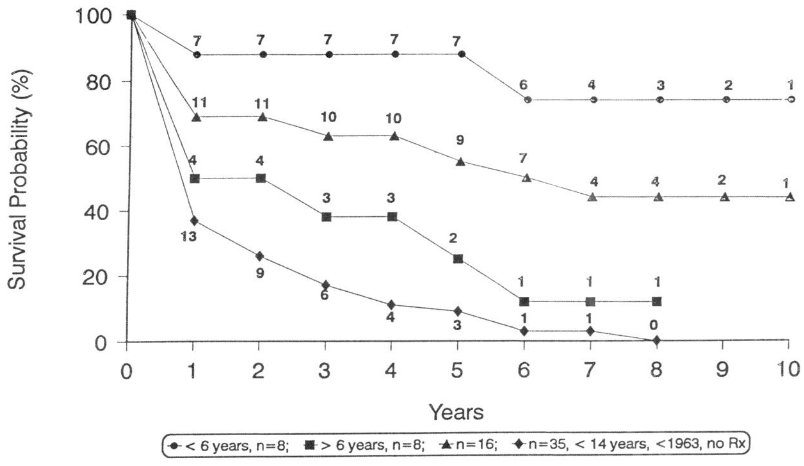

Figure 8 Prolonged vasodilator therapy improved long-term survival in children with primary pulmonary hypertension (n = 16) compared with historical controls (n = 35) who never received vasodilator treatment (5-year survival 55 vs. 9%, respectively; p <0.005). Long-term survival was further increased in the children diagnosed early in life. Five-year survival for the younger children was 88% compared with 25% for patients diagnosed at 6 years of age or older (p <0.02). (From Ref. 69.)

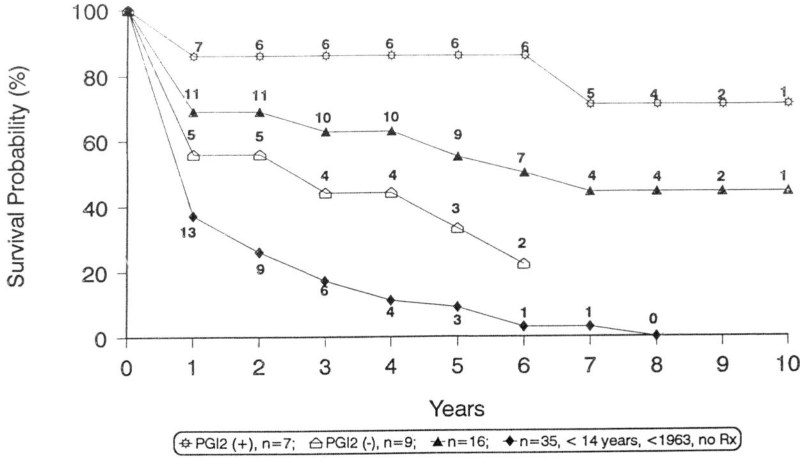

Figure 9 Improved long-term survival in children with primary pulmonary hypertension who had a positive response to acute prostacyclin testing. Five-year survival for children with a positive response to acute prostacyclin testing was 86% compared with 33% for patients who did not respond favorably to such testing (p = 0.06). (From Ref. 69.)

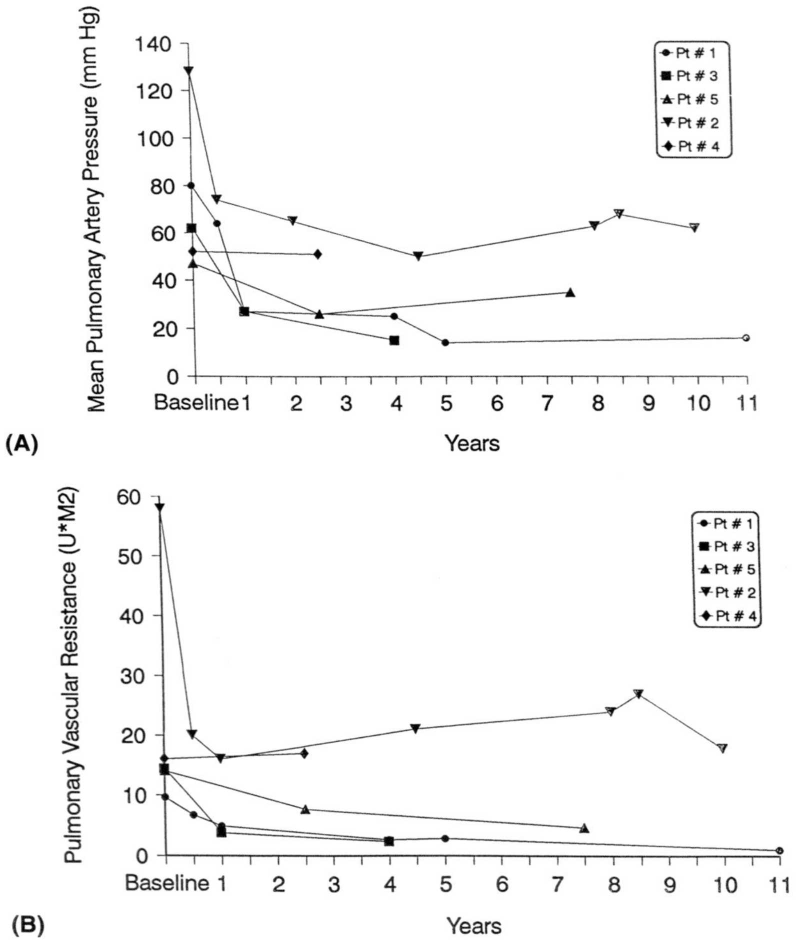

Figure 10 Long-term follow-up (2.6–11 years) in five children with a positive response to acute prostacyclin testing. (A) Mean pulmonary artery pressure and (B) pulmonary vascular resistance index were measured at baseline (before starting vasodilatory therapy) and during serial follow-up hemodynamic studies. (From Ref. 69.)

natives for acute vasodilator testing include adenosine, acetylcholine, prostaglandin E_1, and inhaled nitric oxide.

The following case illustrates an example of the response to extended calcium channel blockade in a child who demonstrated a positive response to acute prostacyclin testing: A 7-year-old boy, referred for evaluation, had a history of recurrent syncope and decreased exercise tolerance and was found to have primary pulmonary hypertension. Acute pulmonary vasodilation was demonstrated with acute prostacyclin testing: pulmonary artery pressure decreased from a baseline of 72/32 (mean 50) mmHg to 29/6 (mean 17) mmHg, with an increase in cardiac output from 3.2 to 5.0 L/min. Nifedipine administered acutely decreased his pulmonary artery pressure from 73/37 (mean 52) to 35/12 (mean 19) mmHg, with an increase in cardiac output from 3.3 to 6.1 L/min. With long-term calcium channel blocker therapy he is asymptomatic, and his exercise capacity has increased from 41% predicted to 80% predicted. His electrocardiogram and echocardiogram before and after 6 months of nifedipine treatment are shown in Figures 11 and 12.

Based on the acute response to vasodilator testing, children who demonstrate active pulmonary vasodilatation without untoward effects are subsequently evaluated with vasodilators that can be administered long-term. Untoward effects include (1) an increase in pulmonary artery pressure, concomitant with an increase in cardiac index, without a decrease in pulmonary vascular resistance; (2) a decrease in cardiac index; or (3) an increase in right atrial pressure. Of all the vasodilators currently being used, calcium channel blockers appear to have the most promise. On occasion, we will use α-adrenergic blockade (phenoxybenzamine) when circulating levels of catecholamines are elevated and a favorable response to acute α-adrenergic blockade testing with phentolamine is seen.

Although the long-term outlook for children who are not acutely responsive does not appear to be as favorable as that for responders, continued vasodilator therapy in nonresponders may be useful palliative therapy while awaiting newer investigational therapeutic options. Chronic oral vasodilator therapy is not continued in nonresponders who complain of nausea, vomiting, dizziness, or orthostatic hypotension when receiving long-term therapy. Unmonitored, empiric treatment with any vasodilator is *strongly discouraged*. If a child has unfavorable hemodynamic effects from the chronic vasodilator therapy, right ventricular work could increase and precipitate or aggravate right-sided heart failure (104). Furthermore, sudden death in patients empirically started on a long-acting vasodilators regimen with undiagnosed fixed pulmonary vascular disease has been reported, underscoring the need for evaluation with acute vasodilator testing at an experienced center (105–114).

Patients unresponsive to chronic oral vasodilator therapy have recently been treated with continuous intravenous prostacyclin, with long-term follow-up studies demonstrating clinical and hemodynamic improvement, as well as increased survival (115–117). Although these studies have primarily involved adult patients, children have also been treated with continuous intravenous prostacyclin. Two examples of long-term follow-up with children receiving continuous prostacyclin are shown in Tables 4 and 5 and Figure 13. Despite maximal standard therapy, a 6-year-old girl, with severe primary pulmonary hypertension, rapidly

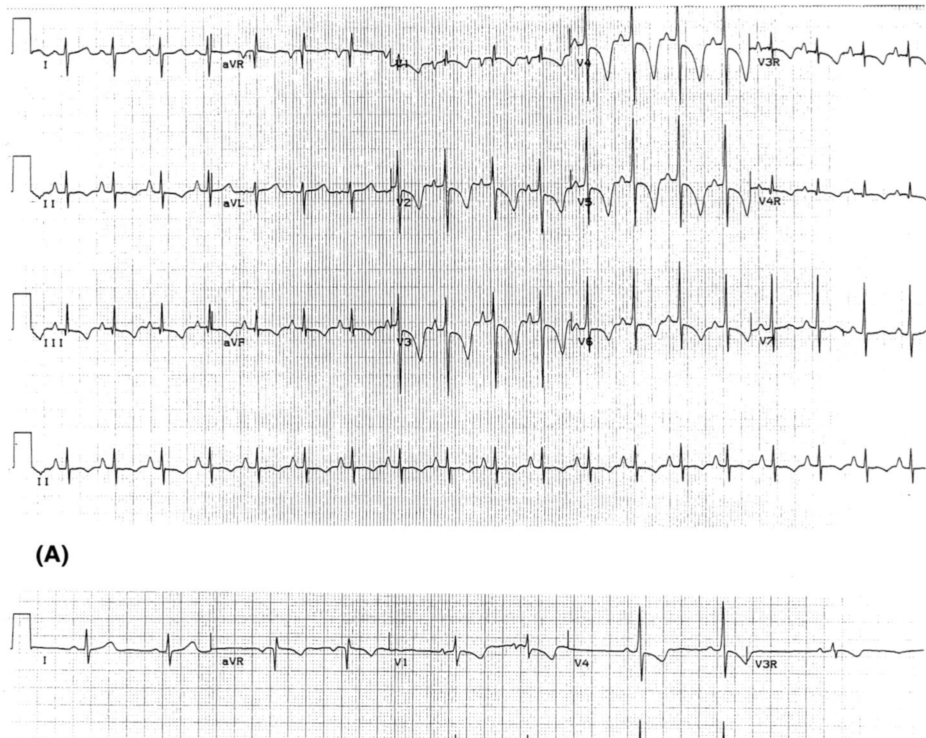

(A)

(B)

Figure 11 Electrocardiograms (A) before and after (B) 6 months of continued calcium channel blockade therapy in a 7-year-old boy. The axis decreased from 120° to 70°, right atrial enlargement resolved, and the decrease in R wave voltage in leads V_1 and V_3R suggests regression of right ventricular hypertrophy. The right ventricular strain pattern also resolved.

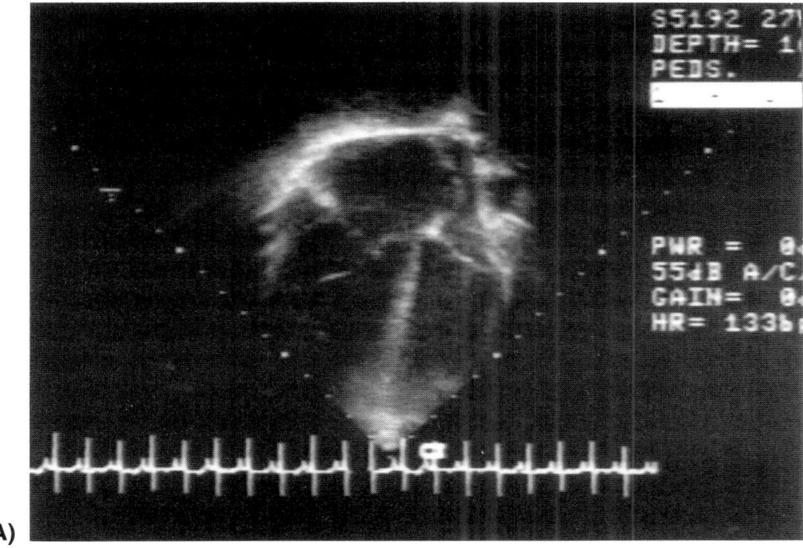

(A)

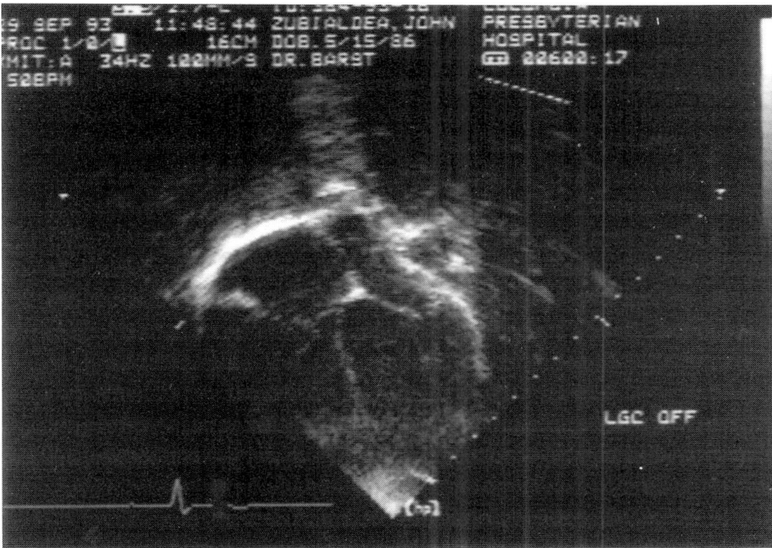

(B)

Figure 12 Two-dimensional (2-D) echocardiograms (A) before and (B) after 6 months of continued calcium channel blockade therapy in a 7-year-old boy. On a nifedipine regimen, the right ventricle decreased in size, the systolic posterior bowing of the interventricular septum resolved, as well as the posterior bowing of the interatrial septum resolving. The estimated peak systolic gradient decreased from 79 to 37 mmHg. The systolic pulmonary artery pressure at the time of the initial 2-D echocardiogram was 72 mmHg. The patient has not had a follow-up cardiac catheterization.

Table 4 Hemodynamic Effects of Long-Term Continuous Intravenous Prostacyclin in a 6-Year-Old Girl with Severe Primary Pulmonary Hypertension who Failed Conventional Vasodilator Therapy

	Baseline	Prostacyclin
Pulmonary artery pressure (mmHg)	102/57 $\overline{76}$	26/6 $\overline{15}$
Systemic arterial pressure (mmHg)	108/64 $\overline{80}$	94/52 $\overline{68}$
Right atrial pressure (mmHg)	18	4
Cardiac index (L/min/M^2)	2.6	7.2
Pulmonary vascular resistance (units/M^2)	25.4	1.1
Mixed venous O_2 saturation (%)	49	78
Systemic arterial O_2 saturation (%)	94	96

Baseline values were obtained prior to starting prostacyclin; prostacyclin values were obtained after 2 years of continuous prostacyclin treatment.

deteriorated while receiving oral vasodilator therapy and was started on a continuous prostacyclin regimen as a bridge to transplantation. Given her marked hemodynamic and clinical improvement (New York Heart Association; NYHA class IV to NYHA class I), she was taken off the transplantation list and continues to be treated with continuous prostacyclin as an alternative to transplantation. Her ECG, echocardiogram, and magnetic resonance imaging studies are shown in Figures 14–16 before starting prostacyclin and after 2 years of treatment. Table 5 and Figure 13 show the hemodynamic response to continuous prostacyclin in a 6-month-old girl with severe primary pulmonary hypertension. Her ECG and echocardiogram before starting the prostacyclin therapy and after 6 months of prostacyclin treatment are shown in Figures 17 and 18. This infant was not

Table 5 Hemodynamic Effects of Continuous Intravenous Prostacyclin in a 6-Month-Old Girl with Severe Primary Pulmonary Hypertension

	Baseline	Prostacyclin
Pulmonary artery pressure (mmHg)	100/50 $\overline{74}$	18/3 $\overline{11}$
Systemic arterial pressure (mmHg)	70/40 $\overline{55}$	100/50 $\overline{69}$
Right atrial pressure (mmHg)	6	0
Cardiac index (L/min/M^2)	2.5	7.2
Pulmonary vascular resistance (units/M^2)	26.5	1.5
Mixed venous O_2 saturation (%)	51	67
Systemic arterial O_2 saturation (%)	90	94

Baseline values were obtained prior to starting prostacyclin; prostacyclin values were obtained after 6 months of continuous prostacyclin treatment.

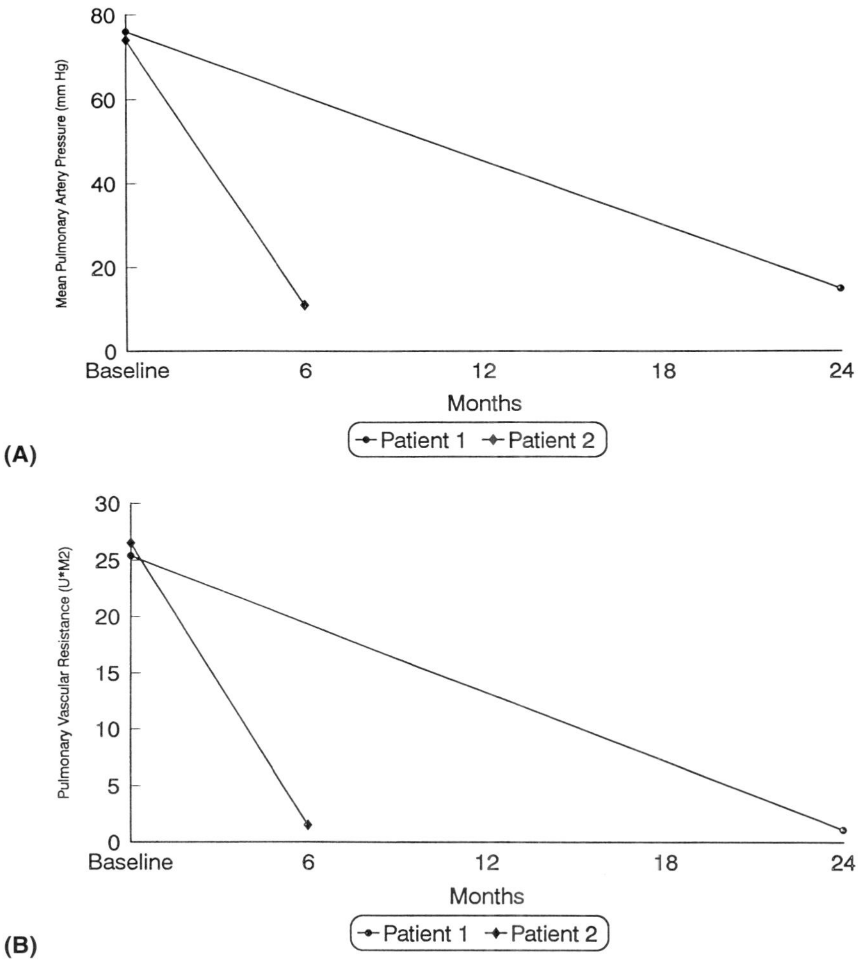

Figure 13 Effects of long-term continuous intravenous infusion of prostacyclin on (A) mean pulmonary artery pressure and (B) on pulmonary vascular resistance index in two children with severe primary pulmonary hypertension. Values shown were measured at baseline (before starting prostacyclin therapy) and at follow-up cardiac catheterization.

evaluated with oral vasodilator therapy before starting prostacyclin owing to the presence of severe right ventricular dysfunction. Long-term prostacyclin therapy significantly improved this infant clinically as well as hemodynamically (Table 5). Indices of right ventricular hypertrophy on ECG were also improved with prostacyclin therapy (Fig. 18). As these two examples demonstrate, prostacyclin

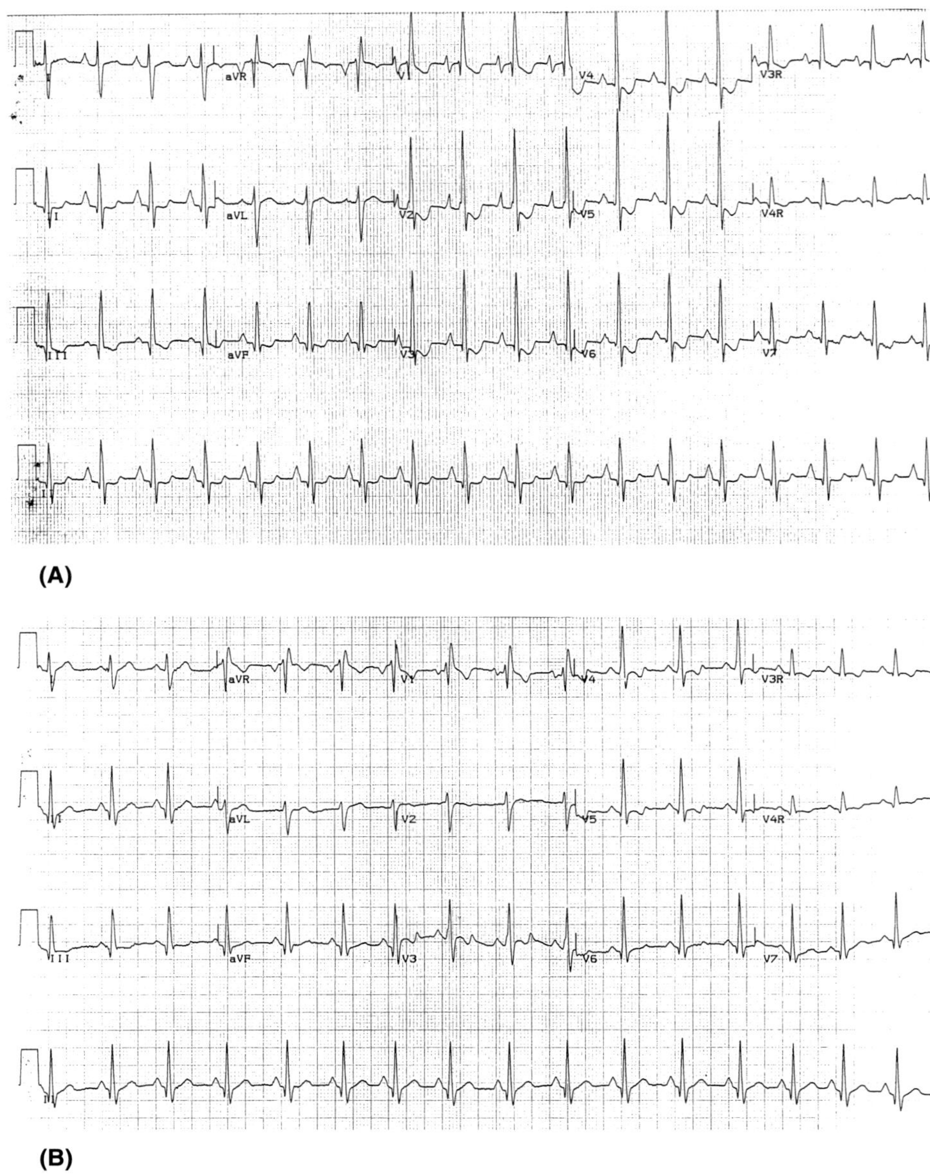

Figure 14 Electrocardiograms (A) before and (B) after 2 years of prostacyclin therapy in a 6-year-old girl. On the prostacyclin regimen, the axis decreased from 110° to 90°, right atrial enlargement resolved, and the decrease in R wave voltage in leads V_1 and V_3R suggests regression of right ventricular hypertrophy. The right ventricular strain pattern also resolved.

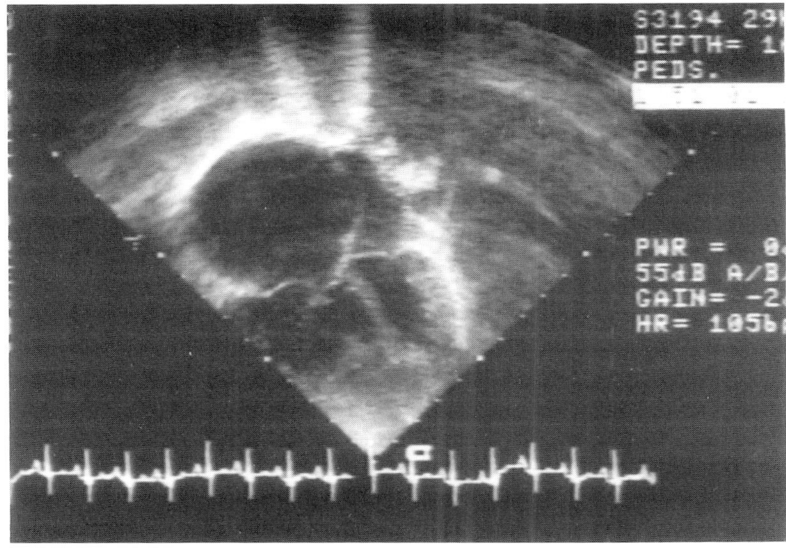

(A)

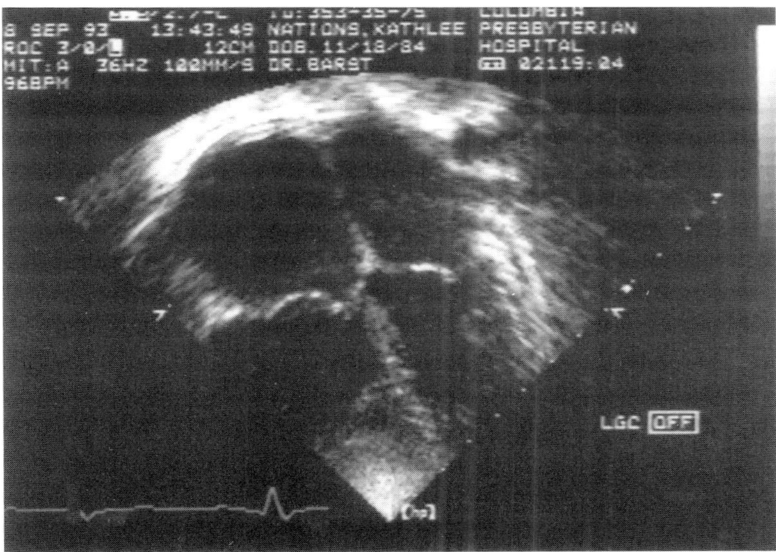

(B)

Figure 15 A 2-D echocardiograms (A) before and (B) after 2 years of prostacyclin therapy in a 6-year-old girl. On the prostacyclin regimen, the right ventricle decreased in size, the systolic posterior bowing of the interventricular septum decreased, and the posterior bowing of the interatrial septum resolved, consistent with her decrease in pulmonary hypertension (see Table 4). The estimated peak systolic gradient decreased from 100 to 27 mmHg (with the measured systolic pulmonary artery pressure decreasing from 102 to 26 mmHg).

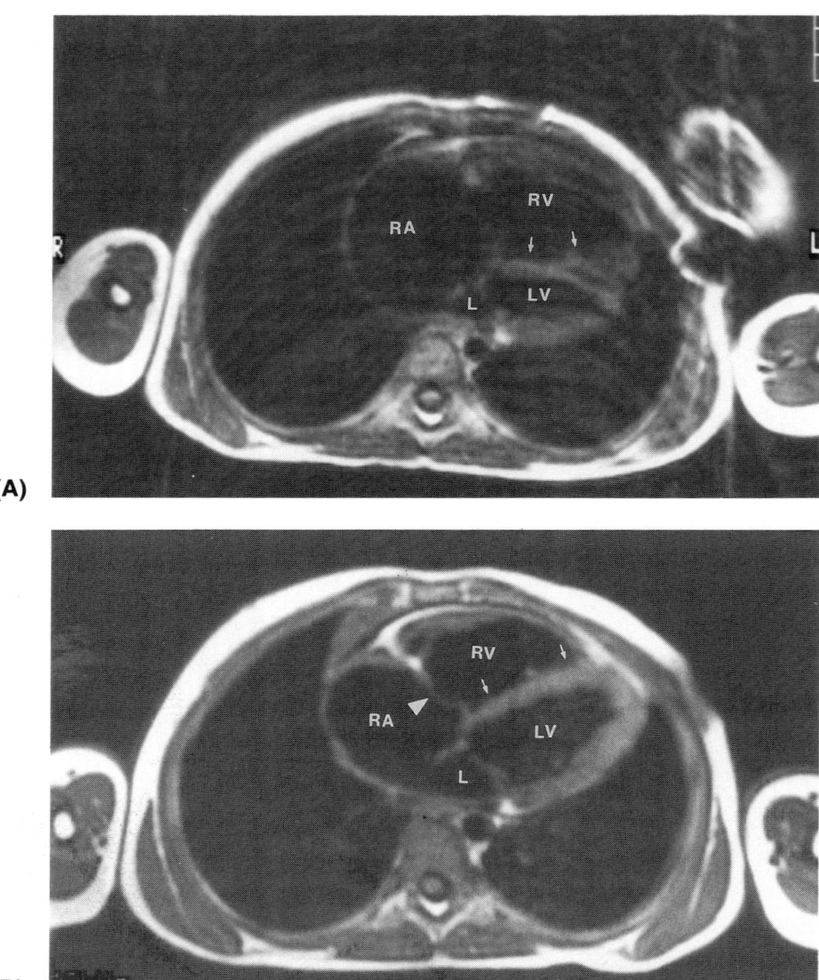

Figure 16 Magnetic resonance imaging studies (A) before and (B) after two years of prostacyclin therapy. (A) ECG-gated spin echo image in axial section obtained at end-diastole. TR (repetition time) = 412 msec; TE (echo time) = 30 msec; slice thickness = 10 mm. The interventricular septum (arrows) is bowed toward the left ventricle (LV). Right ventricular (RV) and right atrial (RA) dilatation secondary to tricuspid regurgitation is evident. The inferior aspect of the left atrium (L) may be seen. (B) End diastolic ECG-gated image at the same level in the heart obtained 2 years later: TR = 618 msec; TE = 20 msec; slice thickness = 10 mm. The interventricular septum (arrows) has returned to its normal convexity toward the right ventricle (RV). Note the tricuspid valve (arrow head).

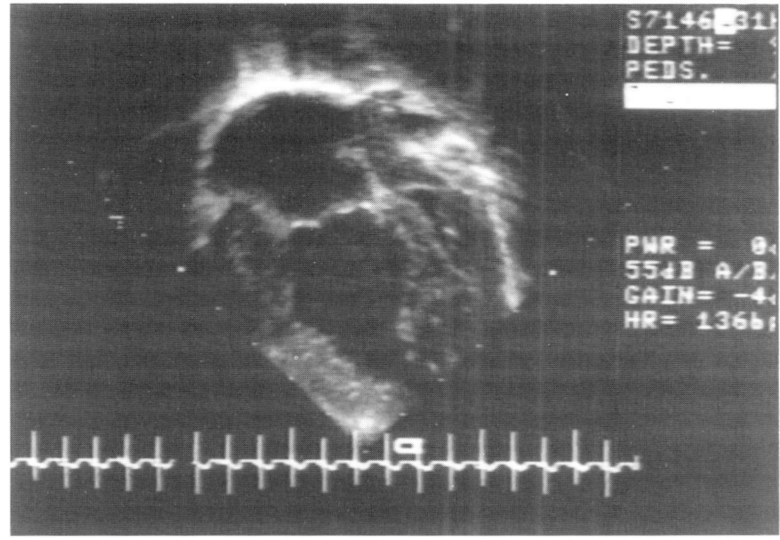

(A)

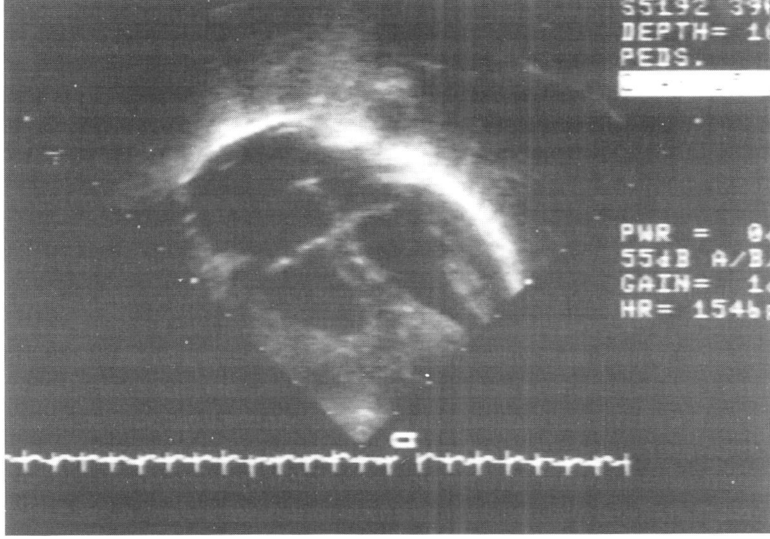

(B)

Figure 17 A 2-D echocardiogram (A) before and (B) after 6 months of prostacyclin therapy in a 6-month-old infant. On a prostacyclin regimen, the right ventricle decreased in size, the systolic posterior bowing of the interventricular septum decreased, and the posterior bowing of the interatrial septum resolved, consistent with her decrease in pulmonary hypertension (see Table 5).

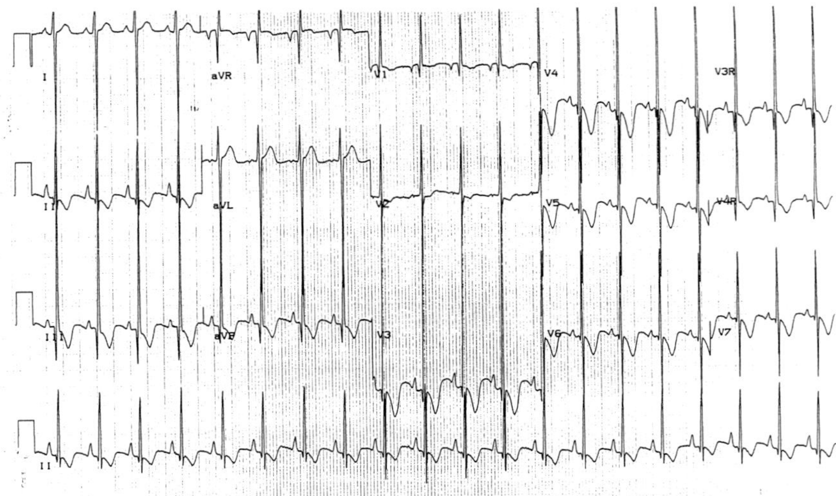

(A)

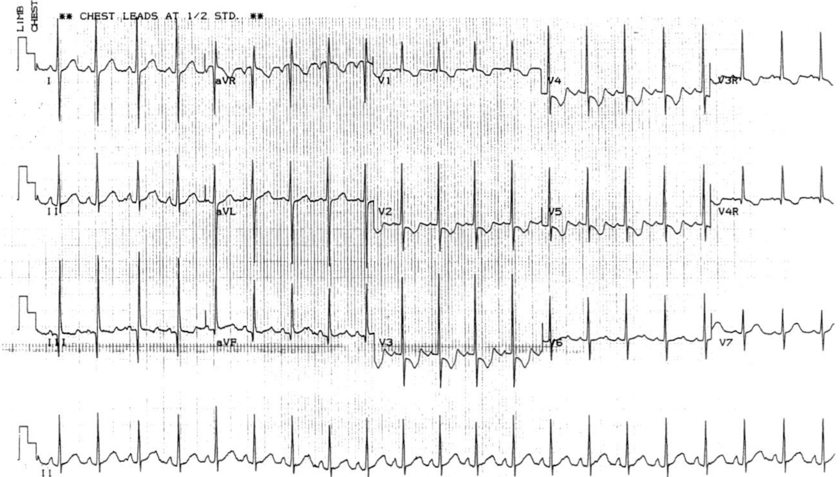

(B)

Figure 18 Electrocardiograms (A) before and (B) after 6 months of prostacyclin treatment in a 6-month-old infant. The rightward axis decreased from 125° to 100°, right atrial enlargement resolved, and the decrease in R wave voltage in leads V_1 and V_3R suggests regression of right ventricular hypertrophy. The right ventricular strain pattern also resolved.

therapy may be a suitable alternative to transplantation in selected children, in addition to being a palliative bridge to transplantation in others. Although the two major pharmacological properties of prostacyclin are inhibition of platelet aggregation (118–120) and a direct vasodilator effect (pulmonary and systemic; 121–126), prostacyclin has many other physiological effects that may play a role in the response to long-term therapy (127–134). Since the risks of transplantation are even less well known in children than in adults, effective clinical palliation now remains the hallmark for treating primary pulmonary hypertension in children.

Nitric oxide is an inhaled vasodilator that exerts selective effects on the pulmonary circulation (135). Preliminary studies reported clinical improvement in infants with persistent fetal circulation treated with inhaled nitric oxide (136,137). Despite the differences between primary pulmonary hypertension and persistent fetal circulation, these studies suggest that inhaled nitric oxide may also be useful in the treatment of PPH. Improvements in gas exchange and pulmonary hemodynamics have been reported with nitric oxide treatment of acute pulmonary hypertension following repair of a ventricular septal defect in a 3-month-old infant (138). Pepke-Zaba et al. (36) compared the immediate effects of inhaled nitric oxide with intravenous prostacyclin in eight patients with PPH and reported similar changes in pulmonary vascular resistance with both agents. Although pulmonary vascular resistance fell after prostacyclin administration, inhaled nitric oxide had no effect on pulmonary vascular resistance. Preliminary reports suggest that nitric oxide may also be useful in treating acute pulmonary hypertension crises (i.e., during an episode of pneumonia). A potential advantage of nitric oxide over prostacyclin is that increased ventilation–perfusion mismatching, with worsening systemic arterial oxygenation, should not occur with nitric oxide, since its effects should be manifest only in adequately ventilated areas of the lung.

The duration of vasodilator treatment in children in whom pulmonary artery pressures decrease to "normal" is unclear. Recurrences of primary pulmonary hypertension after discontinuing vasodilators have been reported in adults (11). From a risk–benefit consideration, we currently recommend continuing long-term vasodilator treatment indefinitely in children who respond favorably to therapy. Whether a child whose pulmonary artery pressure decreases to "normal" on intravenous prostacyclin can be switched to oral vasodilator therapy at some time in the future remains unknown. We now recommend continuing the prostacyclin for at least several years, once pulmonary artery pressure returns to normal, then reevaluating the child to determine the optimal approach.

D. Supplemental Oxygen Therapy

Continuous oxygen has been demonstrated to improve survival in adult patients with chronic lung disease with alveolar hypoxia (139), although the role of oxygen in patients without alveolar hypoxia remains unclear (140). Some children, who remain fully saturated while awake, demonstrate modest systemic arterial oxygen desaturation with sleep, which appears to be due to mild hypoventilation. During these episodes, children may experience severe dyspnea, and syncope with or without hypoxic seizures. Desaturation during sleep usually occurs during the early-morning hours and can be eliminated by using supplemental oxygen.

We recommend that children have supplemental oxygen available at home for emergency use, even if they do not use it on a routine basis. Children should also be treated with supplemental oxygen during significant upper respiratory tract infections if systemic arterial oxygen desaturation occurs, even if the child is treated at home with oral antibiotics. If more than mild oxygen desaturation occurs, the child should be treated in a hospital setting. Children with desaturation due to right-to-left shunting through a patent foramen ovale usually do not improve their oxygen saturation with supplemental oxygen. However, based on a study of children with Eisenmenger's syndrome that demonstrated improved long-term survival with supplemental oxygen (141), children with right-to-left shunting through a patent foramen ovale, who increase their oxygen saturation during sleep with supplemental oxygen, may benefit from treatment with nocturnal oxygen. Supplemental oxygen may also reduce the degree of polycythemia in patients with significant intracardiac right-to-left shunting.

E. Additional Pharmacotherapy

Cardiac Glycosides, Diuretics, Antiarrhythmic Therapy, Inotropic Agents, and Nitrates

Although controversy persists concerning the value of digitalis in primary pulmonary hypertension (142), we believe that children with right-sided heart failure may benefit from digitalis, in addition to diuretic therapy. Diuretic therapy must be instituted cautiously, since patients appear to be extremely dependent on preload to maintain optimal cardiac output. Despite this, relatively high doses of diuretic therapy are commonly needed.

Although malignant arrhythmias are rare in primary pulmonary hypertension, they should be treated if documented. Atrial flutter or fibrillation often precipitates an abrupt decrease in cardiac output and clinical deterioration once atrial systole is lost. As opposed to normal persons, in whom atrial systole is responsible for approximately 25% of the cardiac output, atrial systole in patients with primary pulmonary hypertension often contributes as much as 70% of the cardiac output. Therefore, aggressive treatment of atrial flutter or fibrillation is advised. We recommend treating patients with clinically significant supraventricular tachycardias as well as frequent episodes of nonsustained ventricular tachycardia and complex ventricular arrhythmias, but would be inclined to avoid treatment of lesser grades of arrhythmia.

There are no studies on the usefulness of intermittent or continuous treatment with inotropic agents. We occasionally add dobutamine, for additional inotropic support, to continuous intravenous prostacyclin for a child with severe right ventricular dysfunction until lung transplantation can be performed. We also recommend short-term inotropic support in selected patients before performing an atrial septostomy (see following section). Children have occasionally benefited from short-term inotropic support, using dobutamine or amrinone during an acute pulmonary hypertensive crisis to augment cardiac output during a period of increased metabolic demands.

Oral and topical nitrates have been used to treat some children with PPH, although the experience with these agents remains limited. Children who complain of chest tightness, pressure, or vague discomfort that is responsive to sublingual nitroglycerin, may also benefit from long-term transdermal nitroglycerin therapy.

F. Atrial Septostomy

Patients with recurrent syncope or severe right-sided heart failure have a very poor prognosis (1,2). Exercise-induced syncope is due to systemic vasodilatation, with an inability to augment cardiac output to maintain cerebral perfusion pressure. Thoele et al. reported that patients with PPH and recurrent syncope do not have adequate shunting through a patent foramen ovale (144). If right-to-left shunting through an interatrial communication is present, cardiac output can be maintained or increased as necessary. Furthermore, right-to-left shunting at the atrial level alleviates signs and symptoms of right-sided heart failure by decompression of the right atrium and right ventricle. Increased survival has been reported in patients with a patent foramen ovale (143), although this has been questioned recently (145). Patency of the foramen ovale may improve survival if it allows sufficient right-to-left shunting to occur to maintain cardiac output, as is evidenced by significant systemic arterial oxygen desaturation at rest or during exercise.

Successful palliation of symptoms with a blade balloon atrial septostomy has been reported in patients with advanced pulmonary vascular disease, with variable clinical improvement (146–148). Recently, Kerstein et al. reported significant clinical and hemodynamic improvement in PPH patients with recurrent syncope and right heart failure (149,150). No patient experienced further syncope, and signs and symptoms improved in all patients with right-sided heart failure. Although systemic arterial oxygen saturation decreased, cardiac output and oxygen delivery improved through right-to-left shunting at the atrial level. In addition, the 1- and 2-year survival rates (87 and 76%, respectively) were significantly improved following atrial septostomy, compared with standard therapy (54 and 42% at 1 and 2 years, respectively; Fig. 19). Although blade balloon atrial septostomy does not alter the underlying disease process, it may improve the quality of life. Blade balloon atrial septostomy may be particularly useful as a

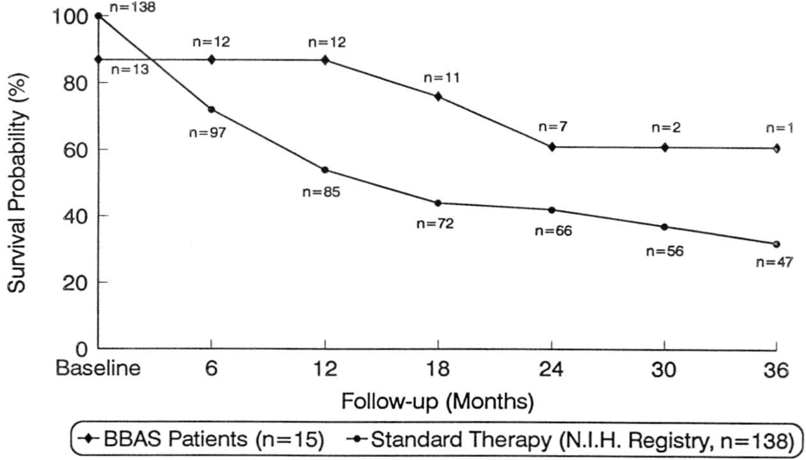

Figure 19 Probability of survival for patients who underwent blade balloon atrial septostomy ($n = 15$) versus patients treated with standard therapy from the NIH Primary Pulmonary Hypertension Registry ($n = 138$). Survival was significantly improved in the blade balloon atrial septostomy patients ($p < 0.01$ at 1 and 2 years; $p < 0.1$ at 3 years). (From Ref. 150.)

palliative bridge to transplantation, although it should be emphasized that this invasive procedure is not without risk and remains investigational at this time. Closure of the septal defect can be performed at the time of transplantation.

G. Transplantation

Heart–lung, single-lung, and bilateral-lung transplantation have been performed successfully for primary pulmonary hypertension (154,155), primarily in adults (see Chapter 12). A role for living, donor-related lung transplantation using the child's parents as donors is theoretically very appealing. Preliminary results suggest parental donor lung transplantation may decrease postoperative morbidity and improve long-term survival.

VII. Conclusions

Primary pulmonary hypertension in children remains a devastating disease, although recent therapeutic advances appear to have significantly improved its natural history. Future developments in vascular biology will help us improve our understanding of the etiology and pathogenesis, as well as provide the rationale for specific medical therapies. We hope that by increasing our understanding of the pathogenesis and pathophysiology of PPH, one day we will be able to prevent or cure this disease, as opposed to providing palliative therapy.

References

1. Thilenius OG, Nadas AS, Jockin H. Primary pulmonary vascular obstruction in children. Pediatrics 1965; 36:75–87.
2. D'Alonzo GE, Barst RJ, Ayres SM, et al. Survival in patients with primary pulmonary hypertension: results from a national prospective registry. Ann Intern Med 1991; 115:343–349.
3. Wagenvoort CA, Wagenvoort N. Primary pulmonary hypertension. A pathological study of the lung vessels in 156 clinically diagnosed cases. Circulation 1970; 42: 1163–1184.
4. Grover RF, Vogel JHK, Averill KH, Blount SG. Pulmonary hypertension. Individual and species variability relative to vascular reacticity. Am Heart J 1963; 66:1.
5. Grover RF, Will DH, Reeves JT, Weir EK, McMurtry IF, Alexander AF. Genetic transmission of susceptibility to hypoxic pulmonary hypertension. Prog Respir Res 1975; 9:112–117.
6. Vogel JHK. Importance of mild hypoxia on abnormal pulmonary vascular beds. Adv Cardiol 1970; 5:159.
7. Vogel JHK, McNamara DG, Blount SG. Role of hypoxia in determining pulmonary vascular resistance in infants with ventricular septal defects. Am J Cardiol 1967; 20:346.
8. O'Neill D, Morton R, Kennedy JA. Progressive primary pulmonary hypertension in a patient born at high altitude. Br Heart J 1981; 45:725.
9. Gersony WM, Duc GV, Sinclair JC. "PFC" syndrome (persistence of the fetal circulation) (abstrt). Circulation 1969; 40S:III:87.
10. Long WA. Persistent pulmonary hypertension of the newborn syndrome. In: Long WA, ed. Fetal and Neonatal Cardiology. Philadelphia: WB Saunders, 1989:627–655.
11. Reeves JT, Groves BM, Turkevich D. The case for treatment of selected patients with primary pulmonary hypertension. Am Rev Respir Dis 1986; 134:342–346.
12. Heath D, Edwards JE. Configuration of elastic tissue of pulmonary trunk in idiopathic pulmonary hypertension. Circulation 1960; 21:59.
13. Roberts WC. The histologic structure of the pulmonary trunk in patients with "primary" pulmonary hypertension. Am Heart J 1963; 65:230.
14. Blieden LC, Moller JH. Small ventricular septal defect associated with severe pulmonary hypertension. Br Heart J 1984; 52:117.
15. Bissett GS III, Hirschfeld SS. Severe pulmonary hypertension associated with a small ventricular septal defect. Circulation 1983; 67:470.
16. Haworth SG. Pulmonary vascular disease in secundum atrial septal defect in childhood. Am J Cardiol 1983; 51:265.
17. Morse JH, Barst RJ, Fotino M. Familial pulmonary hypertension: immunogenetic findings in four Caucasian kindreds. Am Rev Respir Dis 1992; 145:787–792.

18. Rich S, Dantzker DR, Ayres SM, et al. Primary pulmonary hypertension: a national prospective study. Ann Intern Med 1987; 107:216–223.
19. Loyd JE, Primm RK, Newman JH. Familial primary pulmonary hypertension: clinical patterns. Am Rev Respir Dis 1984; 129:194–197.
20. Loyd JE, Atkinson JB, Pietra GG, Virmani R, Newman JH. Heterogeneity of pathologic lesions in familial primary pulmonary hypertension. Am Rev Respir Dis 1988; 138:952–957.
21. Barst RJ. Pharmacologically induced pulmonary vasodilatation in children and young adults with primary pulmonary hypertension. Chest 1986; 98:497–503.
22. Edwards WD, Edwards KE. Clinical primary pulmonary hypertension: three pathologic types. Circulation 1977; 56:884–888.
23. Yamaki S, Wagenvoort CA. Comparison of primary plexogenic arteriopathy in adults and children. Br Heart J 1985; 54:428–434.
24. Rich S, Brundage BH. High dose calcium channel blocking therapy for primary pulmonary hypertension: evidence for long-term reduction in pulmonary arterial pressure and regression of right ventricular hypertrophy. Circulation 1987; 76: 135–141.
25. Rich S, Kaufmann E, Levy PS. The effect of high doses of calcium-channel blockers on survival in primary pulmonary hypertension. N Engl J Med 1992; 327:76–81.
26. Heath D, Whitaker W. Hypertensive pulmonary vascular disease. Circulation 1956; 25:323–343.
27. Rich S, Kieras K, Hart K, Groves BM, Stodo JD, Brundage BH. Antinuclear antibodies in primary pulmonary hypertension. J Am Coll Cardiol 1986; 8:1307–1311.
28. Barst RJ, Flaster ER, Menom A, Fotino M, Morse JH. Evidence for the association of unexplained pulmonary hypertension in children with the major histocompatibility complex. Circulation 1992; 85:249–258.
29. Gurtner HP. Aminorex and pulmonary hypertension. Cor Vasa 1985; 27:160–171.
30. Yamaki S, Horiuchi T, Miura M, Suzuki Y, Ishizawa E, Takahashi T. Pulmonary vascular disease in secundum atrial septal defect with pulmonary hypertension. Chest 1986; 89:694–698.
31. Davies PF. How do vascular endothelial cells respond to flow? Notes Physiol Sci 1989; 4:22–25.
32. Guazzi MD, Alimeato M, Fiorentini C, Pep M, Polese A. Hypersensitivity of lung vessels to catecholamines in systemic hypertension. Br Med J 1986; 293:291–294.
33. Barst RJ, Stalcup SA, Steeg CN, Hall JC, Frosolono MF, Cato AE, Mellins RB. Relation of arachidonate metabolites to abnormal control of the pulmonary circulation in a child. Am Rev Respir Dis 1985; 131:171–177.
34. Montalevscot G, Lowenstein E, Ogletree ML, et al. Thromboxane receptor blockade prevents pulmonary hypertension induced by heparin-protamine reactions in awake sheep. Circulation 1990; 82:1765–1777.
35. Christman BW, McPherson CD, Newman JH, et al. An imbalance between the excretion of thromboxane and prostacyclin metabolites in pulmonary hypertension. N Engl J Med 1991; 327:70–75.
36. Pepke-Zaba J, Higginbottam TW, Dinh-Xuan AT, Stone D, Wallwork J. Inhaled

nitric oxide as a cause of selective pulmonary vasodilatation in pulmonary hypertension. Lancet 1991; 338:1173–1174.
37. Yoshibayashi M, Nishioka K, Nakao K, et al. Plasma endothelin concentrations in patients with pulmonary hypertension associated with congenital heart defects: evidence for increased production of endothelin in pulmonary circulation. Circulation 1991; 84:2280–2285.
38. Rabinovitch M, Andrew M, Thom H, et al. Abnormal endothelial factor VIII associated with pulmonary hypertension and congenital heart defects. Circulation 1987; 76:1043–1052.
39. Geggel RL, Carvalho CA, Hoyer LW, Reid LM. von Willebrand factor abnormalities in primary pulmonary hypertension. Am Rev Respir Dis 1987; 135:294–299.
40. Rosenberg HC, Rabinovitch M. Endothelial injury and vascular reactivity in monocrotaline pulmonary hypertension. Am J Physiol 1988; 255:H1484–1491.
41. Todorovich-Hunter L, Johnson DJ, Ranger P, Keeley FW, Rabinovitch M. Altered elastin and collagen synthesis associated with progressive pulmonary hypertension induced by monocrotaline: a biochemical and ultrastructural study. Lab Invest 1988; 58:184–195.
42. Smith P, Heath D, Yacoub M, et al. The ultrastructure of plexogenic pulmonary arteriopathy. J Pathol 1990; 160:111–121.
43. Ryan US. The endothelial surface and responses to injury. Fed Proc 1986; 45:101–108.
44. Eisenberg PR, Lucore C, Kaufmann E, et al. Fibrinopeptide A levels indicative of pulmonary vascular thrombosis in patients with primary pulmonary hypertension. Circulation 1990; 82:841–847.
45. Scully RE, Mark EJ, McNeely BE. Case records of the Massachusetts General Hospital: weekly clinicopathological exercises. N Engl J Med 1983; 309:1627–1636.
46. Vane JR. The release and fate of vasoactive hormones in the circulation. Br J Pharmacol 1969; 35:209–242.
47. Bakhle YS, Vane JR. Pharmacokinetic function of the pulmonary circulation. Physiol Rev 1974; 1007–1045.
48. Junod AF. Metabolism, production and release of hormones and mediators in the lung. Am Rev Respir Dis 1975; 122:93–108.
49. Gillis CN, Greene NM. Possible clinical implications of metabolism of blood borne substances by the human lung. In: Bakhle YS, Vane JR, eds. Metabolic Functions of the Lung. New York: Marcel Dekker, 1977:173–193.
50. Said SI. Metabolic functions of the pulmonary circulation. Circ Res 1982; 50: 325–333.
51. Barst RJ, Stalcup SA. Endothelial function in clinical pulmonary hypertension. Chest 1985; 88S:216S–220S.
52. Allen SW, Chatfield BA, Koppenhafer SA, Schaffer MS, Wolfe RR, Abman SH. Circulating immunoreactive endothelin-1 in children with pulmonary hypertension: association with acute hypoxic pulmonary vasoreactivity. Am Rev Respir Dis 1993; 148:519–522.
53. Giaid A, Yanagisawa M, Iangleben D, Michel RP, Levy R, Shennib H, Kimura S, Masaki T, Duguid WP, Stewart DJ. Expression of endothelin-1 in the lungs of patients with pulmonary hypertension. N Engl J Med 1993; 328:1732–1739.

54. van Grondelle A, Voelkel NF, Mathias M, et al. Lung prostaglandin production with change in shear stress and vascular distension. Fed Proc 1982; 41:1749.
55. Reeves JT, van Grondelle A, Voelkel NF, et al. Prostacyclin production and lung endothelial cell shear stress. In: Sutton JR, Houston CS, Jones NL, eds. Hypoxia, Exercise, and Altitude: Proceedings of the Third Banff International Hypoxia Symposium. New York: Alan R Liss, 1983:125–131.
56. Rodbard S. Vascular caliber. Cardiology 1975; 60:4–49.
57. Fry DL. Acute vascular endothelial changes associated with increased blood velocity gradients. Circ Res 1968; 22:165–197.
58. Schaub RG, Rawlings CA, Keith JC. Platelet adhesion and myointimal proliferation in canine pulmonary arteries. Am J Pathol 1981; 104:13–22.
59. Celermajer DS, Cullen S, Deanfield JE. Impairment of endothelium-dependent pulmonary artery relaxation in children with congenital heart disease and abnormal pulmonary hemodynamics. Circulation 1993; 87:440–446.
60. Kadowitz PJ, Joiner PD, Hyman AL. Effect of sympathetic nerve stimulation on pulmonary vascular resistance in the intact spontaneously breathing dog. Proc Soc Exp Med 1974; 147:68–71.
61. Lock JE, Olley PR, Coceani F. Enhanced beta-adrenergic-receptor responsiveness in hypoxic neonatal pulmonary circulation. Am J Physiol 1981; 240:H697–H703.
62. Gillis CN, Greene NM, Cronau LH, Hammond GL. Pulmonary extraction of 5-hydroxytryptamine and norepinephrine before and after cardiopulmonary bypass in man. Circ Res 1972; 30:666.
63. Sole MJ, Drobac M, Schwartz L, et al. The extraction of circulating catecholamines by the lungs in normal man and in patients with pulmonary hypertension. Circulation 1979; 60:160–163.
64. Gewitz MH, Pitt BR, Laks H, et al. Reversible changes in norepinephrine extraction by the lungs in children with pulmonary hypertension. Pediatr Pharmacol 1982; 2: 57–63.
65. Zaloga GP, Chernow B, Fletcher JR, et al. Increased circulating plasma norepinephrine concentrations in noncardiac causes of pulmonary hypertension. Crit Care Med 1984; 12:85–89.
66. Barst RJ, Stalcup SA, Mellins RB. Endogenous catecholamines in children with pulmonary hypertension. Am Rev Respir Dis 1984; 129:A340.
67. Ruskin JN, Hutter AM Jr. Primary pulmonary hypertension treated with oral phentolamine. Ann Intern Med 1979; 90:772–774.
68. Robalino BD, Moodie DS. Association between primary pulmonary hypertension and portal hypertension: analysis of its pathophysiology and clinical, laboratory and hemodynamic manifestations. J Am Coll Cardiol 1991; 17:492–498.
69. Barst RJ, Long WA, Gersony WM. Long-term vasodilator treatment improves survival in children with primary pulmonary hypertension. (in press).
70. Asherson RA, Higenbottam TW, Dinh Xuan AT, Khamashta MA, Hughes GRV. Pulmonary hypertension in a lupus clinic: experience with twenty-four patients. J Rheumatol 1990; 17:1292–1298.
71. Stupi AM, Steen VD, Ownes GR, Barnes EL, Rodnan GP, Medsger TA Jr. Primary pulmonary hypertension in the CREST syndrome variant of systemic sclerosis. Arthritis Rheum 1986; 29:515–524.

72. Asherson RA, Morgan SH, Hackett D, Montanes P, Oakley C, Hughes GRV. Rheumatoid arthritis and pulmonary hypertension: a report of three cases. J Rheumatol 1985; 12:154–159.
73. Graziano FM, Friedman LC, Grossman J. Pulmonary hypertension in a patient with mixed connective tissue disease: clinical and pathological findings and a review of the literature. Clin Exp Rheumatol 1983; 1:251–255.
74. Caldwell IW, Atchison JD. Pulmonary hypertension in dermatomyositis. Br Heart J 1956; 18:272–276.
75. Morse JH, Barst RJ, Fotino M. Inheritance of shared parental HLA-DR,D2 (class II) alleles in children with unexplained pulmonary hypertension. Circulation 1993; 88:I-285.
76. Long WA, Groves BM, Rubin LJ, Reeves JT, Barst RJ, Moser KM, Mellins RB, Palevsky HI, Fishman AP, Frosolono MF. Acute hemodynamic effects of prostacyclin in 100 patients with primary pulmonary hypertension. Circulation (in press).
77. Gomez-Sanchez MA, Mestre de Juan MJ, Gomez-Pajuelo C, Lopez JI, Diaz de Atauri MJ, Martinez-Tello FJ. Pulmonary hypertension due to toxic oil syndrome: a clinicopathologic study. Chest 1989; 95:325–331.
78. Gomez-Sanchez MA, Saene de la Calzada C, Gomez-Pajuelo C, Martinez-Tello FJ, Mestre de Juan MJ, James TN. Clinical and pathologic manifestation of pulmonary vascular disease in the toxic oil syndrome. J Am Coll Cardiol 1991; 18:1539–1545.
79. Auger WR, Fedullo PF, Moser KM, Buchbinder M, Peterson K. Chronic major-vessel thromboembolic pulmonary artery obstruction: appearance at angiography. Radiology 1992; 182:393–398.
80. Rabinovitch M, Keane JF, Fellows KG, Castaneda AR, Reid L. Quantitative analysis of the pulmonary wedge angiogram in congenital heart defects. Circulation 1981; 63:152–164.
81. Boxt LM, Katz J, Kolb T, Czegledy FP, Barst RJ. Direct quantitation of right and left ventricular volumes using nuclear magnetic resonance imaging in patients with primary pulmonary hypertension. J Am Coll Cardiol 1992; 19:1508–1515.
82. Katz J, Whang J, Boxt LM, Barst RJ. MRI estimation of right ventricular mass in normals and in patients with primary pulmonary hypertension. J Am Coll Cardiol 1993; 21:L1475–1481.
83. Mikkilineni S, Barst RJ, Cropp GJ. Pulmonary function in primary pulmonary hypertension. Pediatr Res 1990; 27:359A.
84. Rhodes J, Barst RJ, Garofano RP, Thoele DG, Gersony WM. Hemodynamic correlates of exercise function in patients with primary pulmonary hypertension. J Am Coll Cardiol 1991; 18:1738–1744.
85. Speich R, Jenni R, Oprvil M, Pfab M, Russi EW. Primary pulmonary hypertension in HIV infection. Chest 1991; 100:1268–1271.
86. Lockshin MD. Antiphospholipid antibody syndrome. JAMA 1992; 268:1451–1453.
87. Luchi ME, Asherson RA, Lahita RG. Primary idiopathic pulmonary hypertension complicated by pulmonary arterial thrombosis: association with antiphospholipid antibodies. Arthritis Rheum 1992; 35:700–705.
88. McDonnell PJ, Toye PA, Hutchins GM. Primary pulmonary hypertension and cirrhosis: are they related? Am Rev Respir Dis 1983; 127:437–441.
89. Hashim SW, Kay HR, Hammond GL, Kopf GS, Geha AS. Noncardiogenic pulmonary edema after cardiopulmonary bypass. Am J Surg 1983; 147:560–564.

90. D'Angelo A, Della Valle P, Crippa L, Pattarini E, Grimaldi LMG, D'Angelo SV. Autoimmune protein S deficiency in a boy with severe thromboembolic disease. N Engl J Med 1993; 328:1753–1757.
91. Eaton AM, Serota H, Kernodle GW Jr, Uglietta JP, Crawford J, Fulkerson WJ. Pulmonary hypertension secondary to serum hyperviscosity in a patient with rheumatoid arthritis. Am J Med 1987; 82:1039–1045.
92. Badesch DB, Wynne KM, Bonvallet S, Voelkel NF, Ridgway C, Groves BM. Hypothyroidism and primary pulmonary hypertension: an autoimmune pathogenetic link? Ann Intern Med 1993; 119:44–46.
93. Pietra GG, Edward WD, Kay JM, et al. Histopathology of primary pulmonary hypertension: a qualitative and quantitative study of pulmonary blood vessels from 58 patients in the National Heart, Lung, and Blood Institute Primary Pulmonary Hypertension Registry. Circulation 1989; 80:1198–1206.
94. Rubin LJ, Mendoza J, Hood M, McGoon M, Barst R, Williams WB. Treatment of primary pulmonary hypertension with continuous intravenous prostacyclin (epoprostenol). Ann Intern Med 1990; 112:485–491.
95. Barst RJ, Hall JC, Gersony WM. Factors influencing survival among children with primary pulmonary hypertension treated with vasodilator agents. Circulation 1988; 78(suppl 2):293.
96. Fuster V, Steele PM, Edwards WD, Gersh BJ, McGoon MD, Frye RL. Primary pulmonary hypertension: natural history and the importance of thrombosis. Circulation 1984; 70:580–587.
97. Wagenvoort CA, Wagenvoort N. Pathology of Pulmonary Hypertension. New York: John Wiley & Sons, 1977:119–142.
98. Barst R, Long W, Gersony W. Long-term vasodilator treatment improves survival in children with primary pulmonary hypertension. Cardiol Young 1993; 3(S1):89.
99. Permutt S, Riley RL. Hemodynamics of collapsible vessels with tone: the vascular waterfall. J Appl Physiol 1963; 18:924–932.
100. Maseri A, Caldini P, Howard P, Joshir C, Permutt S, Zierler KL. Determinants of pulmonary vascular volume–recruitment versus distensibility. Circ Res 1972; 31: 218–228.
101. Rich S, D'Alonzo GE, Dantzker DR, Levy PS. Magnitude and implications of spontaneous hemodynamic variability in primary pulmonary hypertension. Am J Cardiol 1985; 55:159–163.
102. Rich S, Brundage BH, Levy PS, The effect of vasodilator therapy on the clinical outcome of patients with primary pulmonary hypertension. Circulation 1985; 71: 1191–1196.
103. Rubin LJ, Groves BM, Reeves JT, Frosolono M, Handel F, Cato AE. Prostacyclin-induced pulmonary vasodilatation in primary pulmonary hypertension. Circulation 1982; 66:334–338.
104. Packer M, Medina N, Yushak M. Adverse hemodynamic and clinical effects of calcium channel blockade in pulmonary hypertension secondary to obliterative pulmonary vascular disease. J Am Coll Cardiol 1984; 4:890.
105. Farber HW, Karlinsky JB, Faling LJ. Fatal outcome following nifedipine for primary pulmonary hypertension (letter). Chest 1983; 83:708.

106. Aromatorio GJ, Uretsky BF, Reddy PS. Hypotension and sinus arrest with nifedipine in pulmonary hypertension. Chest 1985; 87:265.
107. Hoit B, Gregoratus G, Shabetai R. Paradoxical pulmonary vasoconstriction induced by nitroglycerin in idiopathic pulmonary hypertension. J Am Coll Cardiol 1985; 6:490.
108. Buch J, Wennevold A. Hazards of diazoxide in pulmonary hypertension. Br Heart J 1981; 46:401.
109. Cohen ML, Kronzon I. Adverse hemodynamic effects of phentolamine in primary pulmonary hypertension. Ann Intern Med 1981; 95:591.
110. Elkayam U, Frishman WH, Yoran C, et al. Unfavorable hemodynamic and clinical effects of isoproterenol in primary pulmonary hypertension. Cardiovasc Med 1978; 3:1177.
111. Kronzon I, Cohen M, Winer HE. Adverse effect of hydralazine in patients with primary pulmonary hypertension. JAMA 1982; 247:3112.
112. Packer M. Vasodilator therapy for primary pulmonary hypertension: limitations and hazards. Ann Intern Med 1985; 103:258.
113. Packer M, Greenberg B, Massie B, Dash H. Deleterious effects of hydralazine in patients with primary pulmonary hypertension. N Engl J Med 1982; 306:1326.
114. Partanan J, Nieminen MS, Luomanmaki K. Death in patient with primary pulmonary hypertension after 20 mg of nifedipine. N Engl J Med 1993; 329:812–813.
115. Jones DK, Higgenbottam TW, Wallwork J. Treatment of primary pulmonary hypertension with intravenous epoprostenol (prostacyclin). Br Heart J 1987; 57:270–278.
116. Barst RJ, Rubin LJ, McGoon MD, Caldwell EJ, Long WA, Levy PS. Survival in primary pulmonary hypertension with long-term continuous intravenous prostacyclin. Ann Intern Med 1994; 121:409–415.
117. Barst RJ, Rubin LJ, Long WA, McGoon MD, Rich S, Badesch DB, Groves BM, Tapson VF, Bourge RC, Brundage BH, Koerner SK, Langleben D, Keller CA, Murali S, Uretsky BF, Clayton LM, Jobsis MM, Blackburn SD, Shortino D, Crow JW. A comparison of continuous intravenous epoprostenol with conventional therapy in primary pulmonary hypertension. N Engl J Med 1996; 334:296–301.
118. Moncada S, Korbut R, Bunting S, Vane JR. Prostacyclin is a circulating hormone. Nature 1978; 273:767.
119. Moncada S, Gryglewski R, Bunting S, Vane JR. An enzyme isolated from arteries transforms prostaglandin endoperoxides to an unstable substance that inhibits platelet aggregation. Nature 1976; 263:663.
120. Moncada S, Vane JR. Arachidonic acid metabolites and the interactions between platelets and blood-vessel walls. N Engl J Med 1979; 300:1142.
121. Gryglewski RJ, Bunting S, Moncada S, et al. Arterial walls are protected against deposition of platelet thrombi by a substance (prostaglandin X) which they make from prostaglandin endoperoxides. Prostaglandins 1976; 12:685.
122. Hintze TM, Martin EG, Messina EJ, Kaley G. Prostacyclin (PGI_2) elicits reflex bradycardia in dogs: evidence for vagal mediation. Proc Soc Exp Biol Med 1979; 162:96.
123. Hyman AL, Kadowitz PJ. Pulmonary vasodilator activity of prostacyclin (PGI_2) in the cat. Circ Res 1979; 45:404.

124. Lock JE, Olley PM, Coceani F, et al. Hemodynamic effects of intravenous (IV) indomethacin (Indo) in unsedated newborn lambs (abstrt). Circulation 1978; 58(suppl 2):II-44.
125. Lock JE, Olley PM, Coceani F, et al. Use of prostacyclin in persistent fetal circulation (letter). Lancet 1979; 1:1343.
126. Starling MB, Neutze JM, Elliott RL. Control of elevated pulmonary vascular resistance in neonatal swine with prostacyclin (PGI_2). Prostaglandins Med 1979; 3:105.
127. Camussi G, Bussolino F, Tetta C, et al. Effect of prostacyclin (PGI_2) on immune-complex-induced neutropenia. Immunology 1983; 48:625.
128. Cassin S, Winikor I, Tod M, et al. Effects of prostacyclin on the fetal pulmonary circulation. Pediatr Pharmacol 1981; 1:197.
129. Coceani F, Olley PM. Prostaglandins and the circulation at birth. In: Herman AG, Vanhoulte, PM, Denolin, H, Goosens, A, eds. Cardiovascular Pharmacology of the Prostaglandins. New York: Raven Press, 1982:303–314.
130. Coceani F, Olley PM, Lock JE. Prostaglandins, ductus arteriosus, pulmonary circulation: current concepts and clinical potential. Eur J Clin Pharmacol 1980; 18:75.
131. Konturek SJ, Brzozowski T, Piastucki I, et al. Role of mucosal prostaglandins and DNA synthesis in gastric cytoprotection by luminal epidermal growth factor. Gut 1981; 22:927.
132. Lefer AM, Ogletree ML, Smith JB, et al. Prostacyclin: a potentially valuable agent for preserving myocardial tissue in acute myocardial ischemia. Science 1978; 200:52.
133. Lefer AM, Tabas J, Smith EF III. Salutory effects of prostacyclin in endotoxin shock. Pharmacology 1980; 21:206.
134. Sterin-Borda L, Canga L, Borda ES, et al. Inotropic effect of prostacyclin (PGI_2) on isolated rat atria at different contraction frequencies. Naunyn-Schmiedebergs Arch Pharmacol 1980; 313:95.
135. Frostell C, Fratacci MD, Wain JC, Jones R, Zapol WM. Inhaled nitric oxide. A selective pulmonary vasodilator reversing hypoxic pulmonary vasoconstriction. Circulation 1991; 83:2038–2047.
136. Roberts JD, Polaner DM, Lang P, Zapol WM. Inhaled nitric oxide in persistent pulmonary hypertension of the newborn. Lancet 1992; 340:818–819.
137. Kinsella JP, Neish SR, Shaffer E, Abman SH. Low-dose inhalational nitric oxide in persistent pulmonary hypertension of the newborn. Lancet 1992; 340:819–820.
138. Sellden H, Winberg P, Gustafsson LE, Lundell B, Book K, Frostell CG. Inhalation of nitric oxide reduced pulmonary hypertension after cardiac surgery in a 3.2 kg infant. Anesthesiology 1993; 78:577–580.
139. Timms RM, Khaja FU, Williams GW, the Nocturnal Oxygen Therapy Trial Group. Hemodynamic response to oxygen therapy in chronic obstructive pulmonary disease. Ann Intern Med 1985; 102:29–36.
140. Morgan JM, Griffiths M, du Bois RM. Hypoxic pulmonary vasoconstriction in systemic sclerosis and primary pulmonary hypertension. Chest 1991; 99:551–556.
141. Boyer JJ, Busst CM, Denison DM, Shinebourne EA. Effect of long-term oxygen treatment at home in children with pulmonary vascular disease. Br Heart J 1985; 55: 385–390.

142. Mathur PN, Powles RCP, Pugsley SO, McEwan MP, Campbell EJ. Effect of digoxin on right ventricular function in severe chronic airflow obstruction. Ann Intern Med 1981; 95:283–288.
143. Rozkovec A, Montanes P, Oakley CM. Factors that influence the outcome of primary pulmonary hypertension. Br Heart J 1986; 55:449–458.
144. Thoele DG, Barst RJ, Gersony WM. Physiologic-based management of primary pulmonary hypertension in children and young adults (abstrt). J Am Coll Cardiol 1990; 15:242A.
145. Nootens MT, Berarducci LA, Kaufmann E, Golibijanki R, Devries S, Rich S. Prevalence and hemodynamic implications of a patent foramen ovale in pulmonary hypertension (abstrt). J Am Coll Cardiol 1993; 2:402A.
146. Rich S, Lam W. Atrial septostomy as palliative therapy for refractory primary pulmonary hypertension. Am J Cardiol 1983; 51:1560–1561.
147. Nihill MR, O'Laughlin MP, Mullins CE. Blade balloon atrial septostomy is effective palliation for terminal cor pulmonale (abstrt). Am J Cardiol 1987; 60(suppl):1.
148. Hausknecht MJ, Sims RE, Nihill MR, Cashion WR. Successful palliation of primary pulmonary hypertension by atrial septostomy. Am J Cardiol 1990; 65:1045–1046.
149. Kerstein D, Garofano RP, Hsu DT, Hordof AJ, Barst RJ. Efficacy of blade balloon atrial septostomy in advanced pulmonary vascular disease (abstrt). Am Rev Respir Dis 1992; 145:A717.
150. Kerstein D, Levy PS, Hsu DT, Hordof AJ, Gersony WM, Barst RJ. Blade balloon atrial septostomy improves survival in patients with severe primary pulmonary hypertension. Circulation 1995; 91:2028–2035.
151. Reitz BA, Wallwork JL, Hunt SA, et al. Heart–lung transplantation: successful therapy for patients with pulmonary vascular disease. N Engl J Med 1982; 306:557–564.
152. Pasque MK, Trulock EP, Kaiser LD, Cooper JD. Single lung transplantation for pulmonary hypertension: three months hemodynamic follow-up. Circulation 1991; 84:2275–2279.
153. UNOS organ procurement and transplantation network data and UNOS Scientific Registry.
154. DeHoyos AL, Patterson GA, Maurer JR, Ramirez JC, Miller JD, Winton TL. Pulmonary transplantation: early and late results: the Toronto Lung Transplant Group. J Thorac Cardiovasc Surg 1992; 103:295–306.
155. McCarthy PM, Kirby TJ, White RD, Rice TW, Rosenkranz ER, Baldyga AP, Vargo R, Mehta AC. Lung and heart–lung transplantation: the state of the art. Cleve Clin J Med 1992; 59:307–316.

9

Diagnosing Primary Pulmonary Hypertension

GILBERT E. D'ALONZO

Temple University Health Science Center
Philadelphia, Pennsylvania

DAVID R. DANTZKER

Long Island Jewish Medical Center
New Hyde Park
and Albert Einstein College of Medicine
Bronx, New York

I. Introduction

Pulmonary hypertension may complicate the course of many pulmonary and cardiac disorders or develop as a result of primary disease of the pulmonary vessels. Whether it is primary or secondary, the pathophysiological alterations caused by pulmonary hypertension usually remain clinically silent until the process is far advanced; then patients often present with severe exercise limitation, signs of right-sided heart failure, or symptoms suggesting decreased left ventricular output. Since a routine screening procedure for this disorder is not available, the physician must have an enhanced index of suspicion when dealing with patients who are at risk for developing pulmonary hypertension.

This chapter will present an approach to the differential diagnosis of pulmonary hypertension, with emphasis on the recognition of primary pulmonary hypertension.

II. Definition and Classification

Pulmonary hypertension is defined as a mean pulmonary arterial pressure greater than 25 mmHg at rest or 30 mmHg during exercise. There are various ways of categorizing the etiologies of this disorder. A useful approach, based on the major pathophysiological mechanism is shown in Table 1. A second classification, organized according to the anatomical site of the underlying disease process, is shown in Table 2. In this system, the two major anatomic categories of pulmonary hypertension are postcapillary, and mixed capillary or precapillary. Postcapillary pulmonary hypertension is, most commonly, due to diseases of the left heart that cause the pulmonary venous pressure to be elevated, with a passive increase in pulmonary arterial pressure. Less common diseases that can cause pulmonary venous obstruction, such as pulmonary veno-occlusive disease and constrictive mediastinitis are also classified as postcapillary. Mixed capillary or precapillary pulmonary hypertension is associated with normal left ventricular end-diastolic pressure, and is secondary to diseases of the lung parenchyma or pulmonary vessels in which the cross-sectional vascular bed surface area is decreased. Pulmonary hypertension may also occur secondary to left-to-right intracardiac shunts, in which the increased pulmonary blood flow is the initial insult, and subsequent anatomical remodeling of the pulmonary vessels accentuates the problem. Extrapulmonary parenchymal diseases, such as severe kyphoscoliosis and fibrothorax, produce distortion of the chest cavity, mechanical compression of

Table 1 Pathophysiological Classification of Pulmonary Hypertension

Type	Mechanism	Examples
Passive	Resistance to pulmonary venous drainage	Mitral stenosis; pulmonary veno-occlusive disease
Hyperkinetic	Increased pulmonary blood flow	Atrial septal defect; ventricular septal defect
Obstructive	Resistance to flow through large pulmonary arteries	Pulmonary thromboembolism; unilateral absence or stenosis of a pulmonary artery
Obliterative	Resistance to flow through small pulmonary blood vessels	Primary pulmonary hypertension; collagen vascular disease
Vasoconstrictive	Resistance to flow from hypoxia-induced vasoconstriction	Chronic mountain sickness; sleep apnea syndrome
Polygenic	Two or more of the mechanisms listed above	Obliterative and vasoconstrictive COPD or interstitial pulmonary fibrosis

Table 2 Classification of Pulmonary Hypertension Based on Anatomical Site of Underlying Disease

Anatomical site	Underlying disease
Postcapillary	Left ventricular dysfunction Mitral valve stenosis Atrial myxoma Constrictive pericarditis Constrictive mediastinits Pulmonary veno-occlusive disease

Mixed capillary and precapillary	Airway and parenchymal disease
	  COPD
	  Interstitial lung disease
	Pulmonary vascular disease
	  Pulmonary embolism
	  Congenital heart disease (left-to-right shunt)
	  Vasculitis
	  Primary pulmonary hypertension
	Chest wall disease
	  Kyphoscoliosis
	  Fibrothorax

Normal or near-normal lungs	High-altitude sickness Chronic alveolar hypoventilation Sleep-disordered breathing Neuromuscular diseases

lung parenchyma, and alveolar hypoventilation. This may lead to a substantial degree of pulmonary hypertension primarily caused by hypoxic vasoconstriction.

Patients with normal or near-normal heart, lungs, or thorax may have pulmonary hypertension secondary to intermittent alveolar hypoxia. Patients with sleep-related breathing disorders or neuromuscular disease, for example, can have transient hypoxemia during sleep and near-normal arterial blood gas concentrations while awake.

Primary pulmonary hypertension (PPH), also referred to as unexplained or idiopathic pulmonary hypertension, can be diagnosed only after all other causes are excluded (1). Although patients with PPH have a characteristic (2–5) pulmonary arteriopathy seen on lung biopsy, none of the pathological findings are diagnostic of the disease. Pulmonary arteriopathy can also be found in patients with congenital heart disease, pulmonary hypertension associated with portal hypertension (6–11), toxin-induced (12,13) and drug-induced (12,14) pulmonary hypertension, and human immunodeficiency virus (HIV)-related pulmonary hypertension (21,23). Several years ago families with PPH were described (24). Fourteen families with PPH were reported in 1984 (25), and the National Institutes of Health (NIH) Registry for Primary Pulmonary Hypertension identified 12 of 187 patients with a familial association (1). Familial associations have also been reported for patients with pulmonary veno-occlusive disease (26,27).

III. History and Physical Examination

The clearest clinical picture of PPH can be gleaned from the data obtained by the NIH registry for PPH, which prospectively evaluated a large cohort of patients with this disease (1). An impressive finding was the long symptomatic period that generally preceded the diagnosis, speaking to the difficulty in making the diagnosis, and partially accounting for the advanced manifestations of pulmonary hypertension at the time of diagnosis. The mean age of the patients was 36 years for both males and females. Although the disease was most common in the third decade for female patients, and the fourth decade for male patients (Fig. 1A), no age range was immune, and 9% of the patients were older than 60 years of age. The female/male ratio was 1.7:1 (although in the African-American patients it was 4.3:1) and was relatively constant for each decade. Female patients tended to have more severe symptoms at presentation, with 75% in New York Heart Association functional class III or IV, compared with 64% for male patients ($p = 0.08$). The distribution of patients by race was similar to the general population, with 12% African-American and 2% Hispanic.

The most commonly reported symptom of PPH was dyspnea, occurring in 60% of patients as an early symptom, and in all patients as the disease progresses (Table 3). Atypical angina was also common, as was easy fatigability (1). Only 10% of the patients reported symptoms of Raynaud's phenomenon, which occurred almost entirely (95%) in the female patients. Although the presence of this phenomenon is of no higher frequency than in the general population, its recognition proved to be a negative prognostic factor for survival. Hoarseness (Ortner's syndrome) and massive hemoptysis have also been reported in patients with PPH, but these findings are uncommon (28–30). The time of onset from the patient's recognition of first symptoms until eventual diagnosis for the patients in the NIH registry was 2 ± 5 years (median 1.3 years), indicating that the diagnosis is often delayed (see Fig. 1B). Although more than 90% of the patients had their illness diagnosed within 3 years of symptom onset, an occasional patient stated that symptoms had been present for up to 20 years before the diagnosis was made.

The mechanism of the dyspnea in patients with PPH is unclear, but it is associated with a characteristic hyperventilation and chronic respiratory alkalosis that is exaggerated during exercise (31). The near syncope and syncope is almost always effort-related and is believed to be due to a limited ability to increase

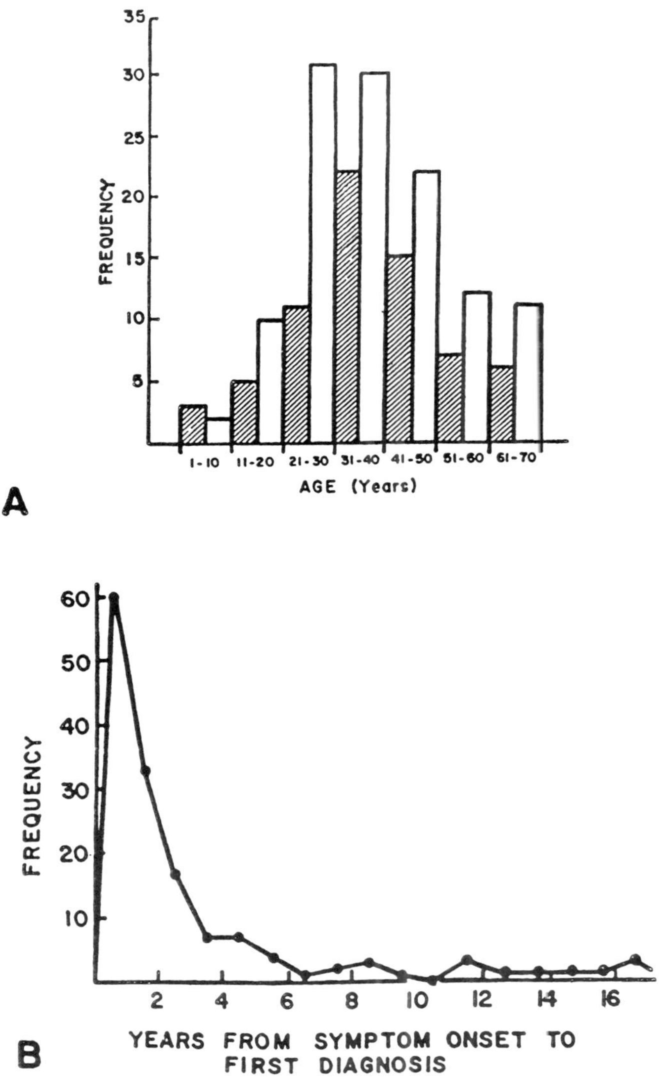

Figure 1 Distribution of patients with pulmonary embolism plotted (A) according to age based on sex, and (B) according to onset of symptoms for both sexes. The disease was most prevalent in age groups in the third and fourth decades, but the female/male ratio of 1.7:1 was not significantly different among decades. The mean time to onset of initial symptoms, 2.03 years (median, 1.27), was similar for both male (shaded bars) and female (open bars) patients. (From Ref. 1.)

Table 3 Frequency of Initial and Late Symptoms in 187 Patients with Primary Pulmonary Hypertension

	Initial %	By the time of diagnosis as PPH %
Dyspnea	60	98
Fatigue	19	73
Chest pain	7	47
New syncope	5	41
Leg edema	3	36
Palpitations	5	33

Source: Ref. 1.

cardiac output in response to increased metabolic demand. In patients who present with syncope at rest, an arrhythmic cause for the syncope should be considered. Given their limited cardiac output, a relatively benign tachyarrhythmia could produce marked systemic hypotension. The angina or atypical chest discomfort associated with PPH is also precipitated by stress, suggesting that it may represent right ventricular ischemia. Biochemical evidence of right ventricular ischemia has been demonstrated in the presence of increased right ventricular afterload in animal studies (32).

The physical examination may be quite helpful in suggesting the presence of pulmonary hypertension (Table 4). The most common physical findings are a loud and occasionally palpable pulmonic valve closing sound and a right ventricular fourth heart sound that waxes and wanes with inspiration and expiration. A

Table 4 Physical Findings That Support a Diagnosis of Pulmonary Hypertension

Loud pulmonic valve closure sound, frequently palpable
Right ventricular third heart sound
Right ventricular fourth heart sound
Sustained left parasternal or epigastric heave or lift (right ventricular heave)
Jugular venous a wave
Prominent jugular V wave
Diminished carotid arterial upstroke
Inspiration-augmented systolic murmur
Soft-blowing diastolic murmur (occasionally harsh)
Signs of right-sided heart failure, such as hepatojugular reflux, tender hepatomegaly (may be pulsatile), ascites, lower extremity edema, anasarca
Central or peripheral cyanosis

sustained left parasternal or epigastric heave or lift may indicate a forcibly contracting hypertrophied right ventricle. A jugular venous A wave is an early sign of reduced right ventricular compliance or an elevated right ventricular pressure. With the onset of right ventricular failure, the right ventricle dilates and often produces tricuspid valve regurgitation; in time, regurgitation causes a prominent V wave in the jugular venous pulse and an inspiration-augmented systolic murmur heard best with auscultation along the left and right sternal borders. In addition, as the right heart dilates, the pulmonary artery annulus is distorted, and regurgitation occurs that is characterized by a soft-blowing diastolic murmur, heard best along the upper left sternal border. The presence of a right ventricular third heart sound is characteristic of right ventricular failure, and it is generally associated with a poor prognosis. It is frequently accompanied by signs of right-sided heart failure, such as a hepatojugular reflux, tender hepatomegaly, ascites, lower extremity edema and, eventually, anasarca. Finally, a thorough examination looking for systemic disease, including musculoskeletal and neurological abnormalities is essential, with particular attention directed toward the subtle findings often associated with collagen vascular disease.

Patients with PPH have physical findings typical of any patient with pulmonary hypertension (1). In the NIH study, an increase in the pulmonic component of the second heart sound was found in 93%, a right ventricular heave and a right-sided fourth heart sound in 38%. More advanced disease was signaled by the presence of a right ventricular third heart sound and tricuspid regurgitation. The presence of an S_3 was associated with elevated right atrial pressure (13 mmHg, compared with 9 mmHg in patients without an S_3; $p<0.001$) and a reduced cardiac index (1.8 compared with 2.4 L min^{-1} m^{-2}; $p<0.0001$). Tricuspid regurgitation was also associated with increased right atrial pressure (12 compared with 8 mmHg; $p<0.0001$) and a reduced cardiac index (1.8 compared with 2.6 L min^{-1} m^{-2}; $p<0.001$). Clubbing is not a feature of PPH and should suggest chronic lung or congenital heart disease.

IV. Diagnostic Evaluation

As with all complex problems, the diagnosis of primary pulmonary hypertension should follow an orderly and logical progression (Figs. 2 and 3).

A. Electrocardiography

An electrocardiogram that suggests right ventricular hypertrophy is a relatively sensitive test of pulmonary hypertension, although the changes do not correlate with the severity of the underlying pressure elevation. Commonly, right axis deviation and right ventricular hypertrophy with secondary T-wave changes are found (33). The national registry on PPH found right axis deviation in 79% of the

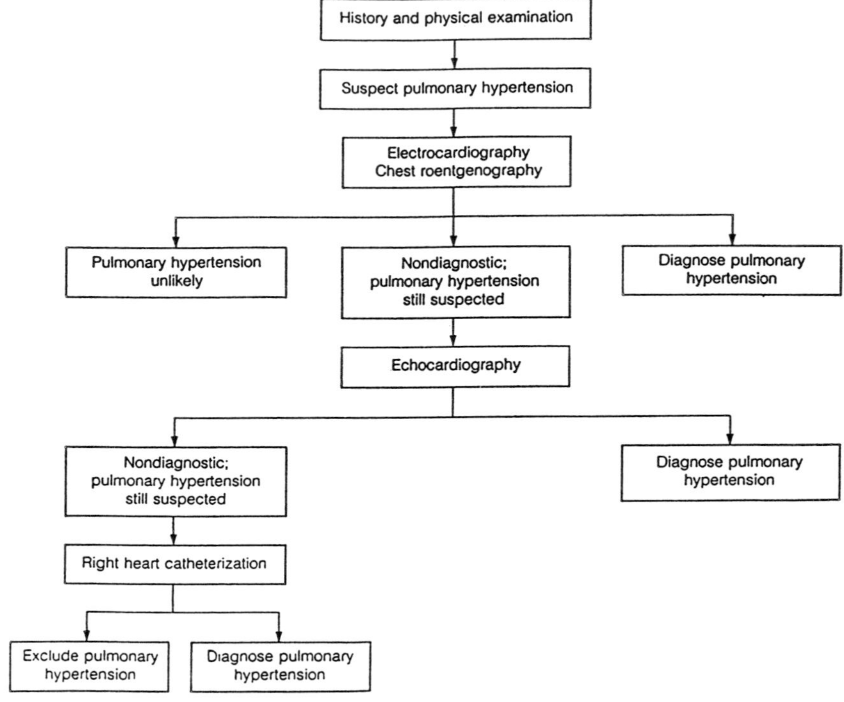

Figure 2 An approach to the diagnosis of pulmonary hypertension.

patients, right ventricular hypertrophy in 87%, and a right ventricular strain pattern in 74% (1).

Unfortunately, mild to moderate pulmonary hypertension may exist with no electrocardiographic findings to suggest it and, thus, the absence of ECG changes suggestive of right ventricular hypertrophy does not rule out its presence. Sinus rhythm seems to be the rule, since no patient with primary pulmonary hypertension and chronic atrial fibrillation has yet been reported. There is a notable disparity concerning the absence of all atrial arrhythmias in patients with PPH when compared with patients with cor pulmonale from lung disease, in whom atrial arrhythmias are common (34). Atrial fibrillation in patients with PPH would not be well tolerated because of the importance of atrial systole to ventricular filling (35,36). On the other hand, patients with chronic lung disease have lesser degrees of pulmonary hypertension and their cardiac outputs are not restricted by excessive right ventricular overload to the same degree.

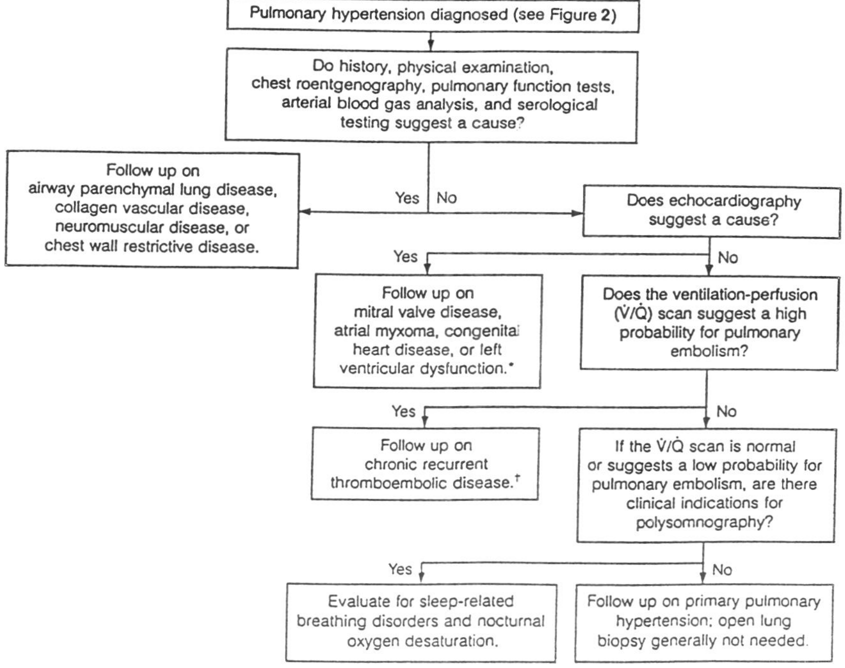

Figure 3 An approach to determining the cause of pulmonary hypertension.

B. Roentgenography

The chest roentgenogram can be helpful in identifying the cause of pulmonary hypertension; therefore, it is an important part of the evaluation process. Parenchymal abnormalities, redistribution of pulmonary blood flow, general or segmental cardiac enlargement, and chest wall and spinal disorders can provide clues to a specific underlying disorder. Most patients with PPH have evidence of pulmonary hypertension on a chest x-ray film (1,37). The two most common findings are prominence of the main pulmonary artery, occurring in 90% of PPH patients, and hilar vessel enlargement with pruning of the peripheral vessels in 80 and 51%, respectively. The presence of all three abnormalities found in 42% of the NIH cohort was associated with a higher mean pulmonary artery pressure (66 compared with 53 mmHg in those without all three findings; $p<0.001$) and lower cardiac index (2.0 compared with 2.4 L mm^{-1} m^{-2}; $p<0.004$). A completely normal chest roentgenogram speaks against the diagnosis, although 6% of patients with PPH in the NIH registry had this finding.

C. Pulmonary Function Testing

Pulmonary function testing is not directly useful as a diagnostic test for pulmonary hypertension. However, spirometry, lung volumes, and carbon monoxide-diffusing capacity are often useful in the diagnostic evaluation of the specific cause of pulmonary hypertension, by demonstrating the presence and degree of obstructive or restrictive lung disease (Fig. 4). Pulmonary function studies may disclose pathophysiological abnormalities that are not otherwise clinically apparent (38).

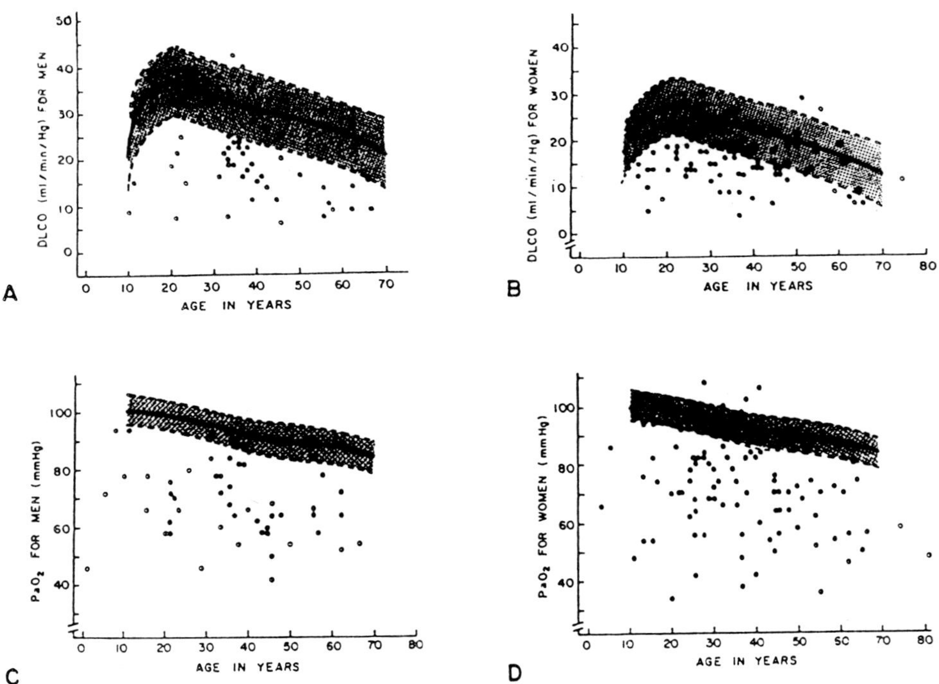

Figure 4 Distribution of findings for diffusing capacity of the lungs for carbon monoxide (DLCO) in (A) men and (B) women is shown, relative to the predicted values (± SD; shaded area based on age and the average American height for the age (7). Distribution of findings of arterial Po_2 with room air for (C) men and (D) women is shown, along with predicted vlaues based on age and sex (10). Diffusing capacity was generally less than predicted, and hypoxemia was almost an ubiquitous finding. (From Ref. 1.)

Patients with PPH generally have abnormal pulmonary function tests (1,39). Mild reduction in lung volumes, reduced diffusion capacity for carbon monoxide, and impaired pulmonary gas exchange are typical (1). Older studies described greater reductions in lung volumes than were seen in the NIH series (40), but most of those patients would have been excluded before entry into the national registry. The presence of a more than mild restrictive (41) or obstructive lung disease should suggest another diagnosis. The reduced diffusing capacity for carbon monoxide has been ascribed to obliteration of the small pulmonary arteries (42), although no significant correlation has been found between DLCO and any index of the severity of pulmonary hypertension (1).

Hypoxemia is commonly associated with disorders associated with pulmonary hypertension and should be ruled out as a precipitating or sustaining factor in its development. Clinically significant hypoxic vasoconstriction usually does not occur until the arterial oxygen tension falls below 60 mmHg. However, in patients who have a sleep-related breathing abnormality, the hypoxemia may occur only during apneic or hypopneic episodes, and blood gases measured while the patient is awake may be only mildly abnormal. Nocturnal episodes of hypoxic vasoconstriction are postulated to be important in the development of pulmonary hypertension in patients with chronic obstructive lung disease, and a variety of restrictive ventilatory diseases as well. Hypercapnia in patients with pulmonary hypertension implies severe parenchymal lung disease or disordered control of breathing.

Patients with PPH have mild-to-moderate abnormalities of pulmonary gas exchange (1,39). One study reported that either a respiratory or a mixed respiratory–metabolic alkalosis—hypoxemia (mean arterial Po_2 of 65 ± 12 mmHg) and a widened alveolar–arterial oxygen gradient (mean 50 ± 12 mmHg)—was present in every patient (39). The national registry reported comparable blood gas parameters with a mean arterial P_{o2} of 71 mmHg and a mean arterial Pco_2 of 31 mmHg (1). The hypoxemia seen with PPH is due to a mild degree of ventilation–perfusion inequality, amplified by the effect of a low mixed venous Po_2, resulting from the inadequate cardiac output (45). Severe hypoxemia can occasionally occur in PPH, usually caused by intracardiac shunting through a patent foramen ovale or, less commonly, a markedly depressed cardiac output. The chronic respiratory alkalosis is attributed to increased afferent activity from intrapulmonary stretch receptors or intravascular baroreceptors (46,47).

A cardiopulmonary exercise test to symptom-limited maximum is useful in the evaluation of patients who complain of dyspnea and in whom no cause is obvious (mystery dyspnea). There is a characteristic pattern of ventilatory and circulatory responses in patients with various forms of cardiac limitations, and the physiological response to exercise has been well described for patients with PPH (31). Cardiopulmonary exercise testing also has potential use as a "noninvasive" method for assessing prognosis, helping to identify patients in need of heart–lung

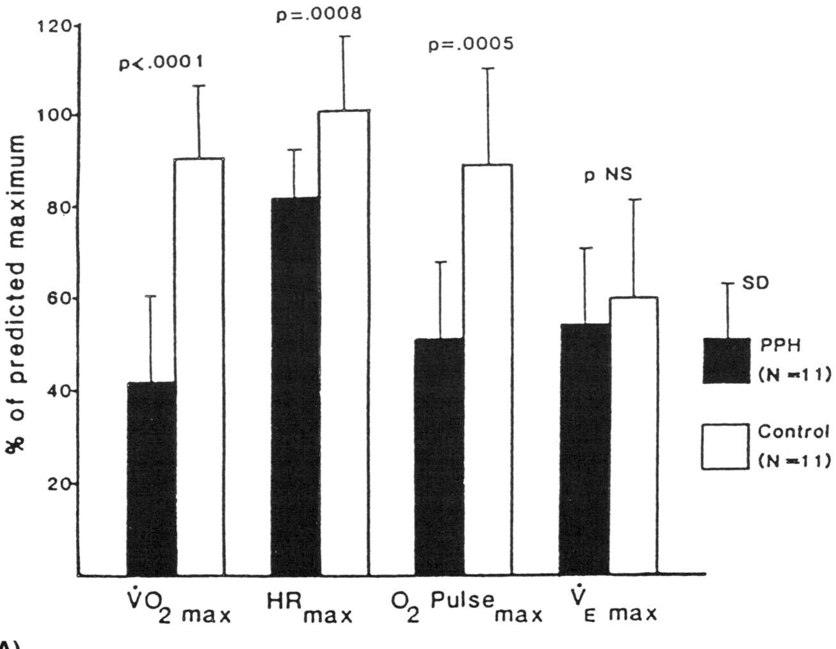

(A)

Figure 5 (A) Comparison of maximal exercise performance between patients with primary pulmonary hypertension (PPH) and control subjects. Both groups had cardiovascular limitation. Functional limitation reflected by the maximal oxygen consumption (Vo_2max), markedly decreased in the PPH group. Reduced O_2 pulse at maximal exercise in the PPH group suggests that these patients were unable to increase stroke volume to the same degree as the control group during exercise, and a greater increase in heart rate was necessary to increase cardiac output. Abbreviation: VE, maximal minute ventilation; HR_{max}, maximal heart rate. (B) Anaerobic threshold (AT) occurred at a lower oxygen consumption (Vo_2) and percentage predicted maximal oxygen consumption in the primary pulmonary hypertension (PPH) group. (From Ref. 31.)

or lung transplantation (48), and for determining the efficiency of therapeutic interventions in patients with PPH (48,49).

Patients with PPH generally have substantial exercise limitation, with marked fatigue and dyspnea on even mild exertion, as well as excessive ventilation at all exercise levels (50,51). These patients usually stop exercising because of dyspnea and lightheadedness during incremental cycle ergometry. A comparison of maximal exercise performance between patients with PPH and control subjects is found in Figures 5A and B. Functional limitation, as determined by the

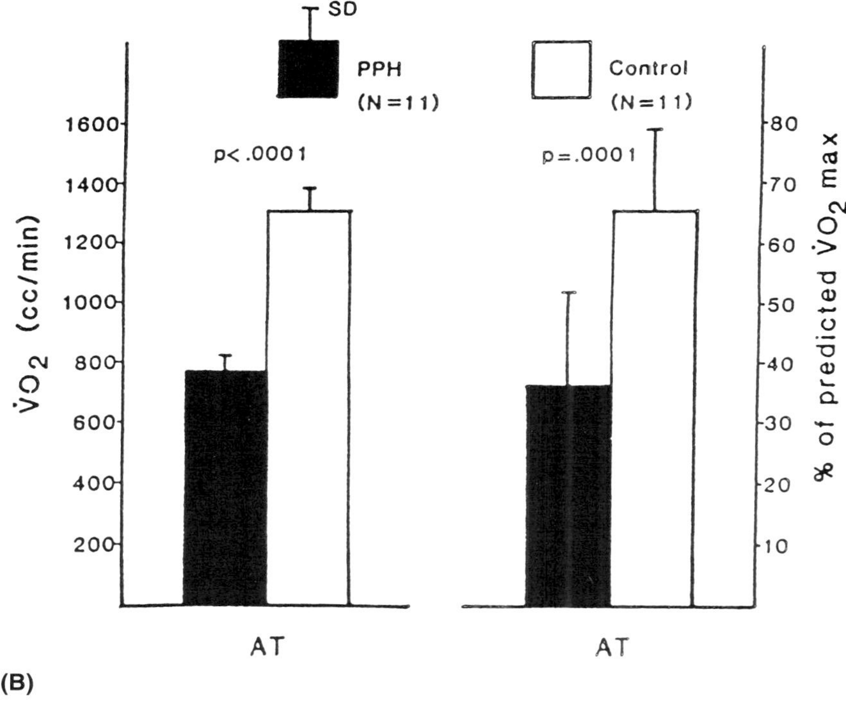

(B)

maximal oxygen consumption, was markedly decreased in the pulmonary hypertensive group (13 ml kg^{-1} min^{-1} versus 28 ml kg^{-1} min^{-1}). The heart rate was higher for any submaximal level of work, expressed as a reduction in the maximum oxygen pulse. Similar to heart rate, the maximal minute ventilation is higher at any submaximal level in the PPH group than in normals. As a consequence, the respiratory alkalosis present at rest in the PPH patients (mean P_{CO_2} 32 ± 5 mmHg) is maintained during moderate exercise (arterial P_{CO_2} 29 ± 3 mmHg). The arterial P_{O_2} at rest varied from 62 to 95 mmHg, but fell in 10 of 11 PPH patients at maximal exercise, whereas the alveolar–arterial oxygen gradient increased in all patients. The increased hypoxemia with exercise is predominately due to the inadequate cardiac response to increased metabolic demands and subsequent exaggerated fall in the mixed venous P_{O_2} (51). The anaerobic threshold (AT) was reached at a lower oxygen consumption in patients with PPH than the control group (see Fig. 5B). A strong positive correlation between the level of AT and maximal oxygen pulse in the PPH patients was found (r = 0.91; p <0.001), suggesting that the reduction in maximal oxygen consumption is due to inadequate cardiac reserve.

D. Echocardiography

Although the echocardiogram is not specific enough to rule out pulmonary hypertension, several findings are consistent with moderate to severe increases in pulmonary artery pressure. These include the presence of a dilated pulmonary artery, right atrial dilation, right ventricular dilation and hypertrophy, paradoxical movement of the interventricular septum, and abnormal pulmonic valve motion (52–54). Midsystolic closure of the pulmonic valve is commonly seen and is demonstrated by Doppler studies to be caused by a reflected pressure wave that is produced by the high pulmonary vascular resistance that results in transient retrograde blood flow (54,55). Of particular diagnostic value is the movement and configuration of the interventricular septum, as seen by two-dimensional echocardiography. As pulmonary hypertension increases, diastolic flattening of the ventricular septum occurs. Eventually, the septum develops a concave configuration relative to the right ventricle (56–58). Doppler studies have also shown an early to late redistribution of left ventricular filling, reflecting reduced left ventricular compliance (35). The echocardiogram can be particularly helpful in establishing whether pulmonary hypertension is caused by left ventricular dysfunction, mitral valve disease, left atrial myxoma, or an intracardiac shunt secondary to congenital heart disease (52).

Exciting developments with Doppler echocardiography makes this mode the noninvasive procedure of choice in determining both the existence and severity of pulmonary hypertension. Several studies have used Doppler echocardiography to estimate mean pulmonary artery pressure. One technique involves measuring the systolic flow velocity across the pulmonic valve or the acceleration of systolic flow velocity in the main pulmonary artery (59–61). The acceleration time is shortened as pulmonary arterial pressure increases. This shortening of the acceleration time correlates with the severity of pulmonary hypertension. It has been reported that this technique could be as high as 70% sensitive for determining the presence of pulmonary hypertension, and 94% specific (62), or perhaps even higher (63).

Since patients with pulmonary hypertension often have tricuspid and pulmonary valve regurgitation, Doppler echocardiography can also use these abnormalities to confirm the presence of pulmonary hypertension. With tricuspid valve regurgitation, the Doppler flow velocity profile can be used to determine the peak right ventricular systolic pressure, since it provides an estimate of the pressure drop from the right ventricle to the right atrium (64,65). When pulmonary valve stenosis is absent, right ventricular systolic pressure provides an accurate estimate of systolic pulmonary arterial pressure. Pulmonary valve insufficiency is frequently seen and certain characteristics indicative of pulmonic regurgitant flow velocity or changes in systolic flow across the pulmonic valve can also be used to estimate pulmonary artery pressure noninvasively (66).

A third technique, using Doppler echocardiography, detects pulmonary hypertension based on abnormal flow characteristics in the inferior vena cava. The advantage of this technique is that it can be used when a more direct echocardiographic study of the heart and pulmonary vasculature is technically difficult, specifically when evaluating patients with chronic obstructive lung disease. An initial study reported an 87% sensitivity and 80% specificity for detecting pulmonary hypertension in patients with chronic obstructive lung disease (67).

Recently, transesophageal echocardiography has been used to evaluate patients with suspected pulmonary hypertension (68). The intracardiac defects, such as a patent foramen ovale, can be better diagnosed with the transesophageal approach (69).

The NIH registry for PPH evaluated M-mode echocardiographic data, which showed a normal to small left ventricular end-diastolic internal dimension in all patients and right ventricular enlargement in 75%. Paradoxic septal motion was described in 59% of the patients and partial systolic closure of the pulmonary valve in 60% (1). Hemodynamic correlations between the calculated pulmonary vascular resistance and echocardiographic findings revealed an inversed relation between left ventricular internal dimension and pulmonary vascular resistance ($r = 0.47$; $p<0.001$), suggesting that underfilling of the left ventricle was a reflection of severity of pulmonary vascular disease. There was no association between right ventricular internal dimension and the level of pulmonary vascular resistance. Right ventricular and right atrial enlargements, with a normal to reduced left ventricular cavity size, have also been reported by others (53). With echocardiographic and Doppler techniques, a marked redistribution of left ventricular filling from early to late diastole in patients with PPH has been reported (35). This may play a destabilizing role in patients with PPH when vasodilator therapy is used, and an increase in cardiac output without a concomitant reduction in pulmonary arterial pressure occurs by causing an increased pulmonary capillary wedge pressure and a worsening of symptoms of orthopnea and dyspnea (70). Finally, the use of serial Doppler studies has been reported to be helpful in following drug therapy that resulted in a reduction pulmonary arterial pressure (71).

E. Lung Imaging

Ventilation–perfusion (V/Q) lung scanning is most useful for distinguishing patients with primary pulmonary hypertension from those with major vessel thromboembolic pulmonary hypertension (39,75–77). The risk associated with lung scans in PPH patients has been overstated; none of the 163 patients who had V/Q lung scans performed in the NIH registry reported any adverse complications.

In PPH, the lung scan is either normal (correlating with predominant plexogenic pulmonary arteriopathy) or low-probability, defined as small, patchy perfusion defects (suggesting thrombotic pulmonary arteriopathy; 78). Conversely, in patients with recurrent thromboembolic pulmonary hypertension, the lung scan demonstrates at least one major V/Q mismatch, but more often, two or more are found. A high-probability scan may not be of high enough specificity, however, and further evaluation with pulmonary angiography may be required for diagnostic confirmation of chronic embolic disease.

F. Pulmonary Angiography

If the lung scan shows one or more segmental, or greater, V/Q mismatches, a pulmonary angiogram is necessary to rule out thromboembolic disease (77). In chronic, recurrent thromboembolic pulmonary hypertension, pulmonary angiography shows smooth, convex-bordered occlusions, stenosis, and intravascular webs (79,80). Signs of large central thrombi, such as filling defects and vessel cutoffs, are also found. In thromboembolic pulmonary hypertension, the clots are actually incorporated into the wall of the pulmonary artery and endothelialized so that the angiogram may underestimate the extent of obstruction. Angioscopy and magnetic resonance imaging (MRI) can be used to further stage these patients. Angioscopy can be helpful, but has limited application because of its technical difficulty and the fact that it is not commercially available, being performed in only one center, which has a considerable experience (82). Magnetic resonance imaging is now being explored as an imaging technique for evaluating thrombi in proximal pulmonary arteries, without the necessity of using an angiographic contrast medium. Patients with PPH by contrast have proximal and hilar vessel dilatation, which then rapidly taper, with marked bilateral symmetric pruning of the distal vessels noted (81).

Pulmonary angiography can be performed safely in patients with severe pulmonary hypertension, although some risk exists (84). In the NIH registry on PPH there were no deaths or sustained morbidity reported among 50 patients who had pulmonary angiograms during the course of their clinical evaluations (1). However, one patient did experience transient hypotension during the procedure. When hypotension occurs, there is generally associated bradycardia (presumably vagal in origin); therefore, pretreatment with 1 mg of intravenous atropine before performing the angiogram has been suggested (84,85). The risk of pulmonary angiography is reduced if the center performing the study has sufficient experience and takes special precautions in patients with severe pulmonary hypertension (84,85). These include catheterization through arm or neck veins, not the femoral vein, a potential sight of thrombus formation; a single injection of nonionic contrast medium into the right and left main pulmonary arteries only; administration of oxygen during the procedure; and review of the large film angiograms after each injection, before moving the catheter. The primary focus is directed at defining anatomical configuration of the main, lobar, and segmental branches of the pulmonary vasculature in patients who are suspected of having chronic thromboembolic pulmonary hypertension. Magnification views and wedge arteriograms are generally avoided because, in this clinical setting, they do not assist in deciding whether the recognized thrombi are surgically accessible.

G. Right Heart Catheterization

Pulmonary artery catheterization, using a thermodilution balloon catheter, remains the gold standard for determining the presence and the severity of pulmonary hypertension. Unfortunately, at times, it can be extremely difficult to pass the catheter into the pulmonary artery in patients with severe pulmonary hypertension because of tricuspid valve regurgitation, a dilated right-sided chamber, and a low cardiac output. This problem is compounded by the lack of stiffness of the ordinary flow-directed balloon-tip catheter. To facilitate the catheter placement process, a catheter with guide wire support has been developed (72). These stiffer catheters virtually eliminate the potential problem of retrograde flipping of the catheter into the right ventricle.

Right heart catheterization may be required to help establish the etiology of the pulmonary hypertension; measurement of the pulmonary capillary wedge pressure distinguishes postcapillary from mixed capillary–precapillary causes (see Table 2). Postcapillary pulmonary hypertension is generally identified by a pulmonary capillary wedge pressure greater than 15 mmHg, whereas mixed capillary–precapillary pulmonary hypertension has a pulmonary capillary wedge pressure of less than 15 mmHg. It should be recognized that left ventricular-filling pressures may increase modestly in severe PPH owing to diastolic dysfunction related to the pulmonary hypertension (73). The finding of an elevated pulmonary capillary wedge pressure necessitates left ventricular catheterization to determine whether there is abnormal left ventricular end-diastolic pressure, mitral valve stenosis, or impairment of left atrial filling by stenosis of the pulmonary venous system. Pulmonary veno-occlusive disease can result in a gradient between the wedge pressure and left ventricular end-diastolic pressure, although the wedge pressure in this unusual form of PPH is usually normal or only mildly elevated. Typical of veno-occlusive disease is the variability in wedge pressure determinations from various sites within the lung.

Measurement of increased oxygen saturation in the central veins, right atrium, right ventricle, and pulmonary artery helps identify the presence and location of a left-to-right shunt. Congenital heart disease can often be missed (especially in patients with ostium secundum–atrial septal defects) if the balloon catheter technique of measuring oxygen saturation is used. A more sensitive method of determining the presence of shunt involves early detection of hydrogen in the right heart after the patient inhales hydrogen gas; this method uses a special electrode-tipped right heart catheter. The presence of a left-to-right shunt may also be demonstrated by injection of indocyanine green into the pulmonary artery, with sampling from the femoral artery; early recirculation is evident on the down-slope of the dye curve.

Particular attention should be paid to the accurate measurement of right atrial pressure, pulmonary artery pressure, and cardiac output, since they are important long-term prognostic indicators in patients with PPH (74). The thermodilution technique seems to be satisfactory for determining cardiac output in most patients with pulmonary hypertension. However, the Fick method, with direct measurement of O_2 consumption, is more accurate in patients with low cardiac output states.

The hemodynamic features of the NIH registry PPH patients are shown in Figure 6. They had severe pulmonary hypertension, with a threefold increase in

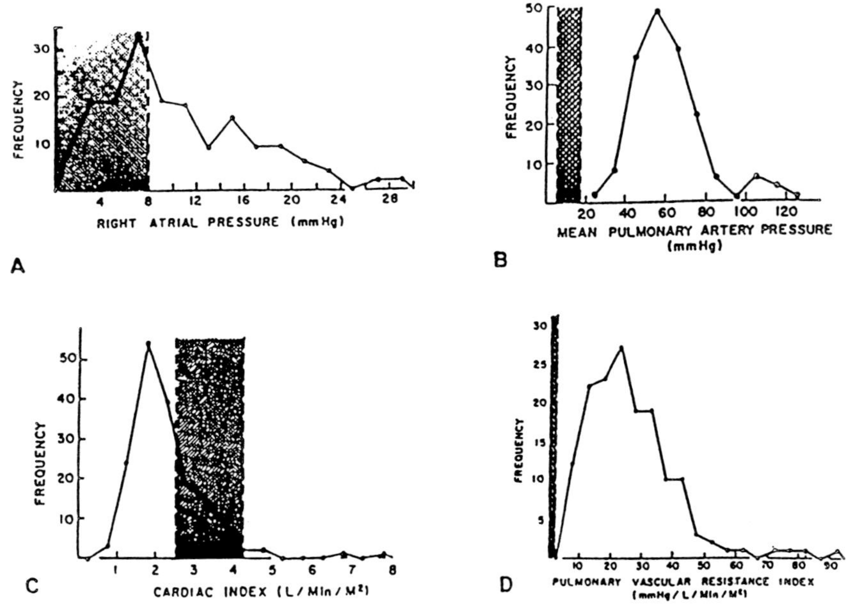

Figure 6 Distribution of hemodynamic finding is shown, in relation to published normal values. (A) The right atrial pressure was elevated 72%. (B) All patients, by definition, had an elevation in mean pulmonary artery pressure, with some having mean pulmonary artery pressures in excess of 100 mmHg. (C) The cardiac index was reduced in 71% and reached a nadir value of 0.9 L mm^{-1} m^{-2}. (D) The pulmonary vascular resistance index averaged 15 times greater than normal. Normal ranges are indicated by shaded regions. (From Ref. 1.)

mean pulmonary atrial pressure (60 ± 18 mmHg; range, 28–127 mmHg), mild-to-moderate elevation in mean right atrial pressure (9 ± 6 mmHg; range, 0–29 mmHg), with normal pulmonary capillary wedge pressures and mildly reduced cardiac indexes (2.27 ± 0.9 L min^{-1} m^{-2}; range, 0.8–7.9 L min^{-1} m^{-2}). Correlations between hemodynamic findings and severity of symptoms were also investigated. Patients with more severe symptoms (functional class III and IV) had higher mean pulmonary arterial pressures (62 compared with 56 mmHg; $p = 0.06$), higher right atrial pressures (11 compared with 7 mmHg; $p = 0.0001$), and lower cardiac indexes (2.06 compared with 2.73 L min^{-1} m^{-2}; $p = 0.0003$) than did their less symptomatic counterparts (functional class II). There was no difference in hemodynamic values among patients when they were analyzed according to duration of symptoms.

H. Serology

The purpose of including serological testing in the evaluation of patients with pulmonary hypertension is to screen for collagen vascular diseases: systemic lupus erythematosus, rheumatoid arthritis, and scleroderma are of concern. A positive antinuclear antigen (ANA) titer is common in patients with primary pulmonary hypertension. Titers ranging from 1:10 to 1:10,000 have been reported, but a specific pattern has not been identified (1,86). A recent study also demonstrated a high incidence of anti-Ku antibodies (87), although the significance of this finding is unclear.

I. Polysomnography

Polysomnography (PSG) is not part of the usual evaluation for pulmonary hypertension; it is used specifically for the diagnosis of sleep-related breathing disorders. Patients with chronic obstructive lung disease (COPD), chronic congestive heart failure, and various neuromuscular diseases are at increased risk for developing sleep-related breathing disorders. Studies performed on large numbers of unselected sleep apneic syndrome patients found the frequency of pulmonary hypertension to be between 12 and 20% (43,44,88). Pulmonary hypertension can increase during sleep in chronic obstructive lung disease patients, exhibiting profound drops in arterial oxygen saturation, particularly during rapid eye-movement (REM) sleep (89–92). This effect is most notable for patients who demonstrate daytime hypoxemia, hypercapnia, and pulmonary hypertension; but similar results have been observed in patients with little or no daytime pulmonary hypertension. The highest pulmonary arterial pressures during sleep can exceed the daytime values by as much as 25 mmHg (92). In COPD patients with little or no daytime hypoxemia we do not yet know if nocturnal hypoxemia can induce permanent pulmonary hypertension. The association of sleep-related breathing problems and the development of pulmonary hypertension in a variety of clinical conditions requires further clinical investigation.

J. Lung Biopsy

In certain patients with unexplained pulmonary hypertension, lung biopsy may be necessary to establish the diagnosis when confounding factors make the diagnosis uncertain. An accurate diagnosis is essential for proper prognosis and management. For example, lung biopsy may distinguish among patients with primary pulmonary hypertension, pulmonary veno-occlusive disease, pulmonary talcosis, and vasculitis (93).

Transbronchial lung biopsy by fiberoptic bronchoscopy is contraindicated because of the risk of hemorrhage owing to elevated pulmonary arterial pressure and because the sample is generally small and does not often include blood vessels. Open-lung biopsy, possibly using a thoracoscope, would be preferred, but this procedure is not without risk, particularly in patients with severe pulmonary hypertension who cannot tolerate the short period of controlled pneumothorax often necessary to permit sufficient visualization of the lung. However, it must be stressed that lung biopsy is not considered essential in making an accurate diagnosis of PPH for most patients with this disease process. Finally, since patients who undergo lung biopsy are usually complex and the histological diagnosis is often difficult, the pathological material should be referred to a pathologist with substantial experience in pulmonary vascular disease.

V. Conclusion

A keen level of suspicion is of paramount importance for the eventual diagnosis of pulmonary hypertension, regardless of the underlying cause. However, once suspected a methodical workup using commonly employed diagnostic interventions generally allows rapid conformation of the presence of pulmonary hypertension and, usually, a specific diagnosis of its etiology. A proper etiologic evaluation is necessary to ensure that the patient's diagnosis is correct and that proper therapeutic intervention can be pursued. For the diagnosis of idiopathic or primary pulmonary hypertension, it is necessary to exclude all secondary causes. The diagnostic approach is, for the most part, noninvasive and safe for the majority of patients with this insidious and devastating disease. A few patients with primary pulmonary hypertension will require more invasive intervention, such as pulmonary angiography or lung biopsy. Reserving these potentially morbid tests for those patients who fall outside of the standard presentation for primary pulmonary hypertension, will reduce the morbidity associated with the diagnostic workup.

References

1. Rich S, Dantzker DR, Ayers SM, et al. Primary pulmonary hypertension: a national prospective study. Ann Intern Med 1987; 107:216–223.
2. Wagenvoort CA, Wagenvoort N. Primary pulmonary hypertension: a pathologic study of the lung vessels in 156 clinically diagnosed cases. Circulation 1970; 42:1163–1184.
3. Bjornsson J, Edwards WD. Primary pulmonary hypertension: a histopathologic study of 80 cases. Mayo Clin Proc 1985; 60:16–25.
4. Palevsky HI, Schloo BL, Pietra GG, et al. Primary pulmonary hypertension: vascular structure, morphometry, and responsiveness to vasodilator agents. Circulation 1989; 80:1207–1221.
5. Pietra GG, Edwards WD, Kay JM, et al. Histopathology of primary pulmonary hypertension: a qualitative and quantitative study of pulmonary blood vessels from 58 patients in the National Heart, Lung, and Blood Institute Primary Pulmonary Hypertension Registry. Circulation 1989; 80:1198–1206.
6. Naeye RL. "Primary" pulmonary hypertension with coexistent portal hypertension. Circulation 1960; 32:376–384.
7. Senior RM, Britton RC, Turino GM, Wood JA, Langer GA, Fishman AP. Pulmonary hypertension associated with cirrhosis of the liver and with portocaval shunts. Circulation 1968; 37:88–96.
8. McDonnell PJ, Toye PA, Hutchins GM. Primary pulmonary hypertension and cirrhosis: are they related? Am Rev Respir Dis 1983; 127:437–441.
9. Edwards BS, Weir EK, Edwards WD, Ludwig J, Dykoski RK, Edwards JE. Coexistent pulmonary and portal hypertension: morphologic and clinical features. J Am Coll Cardiol 1987; 10:1233–1238.
10. Yutani C, Imakita M, Ishibashi-Ueda H, Okuko S, Naito M, Kunieda T. Nodular regenerative hyperplasia of the liver associated with primary pulmonary hypertension. Hum Pathol 1988; 19:726–731.
11. Hadengue A, Behayoun MK, Lebrec D, Benhamou JP. Pulmonary hypertension complicating portal hypertension: prevalence and relation to splanchnic hemodynamics. Gastroenterology 1991; 100:520–528.
12. Gomez-Sanchez MA, Mestre de Juan MJ, Gomez-Pajuelo C, Lopez JI, Diaz de Atauri MJ, Martinez-Tello FJ. Pulmonary hypertension due to toxic oil syndrome: a clinicopathologic study. Chest 1989; 95:325–331.
13. Gomez-Sanchez MA, Saene de la Calzada C, Gomez-Pajuelo C, Martinez-Tello FJ, Mestrede Juan MJ, James TN. Clinical and pathologic manifestation of pulmonary vascular disease in the toxic oil syndrome. J Am Coll Cardiol 1991; 18:1539–1545.
14. Gurtner HP. Aminorex pulmonary hypertension. In: Fishman AP, ed. The Pulmonary Circulation: Normal and Abnormal. Philadelphia: University of Pennsylvania Press, 1990:397–412.
15. Douglas JG, Munro JF, Kitchin AH, Muir AL, Proudfoot AT. Pulmonary hypertension and fenfluramine. Br Med J 1981; 283:881–883.
16. MacMurray J, Bloomfield P, Miller HC. Irreversible pulmonary hypertension after therapy with fenfluramine. Br Med J 1986; 292:239–240.

17. Tazelaar HD, Myers JL, Drage CW, King TE Jr, Aguayo S, Colby TV. Pulmonary disease associated with L-tryptophan-induced eosinophilic myalgia syndrome: clinical and pathology features. Chest 1990; 97:1032–1036.
18. Ellis DA, Capewell SJ. Pulmonary veno-occlusive disease after chemotherapy. Thorax 1986; 41:415–416.
19. Lombard CM, Churg A, Winokur S. Pulmonary veno-occlusive disease following therapy for malignant neoplasms. Chest 1987; 92:871–876.
20. Russell LA, Spehlmann JE, Clarke M, Lillington GA. Pulmonary hypertension in female crack users (abstr). Am Rev Respir Dis 1992; 145:A717.
21. Goldsmith GH, Baily RG, Brettler DB, et al. Primary pulmonary hypertension in patients with classic hemophilia. Ann Intern Med 1988; 108:797–799.
22. Himelman RB, Dohrman M, Goodman P, et al. Severe pulmonary hypertension and cor pulmonale in the acquired immunodeficiency syndrome. Am J Cardiol 1989; 64: 1396–1399.
23. Speich R, Jenni R, Opravil M, Pfab M, Russi EW. Primary pulmonary hypertension in HIV infection. Chest 1991; 100:1268–1271.
24. Dresdale DT, Schultz M, Michtom RJ. Primary pulmonary hypertension: clinical and hemodynamic study. Am J Med 1951; 11:686–705.
25. Loyd JE, Primm RK, Newman JH. Familial primary pulmonary hypertension: clinical patterns. Am Rev Respir Dis 1984; 129:194–197.
26. Voordes CG, Kuipers JRG, Elema JD. Familial pulmonary veno-occlusive disease: a case report. Thorax 1977; 32:763–766.
27. Davies P, Reid L. Pulmonary veno-occlusive disease in siblings: case report and morphometric study. Hum Pathol 1982; 13:911–915.
28. Ortner N. Recurrenslahmung bei Mitral Stenose. Wien Klin Wochenschr 1897; 10: 753–755.
29. Yuceoglu YZ, Dresdale DT, Valensi QJ, Narvas RM, Gottlieb NT. Primary pulmonary hypertension with hoarseness and massive (fatal) hemoptysis. Review of the literature and report of a case. Vasc Dis 1967; 4:290.
30. Nakao M, Sawayama T, Samukawa M, et al. Left recurrent laryngeal nerve palsy associated with primary pulmonary hypertension and patent ductus arteriosus. J Am Coll Cardiol 1985; 5:788–792.
31. D'Alonzo GE, Gianotti LA, Pohil RL, et al. Comparison of progressive exercise performance of normal subjects and patients with primary pulmonary hypertension. Chest 1987; 92:57–62.
32. Vlahakes GJ, Turley K, Hoffman JIE. The pathophysiology of failure in acute right ventricular hypertension: hemodynamic and biochemical correlations. Circulation 1981; 63:87–95.
33. Kanemoto N. Electrocardiogram in primary pulmonary hypertension. Eur J Cardiol 1980; 12:181–193.
34. Shine KI, Kastor JA, Yurchak PM. Multifocal atrial tachycardia. Clinical and electrocardiographic features in 32 patients. N Engl J Med 1968; 279:344–348.
35. Louie EK, Rich S, Brundage BH. Doppler echocardiographic assessment of impaired left ventricular filling in patients with right ventricular pressure overload due to primary pulmonary hypertension. J Am Coll Cardiol 1986; 8:1307–1311.

36. Rich S. Primary pulmonary hypertension. Prog Cardiovasc Dis 1988; 31:205–238.
37. Kanemoto N, Furuya H, Etoh T, Sasamoto H, Matsuyama S. Chest roentgenograms in primary pulmonary hypertension. Chest 1979; 96:45–49.
38. Elper GR, McCloud TC. Normal chest roentgenograms in chronic diffuse infiltrative lung disease. N Engl J Med 1978; 298:934–939.
39. D'Alonzo GE, Bower JS, Dantzker DR. Differentiation of patients with primary and thromboembolic pulmonary hypertension. Chest 1984; 85:457–461.
40. Phipps B, Wang B, Chang CHJ, Dunn M. Unexplained severe pulmonary hypertension in the older age group. Chest 1983; 84:399–402.
41. Williams MH, Adler JJ, Colp C. Pulmonary function studies as an aid in the differential diagnosis of pulmonary hypertension. Am J Med 1969; 47:378–383.
42. Anderson EG, Simon G, Reid L. Primary and thromboembolic pulmonary hypertension: a quantitative pathological study. J Pathol 1973; 110:273–293.
43. Podszus T, Bauer W, Mayer J, Penzel T, Peter JH, Wichert P. Sleep apnea and pulmonary hypertension. Klin Wochenschr 1986; 64:131–134.
44. Weitzenblum E, Krieger J, Apprill M, Vallee E, Ehrhart E, Ratomaharo J, Oswald M, Kurtz D. Daytime pulmonary hypertension in patients with obstructive sleep apnea syndrome. Am Rev Respir Dis 1988; 138:345–349.
45. Dantzker DR, Bower JS. Mechanisms of gas exchange abnormality in patients with chronic obliterative pulmonary vascular disease. J Clin Invest 1979; 64:1050–1055.
46. Guz A, Nobel MIM, Eisele JH, Trenchard D. Experimental results of vagal block in cardiopulmonary disease. In: Porter R, ed. Breathing: Hering–Breuer Centenary Symposium. London: J & A Churchill, 1970:315–329.
47. Jones PW, Huszczuk A, Wassermann K. Cardiac output as a controller of ventilation through changes in right ventricular loading. J Appl Physiol 1982; 53:281–284.
48. Rhodes J, Barst RJ, Garofano RP, Thoele DG, Gersony WM. Hemodynamic correlates of exercise function inpatients with primary pulmonary hypertension. J Am Coll Cardiol 1991; 18:1738–1744.
49. D'Alonzo GE, Gianotti L, Dantzker DR. Noninvasive assessment of hemodynamic improvement during chronic vasodilator therapy in obliterative pulmonary hypertension. Am Rev Respir Dis 1986; 133:380–384.
50. Janicki JS, Weber KT, Likoff MJ, Fishman AP. Exercise testing to evaluate patients with pulmonary vascular disease. Am Rev Respir Dis 1984; 129(suppl):S93–S95.
51. Dantzker DR, D'Alonzo GE, Bower JS, Popat K, Crevey BJ. Pulmonary gas exchange during exercise in patients with chronic obliterative pulmonary hypertension. Am Rev Respir Dis 1984; 130:412–416.
52. Come PC. Echocardiographic recognition of pulmonary arterial disease and determination of its cause. Am J Med 1988; 84:384–394.
53. Goodman J, Harrison DC, Popp RL. Echocardiographic features of primary pulmonary hypertension. Am J Cardiol 1974; 33:438–443.
54. Weyman AE, Dillon JC, Feigenbaum H, et al. Echocardiographic patterns of pulmonic valve motion with pulmonary hypertension. Circulation 1974; 50:905–910.
55. Meltzer RS, Valk NK, Cate F, et al. Contrast echocardiography in pulmonary hypertension: observations explaining early closure of the pulmonic valve. Am Heart J 1983; 106:1394–1398.

56. Shimada R, Takeshita A, Nakamura M. Noninvasive assessment of right ventricular systolic pressure in atrial septal defect: analysis of the end-systolic configuration of the ventricular septum by two-dimensional echocardiography. Am J Cardiol 1984; 53:1117–1123.
57. Visner MS, Arentzen CE, Crumbly AS, et al. The effects of pressure-induced right ventricular hypertrophy on left ventricular diastolic properties and dynamic geometry in the conscious dog. Circulation 1986; 74:410–419.
58. King ME, Braun H, Goldblatt A, et al. Interventricular septal configuration as a predictor of right ventricular systolic hypertension in children: a cross-sectional echocardiographic study. Circulation 1983; 68:68–75.
59. Kitabatake A, Inoue M, Asao M, et al. Non-invasive evaluation of pulmonary hypertension by a pulsed Doppler technique. Circulation 1983; 68:302–309.
60. Kosturakis D, Goldberg SJ, Allen HD, et al. Doppler echocardiographic prediction of pulmonary arterial hypertension in congenital heart disease. Am J Cardiol 1984; 53: 1110–1115.
61. Martin-Duran R, Larman M, Trugeda A, et al. Comparison of Doppler-determined elevated pulmonary arterial pressure with pressure measured at cardiac catheterization. Am J Cardiol 1986; 57:859–863.
62. Kitabatake A, Ito H, Inoue M, Kamada T. Evaluation of pulmonary hypertension by Doppler echocardiography. Practical Cardiol 1986; 12:136–149.
63. Niederle P, Starek A, Jezek V, Hes I. Doppler echocardiography in the diagnosis of pulmonary hypertension. Cor Vasa 1988; 30:272–278.
64. Yock PG, Popp RL. Non-invasive estimation of right ventricular systolic pressure by Doppler ultrasound in patients with tricuspid regurgitation. Circulation 1984; 70:657–662.
65. Berger M, Haimowitz A, Van Tosh A, Berdoff RL, Goldberg E. Quantitative assessment of pulmonary hypertension in patients with tricuspid regurgitation using continuous wave Doppler ultrasound. J Am Coll Cardiol 1985; 6:359–365.
66. Masuyama T, Kodama K, Kitabatake A, Sato H, Nanto S, Inoue M. Continuous-wave Doppler echocardiographic detection of pulmonary regurgitation and its application to non-invasive estimation of pulmonary artery pressure. Circulation 1986; 74:484–494.
67. Laaban JP, Diebold B, LaFay M, et al. Detection of pulmonary hypertension by Doppler echocardiography of the inferior vena cava in chronic airflow obstruction. Thorax 1989; 44:396–401.
68. Blanchard DG, Dittrich HC. Pericardial adaptation in severe chronic pulmonary hypertension: an intraoperative transesophageal echocardiographic study. Circulation 1992; 85:1414–1422.
69. Chen WJ, Kuan P, Lien W, Lin FY. Detection of patient foramen ovale by contrast transesophageal echocardiography. Chest 1992; 101:1515–1520.
70. Packer MB, Greenberg B, Massie B, et al. Deleterious effects of hydralazine in patients with primary pulmonary hypertension. N Engl J Med 1982; 306:1326–1331.
71. Hecht SR, Berger M, Berdoff RL, et al. Use of continuous-wave Doppler ultrasound to evaluate and manage primary pulmonary hypertension. Chest 1986; 90:781–783.
72. Groves BM, Ditchey RV, Reeves JT, et al. Multicenter trial of a new guidewire thermodilution catheter. J Am Coll Cardiol 1984; 3:599 (abstr).

73. Rozkovec A, Montanes P, Oakley CM. Factors that influence the outcome of primary pulmonary hypertension. Br Heart J 1986; 55:449–458.
74. D'Alonzo GG, Barst RJ, Ayres SM, et al. Survival in patients with primary pulmonary hypertension: results from a natural prospective registry. Ann Intern Med 1991; 115: 343–349.
75. Wilson AG, Harris CN, Lavender JP, et al. Perfusion lung scanning in obliterative pulmonary hypertension. Br Heart J 1973; 35:917–930.
76. Chapman PJ, Bateman ED, Benatar SR. Primary pulmonary hypertension and thromboembolic pulmonary hypertension—similarities and differences. Respir Med 1990; 84:485–488.
77. Moser KM, Page GT, Ashburn WL, et al. Perfusion lung scans provide a guide to which patients with apparent primary pulmonary hypertension merit angiography. West J Med 1988; 148:167–170.
78. Rich S, Pietra GG, Kieras K, et al. Primary pulmonary hypertension: radiographic and scintigraphic patterns of histologic subtypes. Ann Intern Med 1986; 105:499–502.
79. Rich S, Levitsky S, Brundage BH. Pulmonary hypertension from chronic pulmonary thromboembolism. Ann Intern Med 1988; 108:425–434.
80. Moser KM, Spagg RG, Utley J, et al. Chronic thrombotic obstruction of major pulmonary arteries: results of thromboendarterectomy in 15 patients. Ann Intern Med 1983; 99:299–304.
81. Anderson G, Reid L, Simon G. The radiographic appearances in primary and thromboembolic pulmonary hypertension. Clin Radiol 1973; 24:113–120.
82. Shure D, Gregoratos G, Moser KM. Fiberoptic angioscopy: role in the diagnosis of chronic pulmonary arterial obstruction. Ann Intern Med 1985; 103:844–850.
83. Posteraro RH, Sostman HD, Spritzer CE, Herfkens RJ. Cine-gradient-refocused MR imaging of central pulmonary emboli. Am J Roentgenol 1989; 152:465–468.
84. Perlmutt LM, Braun SD, Newman GE, Oke EJ, Dunnick NR. Pulmonary arteriography in the high-risk patient. Radiology 1987; 162:187–189.
85. Nicod P, Peterson K, Levine M, Dittrich H, Buchbinder M, Chappuis F, Moser K. Pulmonary angiography in severe chronic pulmonary hypertension. Ann Intern Med 1987; 107:565–568.
86. Rich S, Kieras K, Hart K, et al. Antinuclear antibodies in primary pulmonary hypertension. J Am Coll Cardiol 1986; 1307–1311.
87. Isera R, Yaneva M, Weiner E, Parke A, Rohfield N, Dantzker D, Rich S, Arnett F. Autoantibodies in patients with primary pulmonary hypertension. Am J Med 1992; 93:307–312.
88. Bradley TD, Rutherford R, Grossman RF, Lue F, Zamel R, Moldofsky H, Phillipson EA. Role of daytime hypoxemia in the pathogenesis of right heart failure in the obstructive sleep apnea syndrome. Am Rev Respir Dis 1985; 131:835–839.
89. Boysen PG, Block AJ, Wynne JW, Hunt LA, Flick MR. Nocturnal pulmonary hypertension in patients with chronic obstructive pulmonary disease. Chest 1979; 76: 536–542.
90. Coccagna G, Lugaresi E. Arterial blood gases and pulmonary and systemic arterial pressure during sleep in chronic obstructive pulmonary disease. Sleep 1978; 1:117–124.

91. Fletcher EC, Levin DC. Cardiopulmonary hemodynamics during sleep in subjects with chronic obstructive pulmonary disease; the effect of short and long-term O_2. Chest 1984; 85:6–14.
92. Weitzenblum E, Muzet A, Ehrhart M, Ehrhart J, Sautegeau A, Weber L. Variations nocturnes des gaz du sang et de la pression arterielle pulmonaire ches les brochitiques chroniques insuffisants respiratoires. Nouv Presse Med 1982; 11:1119–1122.
93. Wagenvoort CA. Lung biopsy specimens in the evaluation of pulmonary vascular disease. Chest 1980; 77:614–625.

10

Hemodynamic Evaluation in Primary Pulmonary Hypertension

DEMETRIOS GEORGIOU

UCLA School of Medicine
Saint John's Cardiovascular Research Center
and Harbor–UCLA Medical Center
Torrance, California

TIESHENG CAO

Tangdic Hospital
Fourth Military Medical University
Xian, People's Republic of China
and Harbor–UCLA Medical Center
Torrance, California

SHELLEY M. SHAPIRO, LEONARD E. GINZTON, and BRUCE H. BRUNDAGE

UCLA School of Medicine,
and Harbor–UCLA Medical Center
Torrance, California

I. Introduction

The diagnosis of primary pulmonary hypertension (PPH) is difficult to make in the early stages. Many of the symptoms are nonspecific and, in the early stages, may be mild. Patients themselves may discount or underplay symptoms delaying diagnosis. Initial evaluation should include history, physical examination, electrocardiography, chest x-ray films, and Doppler echocardiography, to look for signs of elevated right-sided pressure and vascular changes in the lungs. However, in the National Institutes of Health (NIH) National Heart, Lung, and Blood Institute registry (1), 6% of the patients had normal chest roentgenograms, echocardiograms, and electrocardiograms, despite the presence of significant pulmonary hypertension on cardiac catheterization. Therefore, if the diagnosis is suspected, right-sided heart catheterization should be performed. With this catheterization, direct measurement of pulmonary pressures can be made, as well as calculation of pulmonary vascular resistance and oxygen saturations can be obtained to exclude systemic-to-pulmonary (PA) shunts. Acquisition of hemodynamic data is useful not only for the diagnosis of this disorder, but also for prognosis. The results from the NIH Patient Registry for Primary Pulmonary Hypertension demonstrated that variables, such as elevated mean right atrial pressure (MRAP), elevated mean pulmonary artery pressure (MPAP), and decreased cardiac index (CI) were associated with poor survival (2). Although catheterization is the most direct technique to obtain hemodynamic data, Doppler echocardiography can be used noninvasively to measure right ventricular (RV) pressures, cardiac output, and right atrial pressure (RAP).

The purpose of this review is to discuss the invasive and noninvasive modalities available for obtaining qualitative as well as quantitative hemodynamic data for the diagnosis of PPH. The hemodynamic assessment of therapy is discussed elsewhere (see Chapter 11).

II. Noninvasive Assessment

A. Echocardiography

Echocardiography has two roles in the identification and assessment of patients with PPH: one is to exclude valvular and other vascular causes for elevated right-sided pressures; the other is to qualitatively and quantitatively estimate the hemodynamic abnormalities associated with PPH. Two-dimensional (2-D) echocardiography can easily identify and quantitate the presence of mitral stenosis and regurgitation, atrial septal defect (ASD), ventricular septal defect (VSD), pulmonic valvular abnormalities, and a variety of congenital abnormalities associated with pulmonary hypertension including aortic-to-pulmonary artery connections. Two-D echocardiography can identify RV hypertrophy, enlargement, and decreased RV function, as indirect markers of elevated pulmonary artery pressure. However, partial anomalous pulmonary venous return, sinus venous ASD, and small VSD can be missed, particularly if the quality of the echocardiographic images is poor. Transesophageal echocardiography (TEE), particularly with the newer multiplane (omniplane) probes, can improve visualization of pulmonary veins and intracardiac structure and may further expand the role of echocardiography in the evaluation of patients with suspected PPH. Use of TEE has not been tested in a prospective way, nor is it clear that it will obviate the need for catheterization.

B. Doppler Echocardiography in the Estimation of Right Ventricular Pressure

Knowledge of pulmonary pressure is critical when the diagnosis of PPH is considered, or when the severity of the process is being evaluated. Until recently, measurements of pulmonary pressures were performed by cardiac catheterization. But with advances in 2-D echocardiography and Doppler, determination of pulmonary pressure has been possible noninvasively (3).

Estimation of pulmonary pressures requires detection of tricuspid or pulmonic regurgitation. Doppler echocardiography is a very sensitive method for the detection of tricuspid regurgitation when the phenomenon is sought meticulously (4,5), using color flow, continuous-, and pulsed-wave techniques. Doppler echocardiographic estimation of RV pressure is based on a formula relating pressure to blood flow velocity: $\Delta p = 4V^2$. By using this formula and the velocity of the tricuspid regurgitation jet, a pressure gradient between RV and RA during systole can be estimated. Right ventricular peak systolic pressure can be expressed by the formula: RVP = Δp + RAP. In the absence of significant pulmonic stenosis, the RVP is equal to the pulmonary artery systolic pressure. An example of a continuous-wave Doppler velocity profile is shown (Fig. 1) in a patient with PPH. The reliability of this estimation has been well documented by several investigators (3,6,11,12). However, there are several potential sources of error in this method. The most important one is that the tricuspid velocity of blood flow differs from the measured velocity by the cosine of the angle between the jet and the ultrasound beam (Fig. 2). Thus, if the angle between the jet and the ultrasound beam is large, RVPs can be severely underestimated. One can use color flow

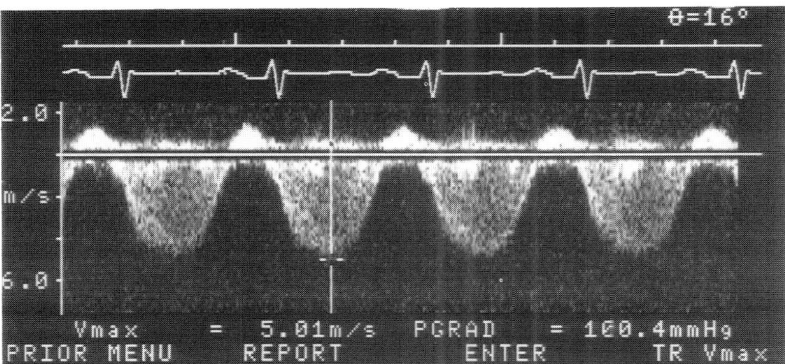

Figure 1 Continuous wave Doppler across the tricuspid valve taken from the apical five-chamber view in a patient with severe primary pulmonary hypertension (PPH) and tricuspid regurgitation. The figure demonstrated velocities of 5 m/sec occurring during systole. By using the modified Bernoulli equation, the estimated right ventricular systolic pressure in this patient with severe PPH is approximately 100 mmHg. The abscissa demonstrates time in 0.2-sec intervals, with the ECG just below the time makers. The ordinate measures velocities in 2-m/sec intervals.

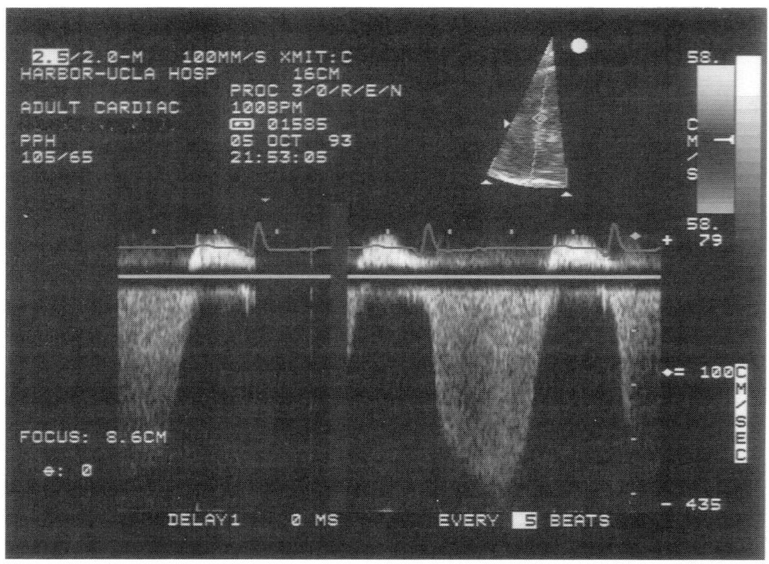
2.5/2.0-M 100MM/S XMIT:C
HARBOR-UCLA HOSP 16CM
PROC 3/0/R/E/N
ADULT CARDIAC 100BPM
01585
PPH 05 OCT 93
105/65 21:53:05
58.
CM/S
58.
+ 79
100 CM/SEC
FOCUS: 8.6CM
θ: 0
- 435
DELAY1 0 MS EVERY 5 BEATS

(A)

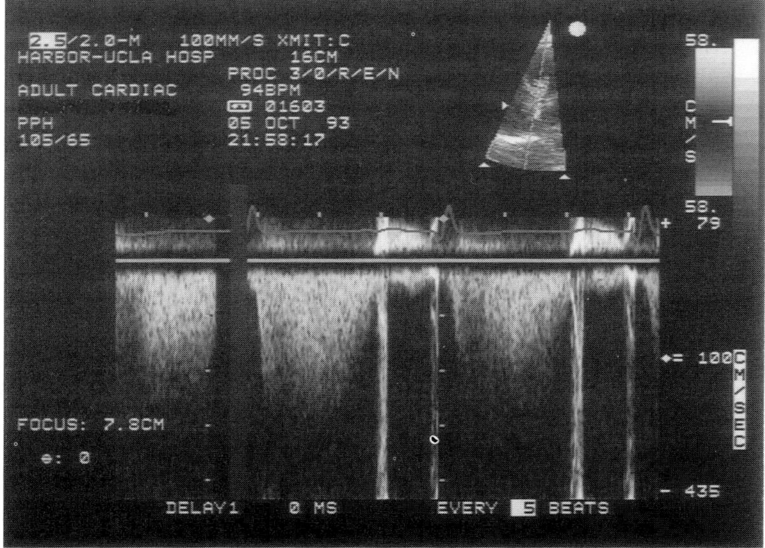
2.5/2.0-M 100MM/S XMIT:C
HARBOR-UCLA HOSP 16CM
PROC 3/0/R/E/N
ADULT CARDIAC 94BPM
01603
PPH 05 OCT 93
105/65 21:58:17
58.
CM/S
58.
+ 79
100 CM/SEC
FOCUS: 7.8CM
θ: 0
- 435
DELAY1 0 MS EVERY 5 BEATS

(B)

Doppler to help localize the jet of tricuspid regurgitation and to improve orientation of the transducer in relation to the regurgitant jet. However, the regurgitant jet is three-dimensional, whereas the echocardiogram scans through a series of 2-D planes. Thus, alignment of the transducer and jet may be difficult if the jet moves out of the plane of the transducer. By using several different views (RV inflow, parasternal short-axis, or apical four-chamber) and modifying the transducer angle to align the color flow or continuous-wave Doppler jet, a maximum regurgitant velocity can be obtained.

The Doppler estimation of pulmonary artery pressure (both systolic and diastolic) incorporates the RAP in the calculation. The estimation of RAP adds another source of error and controversy into the measurement. Some investigators have proposed fixed estimates and suggested adding 10 mmHg, others 5 mmHg, and still others 12 mmHg (6). In patients without RV failure or severe tricuspid regurgitation, these estimates add only a small error to the measurement. However, if the RAP is quite elevated, this approach can cause considerable error. Consequently, direct measurement of the height of jugular venous pulse has been proposed by others (3). Berger et al. (11) used continuous-wave Doppler to predict peak arterial systolic pulmonary pressure, without the estimation of RAP. They found an excellent correlation between the Doppler gradient and the pulmonary artery systolic pressure measured by cardiac catheterization ($r = 0.97$, standard error of the estimate = 4.9 mmHg). Estimating RAP clinically and adding it to the Doppler-determined RV-to-RAP gradient was not necessary to achieve accurate results in patients without right-sided heart failure. However, when Doppler is used to evaluate a diverse group of patients with pulmonary hypertension, we recommend that estimation of RAP from the jugular venous pulse in the individual patient is valuable to more accurately estimate pulmonary pressure.

The appearance of the proximal inferior vena cava (IVC) on an echocardiogram is directly related to the RAP (7,8; Fig. 3). Several investigators have proposed using changes in the diameter of the inferior vena cava to estimate RA

Figure 2 Figures A and B demonstrate the tricuspid regurgitation velocities measured by continuous-wave Doppler taken from the apical four-chamber view in the same patient at close intervals. (A) The transducer is aligned with the jet yielding a maximum velocity of close to 4 m/sec. The density of the signal and the quality of the envelope suggest it is fairly well aligned. (B) The jet is not well aligned, and the measured velocity is closer to 3 m/sec. Note that the Doppler envelope is indistinct and the density of the signal is less. The minor shift in transducer angle resulted in an artifactual reduction of velocity and, therefore, estimated pressure. This is a black and white version from the original color flow velocity map of tricuspid regurgitation. Note that the color velocity map is lost, but the angle between the transducer and the velocity jet is still visible.

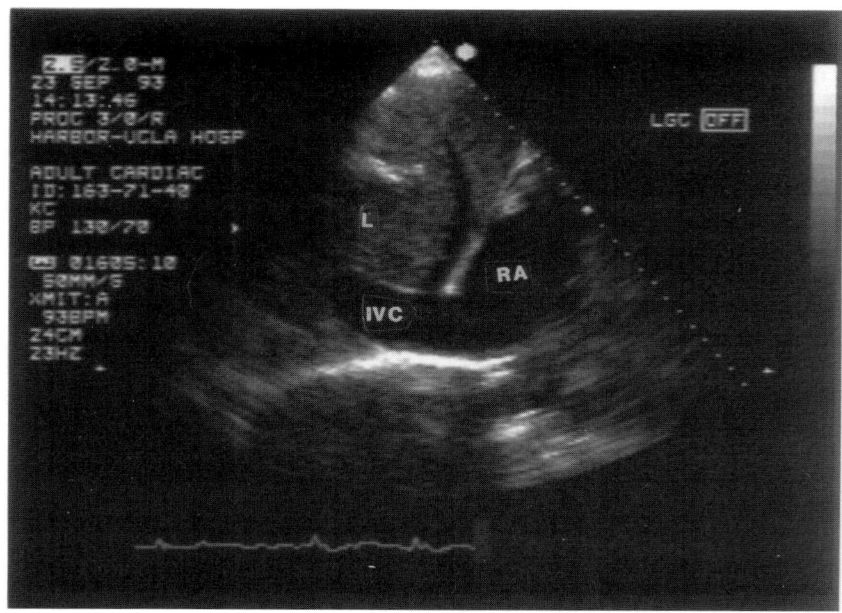

Figure 3 A still frame 2-D echocardiographic image of the liver (L), inferior vena cava (IVC), and right atrium (RA) obtained from a subcostal window. The IVC is quite dilated, consistent with high right atrial pressures and tricuspid regurgitation.

pressure. Schiller has proposed that the RAP is normal if, during inspiration, the IVC collapses, or at least reduces its diameter by 50% or more (9). An RAP greater than 15 mmHg is associated with inspiratory collapse of the IVC that is less than 50% of its original diameter or entirely absent. Shiller and Sahn (10) estimate RAP by recording the behavior of the IVC both during quiet respiration and during voluntary deep inspiration. When the IVC is small and collapses during spontaneous respiration, hypovolemia or obstructive lung disease should be suspected. When the IVC is of normal size and collapses more than 50% during a voluntary deep inspiration, then RAP is less than 10 mmHg. If the IVC does not collapse to 50% of its original diameter, then the RAP is between 15 and 20 mmHg. Use of the IVC diameter in estimating RVP in patients with PPH has not been tested prospectively, and it is not clear that it will improve the accuracy of the technique.

It is also possible to estimate pulmonary artery end-diastolic pressure (PAEDP) using the Doppler velocities generated by the jet of pulmonic regurgitation. Both pulmonic and tricuspid regurgitation can be identified by Doppler in a significant number of normal subjects, as well as in patients with elevated right-sided pressures. In fact, Masuyama et al. (3) detected pulmonary regurgitation with continuous-wave Doppler in about half of the patients without pulmonary hypertension. End-diastolic pressure can be determined by applying the modified Bernoulli equation to the end-diastolic pulmonary regurgitation velocity (13). The PAEDP is equal to the summation of the RAP and the end-diastolic gradient between the pulmonary artery and the RV outflow tract. The peak velocity of the signal occurs just after the onset of diastole, with progressive deceleration throughout diastole.

Although potentially of great value, it has not been established that Doppler echocardiography is sensitive enough in detecting small changes in PAP systolic and diastolic pressure to be reliably used for serial evaluations during therapy.

C. Estimation of Cardiac Output

Cardiac output can be calculated using 2-D and Doppler echocardiography by applying the continuity equation. The flow through the aorta is measured and integrated over systole (velocity times integral). The aortic root or LVOT area can be calculated by measuring the diameter. If one knows the heart rate, one can then determine the cardiac output. The major source of error in this measurement is the use of the aortic root area in determining stroke volume. The assumption made is that flow is laminar through the aortic root. If the measured aortic root area does not represent an accurate area through which flow occurs, the estimation of cardiac output will be wrong. Several studies have used and validated cardiac output determined echocardiographically and shown a reasonable correlation with catheterization data (14,15). Cardiac output derived in this way may permit noninvasive follow-up of patients with PPH undergoing therapy, awaiting transplant, or being followed, and could reduce the need for repeated cardiac catheterization.

D. Qualitative Echocardiographic Assessment

Qualitative assessment of pulmonary hypertension has also been attempted using echocardiographic findings. Pulmonic valve profile in patients with PPH, such as rapid-opening slope in systole (16,17), attenuation or absence of a "dip" of the pulmonic valve profile by Doppler (16,18), prolongation of the ratio of RV preejection period (RVPEP) to RV ejection time (RVET; 17,19), and midsystolic semiclosure of the pulmonic valve (16–18), have been employed with promising results. Kitabatake et al. (20) evaluated the blood flow characteristics in the RV outflow tract in patients with PPH by pulse Doppler technique. They found that midsystolic notching was observed in only 53% of the patients with pulmonary hypertension. Therefore, they concluded that midsystolic notch is not always associated with elevated pulmonary artery pressure. The acceleration time (AcT) of the pulmonic flow or the ratio of AcT to RVET (Act/RVET) decreased with increase in mean pulmonary artery pressure, with a very high correlation ($r = -0.90$) between AcT/+RVET and $\log_{10}$ of mean pulmonary pressure.

E. Evaluation of Left Ventricular Hemodynamics in Patients with Elevated Right Ventricular Pressure

In patients with PPH there are significant geometric alterations in the architecture and filling of the right ventricle (RV) that impinge on the filling pattern and geometry of the left ventricle (LV; Fig. 4). These alterations may affect LV diastolic-filling pressures. Competition between RV and LV for limited pericardial space may be a factor in flattening of the ventricular septum late in systole and early in diastole (21). We used Doppler echocardiography to investigate the relation between the geometric distortions and the filling dynamics in PPH (21). In this study, looking at nine patients with PPH compared with normal controls, transmitral flow was measured with pulsed Doppler. It showed a reduction in early

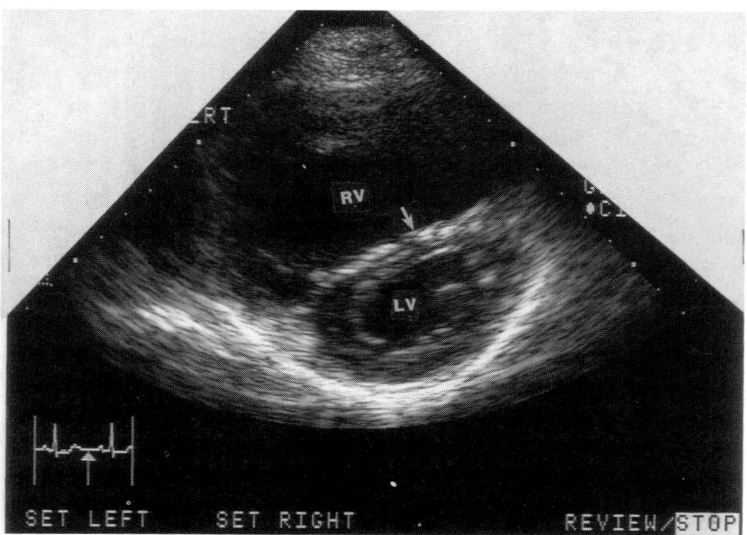

Figure 4 This still frame 2-D echocardiographic image taken from the parasternal short-axis view demonstrates marked flattening of the interventricular septum in a patient with severe pulmonary hypertension. The septum is marked with an arrow. Right ventricle (RV); left ventricle (LV). Note the ECG in the lower left-hand corner of the figure. The arrow marks the part of the cardiac cycle in which the frame occurs. The arrow indicates that the image is from early diastole and the flattening is compromising early LV filling.

diastolic filling and a change in the ratio of early to late filling. The LV isovolumic relaxation time was significantly prolonged, and early diastolic cavity expansion was also reduced. The curvature of the septum in patients with PPH was also distorted and abnormally flattened toward the LV during late systole, and it remained flattened well into diastole. These observations led to the conclusion that, in patients with PPH, late diastolic filling and atrial systole may have a major role in contributing to LV filling and maintaining adequate preload, and that the distortion of the septal geometry by the pressure-overloaded RV results in the abnormal diastolic filling. The differential effect of RV pressure versus RV volume overload on LV geometry and filling were also studied (22). In contrast with patients with pressure overload, those with volume overload and a leftward shift of the septum occurred early in systole and did not affect septal position in early diastole. The duration of isovolumetric relaxation was not prolonged, and the atrial contribution to LV filling was reduced, rather than increased, in patients with RV volume overload. Thus, the position and curvature of the LV septum are affected differently in RV pressure and volume-overloaded states, and these differences result in changes in LV filling. Many patients with PPH have both volume and pressure overload, with the development of RV failure and severe tricuspid regurgitation. In those patients, LV filling may be negatively affected by the combined distortions in architecture.

Relying on late diastolic filling and atrial systole to maintain LV preload in PPH may have significant implications for the use of vasodilator therapy in this disorder. For example, a decrease in pulmonary vascular resistance (PVR) with vasodilator therapy may cause augmentation of pulmonary blood flow, without a concomitant decrease in mean pulmonary pressure, resulting in increased volume loading of the LV at a time when early filling dynamics are still impaired because of flattening of the LV septum toward the LV cavity. This, in turn, may lead to serious side effects, such as pulmonary edema or systemic hypotension.

III. Exercise Testing in Primary Pulmonary Hypertension

Exercise testing may be a useful addition to the noninvasive hemodynamic evaluation of patients with PPH. In a recent report, Rhodes et al. (23) studied the hemodynamic correlates of exercise function in patients with PPH to further define the role of exercise testing in the evaluation of these patients. Exercise and catheterization data were collected prospectively and were analyzed. Mean RAP correlated best with exercise capacity ($r = 0.83$; $p < 0.0001$). Exercise capacity greater than 75% of the predicted value identified the two patients who had a positive response to acute pulmonary vasodilator drug testing. An exercise capacity of less than 10% of predicted value was associated with a high mortality and identified the three patients who died during or soon after cardiac catheterization.

The investigators concluded that the ability of exercise testing to identify patients at high risk was superior to that of other noninvasive variables.

IV. Invasive Evaluation of Hemodynamic Data with Right-Sided Heart Catheterization

Cardiac catheterization is an integral part of the initial evaluation of patients with PPH. There are three major goals of catheterization: First, to directly measure the level of pulmonary artery pressure and estimate pulmonary vascular resistance; second, to exclude any left-to-right shunts or any other significant cardiac disorders affecting the left side of the heart; and third, to test the response to therapeutic agents.

The development of the balloon flotation catheter has made it possible both to rapidly determine and to continuously monitor the pressures in the RV, RA, PA, and to measure the pulmonary capillary wedge pressure (PCWP), as an estimation of LVEDP (24,25). By the time patients with PPH present for cardiac catheterization, the mean pulmonary artery pressures are frequently between 50 and 60 mmHg, with increases in RAP (1,2; Fig. 5A–D). An example of typical hemodynamic recordings in a patient with PPH is shown in Figure 6. Instrumentation of the pulmonary artery in patients with PPH, however, may be very difficult because of significant tricuspid regurgitation, dilatation of the right-sided chambers, severely elevated PA pressures, and low cardiac output. In patients with severe PPH, advancement of the soft flow-directed balloon catheters into the pulmonary artery or wedge position may be virtually impossible. In our experience, the use of a balloon flotation catheter stiffened with a 0.028-cm guide wire (Swan–Ganz guidewire TD catheter) has greatly facilitated the catheterization of the pulmonary artery. To obtain an accurate wedge pressure in these patients may be difficult because of the dilatation of the proximal pulmonary arteries and the marked tapering. One approach to this is, after floating the inflated balloon as far distally as it will go, deflate the balloon and advance the catheter further until there is slight resistance. The balloon can then be carefully reinflated to 0.75–1.0 ml to achieve an accurate wedge measurement. Typically, patients with PPH have low or normal PCWP (1). In the presence of a substantially elevated wedge pressure, left heart catheterization should be performed to measure the LVEDP directly and to exclude pulmonary veno-occlusive disease, mitral stenosis, or left ventricular dysfunction.

When the hemodynamic data are recorded, particular attention should be paid to the RAP and RV end-diastolic pressures. In fact, mean RAP and decreased cardiac index were the most important predictive variables for survival in patients with PPH in the NHLBI registry (2). Therefore, MRAP and RV stroke volume have important prognostic implications. Measurements of all right-sided pressures are properly made at normal end expiration, to avoid underestimation by incorporating negative intrathoracic pressures.

The best method for determining cardiac output in patients with low cardiac output states and with significant tricuspid regurgitation is the Fick method (26). By measuring oxygen saturation, the true forward flow can be determined. When performed in the catheterization laboratory, oxygen consumption should be measured directly, instead of estimated, since the estimations are based on assumptions that may not apply to seriously ill patients with PPH and may introduce significant errors in the calculation. In our experience, determination of cardiac output by thermodilution techniques is usually satisfactory for the adjustment of medication. One can obtain a Fick-derived cardiac output at baseline for comparison.

Understanding the relation between pressure and flow in the pulmonary circulation includes taking into account both steady-state and pulsatile hemodynamic factors. Recently, Laskey et al. (27) compared steady and pulsatile pulmonary hemodynamics at rest and during exercise in eight patients with PPH and in normal controls, using right heart catheterization. They demonstrated that alterations in pulmonary artery vascular hydraulic load are present in the resting state in patients with PPH, and that these abnormalities persist during exercise. These findings indicate that, in patients with PPH, proximal pulmonary artery distensibility is impaired. Both steady and pulsatile components of pulmonary artery vascular hydraulic load have considerable effect on exercise response. During exercise, there was an increase in PAP and no significant change in pulmonary vascular resistance. Although cardiac output increased during exercise, this increase was achieved solely as a result of exercise-induced increase in heart rate, with no change in stroke volume. Because stroke volume does not increase with exercise in PPH patients, the resting stroke volume is an important factor in the total exercise cardiac output. The strongest correlates of the exercise stroke volume response in PPH were resting levels of pulmonary artery diastolic pressure, PVR, and the reflection factor (a component of the pulsatile portion of the load). This relation underscores the importance of considering the total vascular hydraulic load encountered by the ejecting RV.

V. Other Noninvasive Techniques

Other diagnostic modalities, such as nuclear right ventriculography (RVG), computed tomography (CT), and magnetic resonance imaging (MRI), have been used in the noninvasive hemodynamic assessment of pulmonary hypertension.

The RV ejection fraction is inversely proportional to the pulmonary artery pressure (28) and, therefore, estimation of the degree of pulmonary hypertension from RVG has been used by some centers. However, the sensitivity and specificity of this technique in estimating pulmonary artery pressure is poor (29,30). Further-

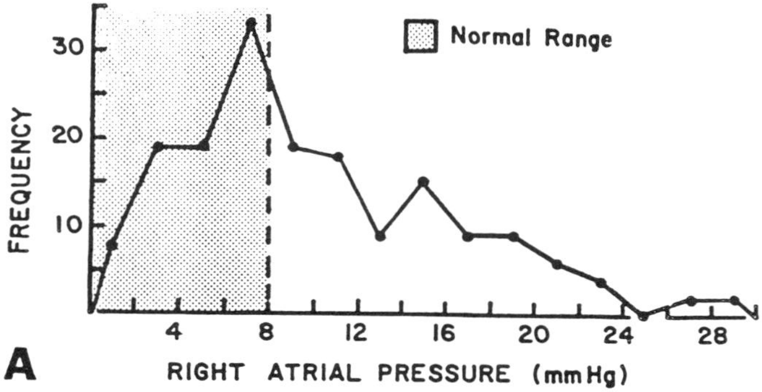

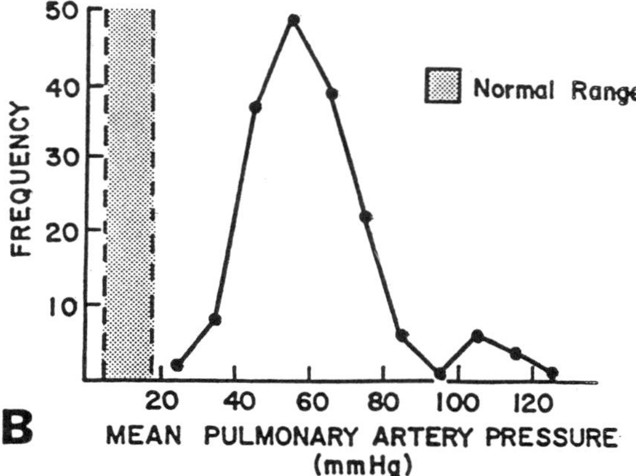

Figure 5 Distribution of hemodynamic findings is shown in relation to published normal values. (A) The right atrial pressure was elevated in 72%. (B) All patients, by definition, had an elevation in mean pulmonary artery pressure, with some having mean pulmonary pressures in excess of 100 mmHg. (C) The cardiac index was reduced in 71% and reached a nadir value of 0.9 L min^{-1} m^{-2}. (D) The pulmonary vascular resistance averaged 15 times higher than normal. Normal ranges are indicated by shaded regions. (From Ref. 1.)

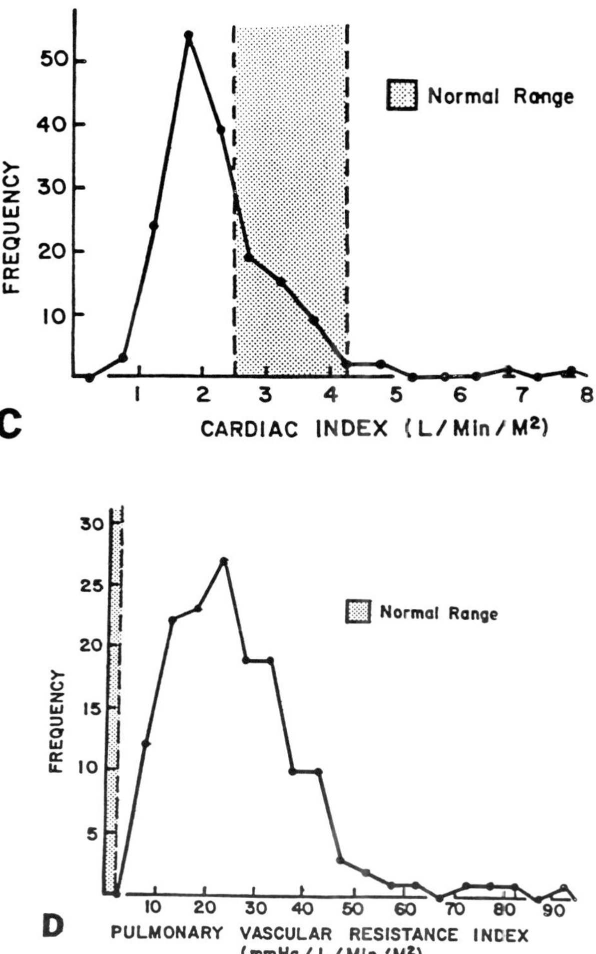

more, the overlap of an enlarged right atrium and RV results in underestimation of RV ejection fraction.

Computed tomography and MRI have been used in the diagnosis of pulmonary hypertension. The measurement of the diameter of the pulmonary artery can be made precisely and noninvasively (31,32). The PA diameter can be correlated with PA pressures, yielding an estimate of the severity of PPH. Advanced cardiac-imaging techniques, such as ultrafast (UF) CT and MRI, also provide very accurate methods for quantitation of LV and RV mass and function at rest and during exercise (32–34). We have measured RV free wall mass by UFCT and

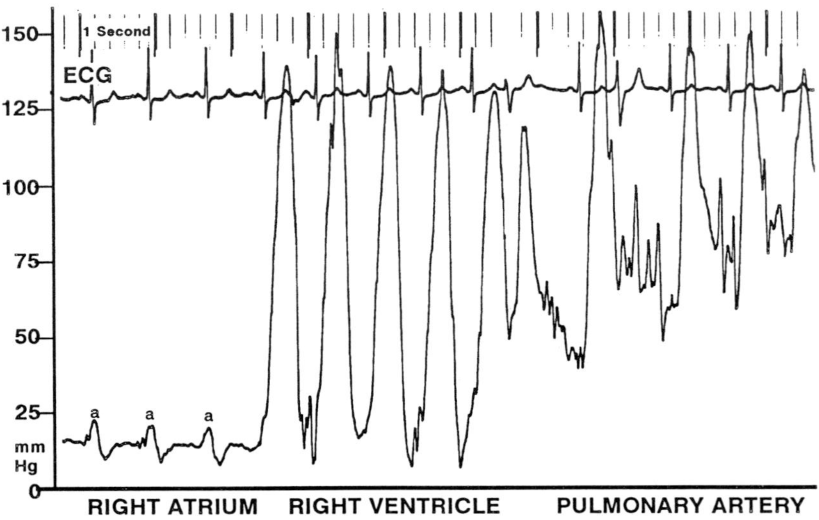

Figure 6 Hemodynamic tracings obtained during right heart catheterization. It is evident that the right ventricular and pulmonary artery systolic pressures are elevated at systemic levels. Right atrial pressure is also markedly elevated. (Courtesy of Dr. John Michael Criley, Saint John's Cardiovascular Research Center, Torrance, California.)

validated our measurements in 20 autopsy specimens with excellent correlation ($r = 0.92$; $p = <0.001$; SEE = 7.4 g); ultrafast CT RV free wall mass 53.9 ± 18.4 g versus anatomical RV free wall mass 55.8 ± 18.4 g (35). Both MRI and ultrafast CT have been used to provide information on pulmonary blood flow (36,37). Tajik et al. (36), using an animal model, were able to demonstrate a decrease in pulmonary flow in the area of pulmonary embolism using ultrafast CT.

Both MRI and ultrafast CT are likely to improve our understanding of RV function and help in the assessment of monitoring of patients with PPH. Both techniques are expensive and are not yet widely available. Therefore, although noninvasive tests, such as echocardiography, electrocardiography, and chest roentgenography, may not identify patients with early PPH, the use of the newer-imaging modalities that have potentially higher sensitivities is still limited.

VI. Conclusions

Frequently, the diagnosis of PPH is a diagnosis of exclusion and is arrived at by performing several diagnostic tests. Doppler and 2-D echocardiography provide quantitative and qualitative information about cardiac hemodynamics and anatomy. When used together, they can noninvasively diagnose and assess the severity of pulmonary hypertension, measure pulmonary artery pressures and cardiac output, and exclude other potential cardiac causes for the patient's clinical findings. Doppler and echocardiographic measurements have technical limitations and are dependent on the quality of the equipment and the skills of those performing and interpreting the studies. The sensitivity of echocardiography for diagnosing PPH falls off with lower levels of pulmonary artery pressures (38). The identification and measurement of the tricuspid regurgitant velocities are essential to the measurement of pulmonary artery pressures. In patients with mild pulmonary hypertension, the absence of tricuspid regurgitation, as well as the absence of significant hypertrophy or enlargement of the RV, may make echocardiography diagnostically useless. Given the data from the NIH registry for patients with PPH (1) in which 6% of patients had normal echocardiograms, despite the fact that they had PPH and the limitations of Doppler and 2-D echocardiography, right heart catheterization is essential in making the diagnosis of PPH. Hemodynamic data obtained at catheterization in combination with exercise testing may help better identify patients at high risk. Despite these limitations, Doppler echocardiography is a useful technique and should be employed first when the clinician is confronted with a patient suspected to have PPH.

Although right heart catheterization is an invasive procedure, it should be part of a complete evaluation, especially when therapeutic interventions are contemplated, such as vasodilator therapy. Advanced cardiac imaging techniques, such as ultrafast CT and MRI, look promising in expanding our understanding of RV function.

References

1. Rich S, Dantzker DR, Ayres SM, Bergofsky EH, Brundage BH, Detre KM, Fishman AP, Goldring RM, Groves BM, Koerner SK, Levy PC, Reid LM, Vreim CE, Williams GW. Primary pulmonary hypertension: a national prospective study. Ann Intern Med 1987; 107:216–223.
2. D'Alonzo GE, Barst RJ, Ayres SM, Bergofsky EH, Brundage BH, Detre KM, Fishman AP, Goldring RM, Groves BM, Kernis JT, Levy PS, Pietra GG, Reid LM, Reeves JT, Rich S, Vreim CE, Williams GW, Wu M. Survival in patients with primary pulmonary hypertension: results from a national prospective registry. Ann Intern Med 1991; 115:343–349.
3. Yock PG, Popp RL. Noninvasive estimation of right ventricular systolic pressure by Doppler ultrasound in patients with tricuspid regurgitation. Circulation 1984; 70:657–662.
4. Berger M, Hect S, VanTosh A, Lingam U. Pulsed and continuous wave Doppler echocardiographic assessment of valvular regurgitation in normal subjects. J Am Coll Cardiol 1989; 13:1540–1545.
5. Choong C, Abascal V, Weyman J, Levine RA, Gentile F, Thomas JD, Weyman AE. Prevalence of valvular regurgitation by Doppler echocardiography in patients with

structurally normal hearts by two dimensional echocardiography. Am Heart J 1989; 117:636–642.

6. Masuyama T, Kodama K, Kitabatake A, Sato H, Nanto S, Inoue M. Continuous wave Doppler echocardiographic detection of pulmonary regurgitation and its application to noninvasive estimation of pulmonary artery pressure. Circulation 1986; 74: 484–492.
7. Moreno FLL, Hagan AD, Holmen JR, Pryor TA, Strickland RD, Castle CH. Evaluation of size and dynamics of the inferior vena cava as an index of right-sided cardiac function. Am J Cardiol 1984; 53:579–584.
8. Natori H, Tamaki S, Kira S. Ultrasonographic evaluation of ventilatory effect on inferior vena cava configuration. Am Rev Respir Dis 1979; 120:421–427.
9. Kircher B, Himelman RB, Shiller NB. Right atrial pressure estimation from respiratory behavior of the inferior vena cava. Circulation 1988; 78:II-550.
10. Shiller NB, Sahn DJ. Pulmonary pressure measurement by Doppler and two-dimensional echocardiography in adult and pediatric populations. In: Weir EK, Archer SL, Reeves JT, eds. The Diagnosis and Treatment of Pulmonary Hypertension. Mount Kisco, NY: Futura Publishing, 1992:41–59.
11. Berger M, Haimowitz A, VanTosh A, Berdoff RL, Goldberg E. Quantitative assessment of pulmonary hypertension in patients with tricuspid regurgitation using continuous wave Doppler ultrasound. J Am Coll Cardiol 1985; 6:359–365.
12. Currie PJ, Seward JB, Chan KL, Fyfe DA, Hagler DJ, Mair DD, Reeder GS, Nishimura RA, Tajik AJ. Continuous wave Doppler determination of right ventricular pressure; a simultaneous Doppler–catheterization study in 127 patients. J Am Coll Cardiol 1985; 6:750–756.
13. Isaaz K, Camacho A, Webb J, Chatterjee K, Schiller NB. Noninvasive computer reconstruction of the pulmonary artery pressure waveform using Doppler echocardiography. J Am Coll Cardiol 1989; 13:225A.
14. Ihlen H, Amlie JP, Dale J, Forfang K, Nitter-Hauge S, Otterstad JE, Simonsen S, Myhre E. Determination of cardiac output of Doppler echocardiography. Br Heart J 1984; 51:54–60.
15. Stewart WJ, Jiang L, Mich R, Pandian N, Guerrero JL, Weyman AR. Variable effects of changes in flow rate through the aortic, pulmonary and mitral valves on valve area and flow velocity: impact on quantitative Doppler flow calculations. J Am Coll Cardiol 1985; 6:653–662.
16. Nanda NC, Gramiak R, Robinson TI, Shah PM. Echocardiographic evaluation of pulmonary hypertension. Circulation 1974; 50:575.
17. Lew W, Karliner JS. Assessment of pulmonary valve echocardiogram in normal subjects and in patients with pulmonary arterial hypertension. Br Heart J 1979; 42:147.
18. Weyman AE, Dillon JC, Feigenbaum H, Chan S. Echocardiographic patterns of pulmonic valve motion with pulmonary hypertension. Circulation 1974; 50:905.
19. Hirshfeld S, Meyer R, Schwartz DC, Korfhagen J, Kaplan S. The echocardiographic assessment of pulmonary artery pressure and pulmonary vascular resistance. Circulation 1975; 52:1975.

20. Kitabatake A, Inoue M, Asao M, Masuyama T, Tanouchi J, Morita T, Mishima M, Uematsu M, Shimazu T, Hori M, Abe H. Noninvasive evaluation of pulmonary hypertension by a pulsed Doppler technique. Circulation 1983; 68:302–309.
21. Louie EK, Rich S, Brundage BH. Doppler echocardiographic assessment of impaired left ventricular filling in patients with right ventricular pressure overload due to primary pulmonary hypertension. J Am Coll Cardiol 1986; 8:1298–1306.
22. Louie EK, Rich S, Levitsky S, Brundage BH. Doppler echocardiographic demonstration of the differential effects of right ventricular pressure and volume overload on left ventricular geometry and filling. J Am Coll Cardiol 1992; 19:84–90.
23. Rodes J, Barst RJ, Garofano RP, Thoele DG, Gersony WM. Hemodynamic correlates of exercise function in patients with primary pulmonary hypertension. J Am Coll Cardiol 1991; 18:1738–1744.
24. Swan HJC, Ganz W, Forrester J, Markus H, Diamond G, Chonette D. Catheterization of the heart in man with use of flow-directed balloon-tipped catheter. N Engl J Med 1970; 283:447–451.
25. Batson GA. Measurement of pulmonary wedge pressure by the flow directed Swan–Ganz catheter. Cardiovasc Res 1972; 6:748–752.
26. Guyton AC, Jones CE, Coleman TG. Circulatory Physiology Cardiac Output and Its Regulation. 2nd ed. Philadelphia: WB Saunders, 1973.
27. Laskey WK, Ferrari VA, Palevsky HI, Kussmaul WG. Pulmonary artery hemodynamics in primary pulmonary hypertension. J Am Coll Cardiol 1993; 21:406–412.
28. Brent BN, Berger HJ, Matthay R, Mahler D, Pytlik, Zaret BL. Physiologic correlates of right ventricular ejection fraction in COPD: a combined radionuclide and hemodynamic study. Am J Cardiol 1982; 50:255–262.
29. Korr KS, Gandsman EJ, Windler ML, Shulman RS, Bough EW. Hemodynamic correlates of right ventricular ejection fraction measured with gated radionuclide angiocardiography. Am J Cardiol 1982; 49:71–77.
30. Marmor AT, Mijiritsky Y, Plich M, Frenkel A, Front D. Improved radionuclide method for assessment of pulmonary artery pressure in COPD. Chest 1986; 89:64–69.
31. Kiriyama K, Gamsu G, Stern RG, Cann CE, Herfkens RJ, Brundage BH. CT-determined pulmonary artery diameters in predicting pulmonary hypertension. Invest Radiol 1984; 19:16–22.
32. Bouchard A, Higgins CB, Byrd BF, Amparo EG, Osaki L, Axelrod R. Magnetic resonance imaging in pulmonary arterial hypertension. Am J Cardiol 1985; 56: 938–942.
33. Hajduczok ZD, Weiss RM, Stanford W, Marcus ML. Determination of right ventricular mass in humans and dogs with ultrafast cardiac computed tomography. Circulation 1990; 82:202–212.
34. Boxt LM, Katz J, Kolb T, Czegledy FP, Barst RJ. Direct quantitation of right and left ventricular volumes with nuclear magnetic resonance imaging in patients with primary pulmonary hypertension. J Am Coll Cardiol 1992; 19:1508–1515.
35. Cutrone JA, Georgiou D, Khan S, Pollak A, Laks MM, Brundage BH. Right ventricular mass measurement by ultrafast computed tomography: validation with autopsy data. Invest Radiol 1995; 30:64–68.

36. Schultness GK, Fisher MR, Higgins CB. Pathologic blood flow in pulmonary vascular disease as shown by gated magnetic resonance imaging. Ann Intern Med 1970; 103: 317–323.
37. Tajik JK, Kugelmass SD, Hoffman EA. An automated method for relating regional pulmonary structure and function: integration of dynamic multislice CT and thin slice high resolution CT. SPIE Electronic Imaging Sci Technol 1993; 339–350.
38. Serwer GA, Cougle AG, Eckerd BM, et al. Factors affecting use of the Doppler-determined time from flow onset to maximal pulmonary artery velocity for measurement of pulmonary artery pressure in children. Am J Cardiol 1986; 58:352–356.

11

Medical Management

LEWIS J. RUBIN

University of Maryland School of Medicine
Baltimore, Maryland

STUART RICH

University of Illinois at Chicago
Chicago, Illinois

I. Introduction

For nearly three decades after its initial clinical description (1), primary pulmonary hypertension (PPH) had been considered an untreatable and uniformly fatal disease. Although there remains no cure for PPH, the past decade has witnessed considerable developments in its management, which translate to significant improvement in morbidity and prolonged survival for many patients. This chapter will review the current nonsurgical management options for PPH.

II. General Measures

A diagnosis of PPH does not necessarily preclude an active and fulfilling lifestyle, but certain measures and precautions should be considered. PPH is a lifelong illness which can be aggravated by a variety of factors, most of which are avoidable. Both patients and their physicians should be familiar with these factors since hemodynamic deterioration can be life-threatening and not easily reversible.

A. Physical Activity

Once a diagnoses of PPH has been established, it is important to counsel the patient regarding physical activity. We generally advise our patients to engage in activities to the extent of their physical capabilities. Since physical activity can be associated with marked increases in pulmonary artery pressure (2), patients should avoid performing isometric exercises and activities that produce dangerous symptoms, such as chest pain, presyncope, or syncope. A supervised cardiopulmonary rehabilitation program may be of benefit to promote conditioning. Many patients with PPH report having "good and bad days," and we encourage patients to respond to these signals by resting when needed.

B. Concomitant Medications

While most medications that are frequently used to treat coexistent illnesses are safe for use in patients with PPH, care should be taken both in prescribing medicines and in using over-the-counter drugs. Decongestants with α-adrenergic properties should be avoided since they can exert cardiovascular effects that are poorly tolerated. Nonsteroidal anti-inflammatory agents (NSAIDs) should be used with caution since their maternal use has been implicated in the pathogenesis of pulmonary hypertension of the newborn (PPHN) (3,4) and they may increase the risk of gastrointestinal hemorrhage when oral anticoagulants are used. Although most antibiotics can be administered safely to patients with PPH, it is preferable, when possible, to avoid agents that interact with warfarin.

C. Birth Control and Pregnancy

Pregnancy and parturition produce dramatic hemodynamic and hormonal changes that are poorly tolerated by PPH patients, and abrupt deterioration and death can occur, particularly during the postpartum period (5–7). Accordingly, we strongly advise our patients to avoid pregnancy by practicing a safe and effective method of contraception. Unfortunately, oral contraceptive agents should also be avoided since they can produce prothrombotic changes that could potentially aggravate pulmonary hypertension (8,9). The most effective form of contraception for most patients is surgical sterilization.

If PPH is diagnosed during pregnancy, the patient should be immediately referred to a specialist and should undergo a thorough assessment including hemodynamic evaluation with right heart catheterization. It is critical that the patient be placed in the most optimum medical condition, which may necessitate the use of high doses of calcium channel blockers (10) or continuous intravenous prostacyclin. In addition, even if labor and delivery are uneventful the patient should be closely monitored for 48–72 hr to avoid the syndrome of postpartum circulatory collapse that has been known to occur.

D. Altitude

Hypoxia is a potent pulmonary vasoconstrictor and plays a major role in the pathogenesis of pulmonary vascular disease in the setting of parenchymal lung disease and altitude sickness (11,12). Patients with PPH are at risk for decompensation upon exposure to hypoxic environments, owing to both the vasoconstrictor effects and the resultant decrease in oxygen-carrying capacity. Thus, patients should be advised to avoid conditions in which the ambient oxygen concentration may be decreased, such as altitude and travel in nonpressurized airplane cabins. If exposure to these environments is necessary, supplemental oxygen should be used. Since most commercial airplanes are pressurized, travel on these is usually safe, although mild reductions in arterial oxygen content can be expected. Thus, patients with marginal gas exchange may benefit from the use of supplemental oxygen during airplane flights, and this can usually be arranged in advance with most commercial air carriers.

III. Specific Measures

A. Anticoagulation

In situ thrombosis appears to be a major pathophysiological mechanism in the development of PPH. In addition, patients with PPH are predisposed to the development of deep venous thrombosis because of venous stasis resulting from right heart dilation, sluggish pulmonary blood flow, and a sedentary life-style. The inability of the hypertensive pulmonary vascular bed to recruit unused vasculature or dilate existent vessels in response to an additional vascular insult places the patient with PPH in jeopardy if a thromboembolic event occurs. Indeed, intravascular thrombosis is frequently seen at autopsy in PPH, and thromboembolism is presumed to be one of several mechanisms responsible for the sudden death that occurs in this population (13).

Although there are no controlled trials of anticoagulation in PPH, two studies suggest that oral anticoagulant therapy prolongs life. Fuster et al. (13), in a retrospective analysis from the Mayo Clinic, demonstrated improved survival in patients who were treated with warfarin (Fig. 1A). In a small prospective study, Rich and his colleagues (14) have shown that patients who did not respond to calcium channel blockers and who were treated with warfarin had improved survival compared with those who were not anticoagulated (1-year survival 91% vs. 62%, and 3-year survival 47% vs. 31%, Fig. 1B).

Warfarin is the anticoagulant of choice, with the recommended dose adjusted to achieve an International Normalized Ratio (INR) of the prothrombin time between 1.5 and 2.5 based on trials of deep venous thrombosis. Heparin administered subcutaneously in doses of 5000–10,000 units twice daily may be a suitable alternative to warfarin in patients who experience adverse effects with the

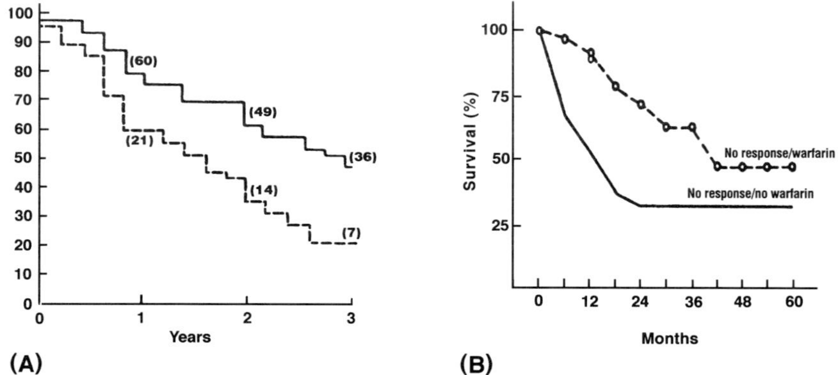

Figure 1 Effects of anticoagulation on survival in PPH. (A) Retrospective series from Mayo Clinic. (From Ref. 13, with permission.) (B) Prospective series from the University of Illinois. (From Ref. 14, with permission.)

latter or in whom the risk of bleeding is considered to be increased, although the long-term side effects of heparin, such as osteopenia and thrombocytopenia, can be troublesome (15). The target aPPT with heparin therapy should be 1.3–1.5 times control.

In addition to the general risk of hemorrhage associated with chronic anticoagulation for cardiovascular diseases, anticoagulant therapy in patients with PPH poses additional, disease-specific problems: Right ventricular failure, which can develop over a relatively brief period of time, can result in hepatic congestion and impaired synthesis of clotting factors. Rupture of atherosclerotic pulmonary vessels can produce life-threatening hemoptysis (16), particularly when anticoagulants have been administered. Despite these risks, we believe that all patients with PPH should be treated with anticoagulants unless a strong contraindication exists.

B. Supplemental Oxygen

Patients with hypoxemic lung disease and secondary pulmonary hypertension manifest improved pulmonary hemodynamics and prolonged survival with the administration of low-flow supplemental oxygen therapy (17–19). In this setting, pulmonary hypertension is due, at least in part, to the pulmonary vasoconstrictive and vasoproliferative effects of alveolar hypoxia. In contrast, hypoxemia is not generally a prominent feature of PPH until late in its course or shunting is present through a patent foramen ovale; hence, supplemental oxygen does not usually produce substantial hemodynamic or symptomatic benefit in most PPH patients (20).

Chronic hypoxemia in PPH is the result of two mechanisms, both of which signify advanced disease: impaired cardiac output, resulting in mixed venous (and, therefore, arterial) hypoxemia, and right-to-left shunting through a patent foramen ovale as right ventricular dysfunction causes right atrial pressure and volume overload. The earliest manifestation of the former may be exercise-induced oxygen desaturation, which can be alleviated or blunted with ambulatory portable oxygen therapy. In contrast, the hallmark of shunt-induced hypoxemia is the absence of substantial improvement of arterial oxygenation with supplemental oxygen. While oxygen therapy may be tried in these patients (15), other pharmacological measures will be necessary in attempting to reduce the extent and consequences of the increased venous admixture (see below).

C. Diuretics and Cardiac Glycosides

Right heart failure results in the same consequences of salt and water retention as left ventricular dysfunction with the exception of pulmonary vascular congestion, and diuretics can be useful in reducing right ventricular preload and alleviating its congestive symptoms such as edema, hepatic distention, and dyspnea. In some patients small doses of loop diuretics such as furosemide are adequate, while others require larger doses of more potent diuretics administered orally or parenterally. Since the calcium channel blocking agents frequently cause salt and water retention, it is often useful to initiate diuretics with the introduction of calcium blocker therapy, even in the absence of clinically apparent right heart failure. As with all patients who are treated with diuretics, careful monitoring of serum electrolytes is necessary, and potassium-sparing agents, such as spironolactone may be useful as adjunctive therapy.

The value of cardiac glycosides in treating isolated right heart dysfunction is controversial. Studies in cor pulmonale suggest that these agents are most useful when left ventricular failure is also present (21). Although glycosides increase tension in isolated pulmonary artery rings, presumably by inhibition of the Na^+ pump and increasing intracellular Ca^{2+} via the Na^+-Ca^{2+} antiporter (22), there is no evidence that their clinical use is detrimental. Some authorities have advocated administering glycosides to patients with PPH who are also receiving calcium channel blockers to counteract the negative inotropic effects of the latter agents (23). Since neurohormonal activation has now been demonstrated in PPH (24), digoxin also has the potential to be of value due to its sympatholytic properties (25).

D. Vasodilator Therapy

Although the earliest clinical reports detailing the hemodynamic derangements in PPH include descriptions of attempts to vasodilate the pulmonary circuit (1,26), it was not until nearly 40 years later, with the development of potent systemic antihypertensive agents, that clinical trials using vasodilators were reported. As

Table 1 Hemodynamic Assessment of Vasodilators in Pulmonary Hypertension

Parameter measured	Desired acute changes	Comments
Mean pulmonary artery pressure	>25% fall; ideally the mean PAP below 30 mmHg	There must not be any associated significant fall in systemic blood pressure.
Pulmonary vascular resistance	>33% fall; ideally the PVR below 6 units	Should be associated with fall in PA pressure *and* increase in cardiac output. An increase in cardiac output alone may lead to future RV failure.
Right atrial pressure	No change, or fall	An increase in RA pressure signals impending RV failure.
Pulmonary capillary wedge pressure	No change	An increase in wedge pressure suggests pulmonary veno-occlusive disease or coexisting LV dysfunction.
Systemic blood pressure	Minimal fall, mean arterial pressure should remain above 90 mmHg	A significant hypotensive response makes chronic vasodilator therapy contraindicated.
Cardiac output	Increase	The increase should be related to increased stroke volume and not solely due to increased heart rate.
Heart rate	No significant change	A chronic increased heart rate will result in RV failure. Watch for bradycardia if high doses of diltiazem are used.
Systemic arterial oxygen saturation	Increase if reduced on room air, little change if normal	A fall in systemic arterial oxygen saturation suggests lung disease or right-to-left shunting and prohibits chronic usage.
Pulmonary artery (mixed venous) oxygen saturation	Increase	Should reflect the increase in cardiac output and improved tissue oxygenation.

our understanding of vascular biology has grown, newer and more selective pulmonary vasodilator agents have been studied, although rarely can the hemodynamic abnormalities of PPH be normalized. It should be appreciated that there are no prospective randomized trials of oral vasodilators in the treatment of primary pulmonary hypertension. The possibility exists that in some patients they may not only fail to be beneficial, but may indeed be harmful and lead to accelerated death. Consequently, we need to emphasize that they should be used with extreme caution, following established hemodynamic guidelines, and with close outpatient follow-up. The empiric use of vasodilators in patients with PPH should be condemned. Despite these important caveats, vasodilator therapy may be useful for many patients, either as definitive treatment or as supportive therapy until transplantation can be performed.

The rationale for using vasodilators to treat PPH was based on the hypothesis that vasoconstriction was an early feature of the disease and could, potentially, be reversed or modified by the use of drugs that exerted pulmonary vascular smooth muscle relaxant effects. This hypothesis was supported initially by pathological studies of "early" pulmonary hypertension, which demonstrated hypertrophy of the smooth muscle in the small and medium-sized pulmonary arteries (27). Subsequently, a number of studies suggested that altered expression or clearance of a variety of vasoactive substances may contribute to the pathogenesis of PPH (28–30). Several potent vasodilator agents that are used to treat systemic hypertension and left ventricular failure have pulmonary vasodilator properties in experimental conditions, although none of the commercially available oral or topical agents consistently exert selective pulmonary vasodilator effects.

Early reports described the acute effects of parenterally administered vasodilators in PPH, including acetylcholine, tolazoline, and isoproterenol (1,26,31). Subsequently, phentolamine, diazoxide, and hydralazine administered orally were reported to produce chronic hemodynamic responses in case reports or small series of patients (32–36), although adverse systemic effects limited their usefulness (35–37). Nevertheless, these preliminary reports established the potential for treating some patients with vasodilators.

Studies in isolated lung preparations, vascular ring segments, and single smooth-muscle cells suggested that membrane-bound calcium channels are involved in the pulmonary vasoconstrictor responses to hypoxia and other agonist stimuli, and that these responses could be altered by the application of calcium-channel blocking agents (38,39). Subsequent studies in primary and secondary forms of pulmonary hypertension demonstrated sustained hemodynamic improvement in some patients treated with calcium-channel blocking agents, which led to their widespread and indiscriminate use (40–43). Unfortunately, these drugs can also produce significant adverse effects including systemic hypotension, worsening gas exchange, or depressed ventricular function (44–46). These untoward effects, which can occur acutely or with chronic therapy, can be life-threatening in patients with a severely compromised hemodynamic state; experience from the NIH Registry on PPH suggests that patients with severely depressed right ventricular function are at the greatest risk of a fatal outcome when vasodilators are administered acutely (47). The most widely used vasodilators to treat PPH are shown in Table 2.

Table 2 Dose Ranges, Route of Administration, and Half-Lives of the Most Frequently Used Vasodilators

Drug	Route	Dose range	Half-life
Prostacyclin[a]	Intravenous	2–24 ng/kg/min	3 min
Prostaglandin E_1	Intravenous	0.005–0.03 μg/kg/min	2–4 min
Adenosine	Intravenous	50–200 ng/kg/min	5–10 sec
Nitric oxide	Inhaled	10–80 ppm	15–30 sec
Nifedipine[b]	Oral	30–240 mg/day	2–5 hr
Diltiazem[b]	Oral	120–900 mg/day	2–4.5 hr

[a]Dose range is for acute infusion; dose requirements and tolerance in patients receiving long-term infusions have increased over time, often exceeding 100–150 ng/kg/min.
[b]Sustained-release preparations (Procardia XL and Cardizem CD) may be administered once daily; half-life shown refers to conventional preparations.

E. Testing of Acute Vasoreactivity

The concept of acutely testing for vasoreactivity prior to embarking on a course of chronic therapy is intended to reduce the risk of adverse events with vasodilators by identifying those patients who are likely to benefit from long-term therapy. Acute pharmacological testing should be performed under invasive hemodynamic monitoring by clinicians who have experience with these agents and with PPH. Several short-acting vasodilators have been used to test for vasoreactivity (48–52), including acetylcholine, prostaglandins E_1 and I_2, and adenosine, and the responses to these agents have generally been useful in predicting the likelihood of response to longer-acting oral agents (53–55). The advantage of acute testing lies in its safety: adverse effects can usually be reversed quickly by discontinuing the infusion, owing to the short half-life of these drugs in the circulation. The agents most commonly used to test acute vasoreactivity and their recommended dosing regimens are shown in Table 1. At present, the most widely used agents are nitric oxide (NO), adenosine, and PGI_2.

Adenosine

Adenosine is an intermediate product in the metabolism of adenosine triphosphate. It has been demonstrated to have potent systemic and pulmonary vasodilator properties. Because of the extremely short half-life (less than 5 sec), it likely works as a local mediator of vascular tone. It is believed that adenosine stimulates endothelial and vascular smooth-muscle receptors of the A2 type, which then induces vascular smooth muscle relaxation by stimulating cyclic AMP. Adenosine has been tested as a pulmonary vasodilator in patients with PPH and found to be predictive of the effects of intravenous prostacyclin and oral calcium channel blockers (55,56). It is administered intravenously in doses of 50 ng/kg/min and titrated upward every 2 min until the patient develops uncomfortable symptoms such as chest tightness or dyspnea. The short half-life provides a measure of safety so that any untoward effects of the medication would be dissipated within moments of its discontinuation. Adenosine is given as an infusion, and not as an intravenous bolus as it is used to treat supraventricular tachyarrhythmias.

Nitric Oxide

Nitric oxide (NO) is produced by vascular endothelium from L-arginine and produces vasorelaxation by increasing cyclic GMP in vascular smooth muscle. Of the short-acting vasodilators, inhaled nitric oxide (NO) may be the safest since it is inactivated by hemoglobin binding in the pulmonary capillaries; thus, inhaled NO has virtually no systemic vasodilator effect (50). Recent experience suggests that the acute responses to inhaled NO, like prostacyclin, are useful in predicting the likelihood of responsiveness to orally active agents (57). Unfortunately, the other nitrovasodilators, nitroglycerin and nitroprusside, are generally less potent and less selective than NO (43,47).

Prostacyclin

Prostacyclin, or prostaglandin I_2 (epoprostenol), is a product of the arachidonic acid cascade of prostanoid metabolism which has potent vasodilator and platelet antiaggregating properties. Prostacyclin tends to produce dose-dependent reductions in systemic vascular resistance when administered acutely, but serious adverse effects are uncommon and most of the side effects are dose-related and short-lived once the dose is decreased or the infusion is discontinued (48,50). Studies comparing the acute effects of nitric oxide and prostacyclin suggest that they are equipotent in their pulmonary vasodilator effects (57), although some patients may have a greater response to one than to the other.

F. Recommended Approach

Our recommended approach to acute vasoreactivity testing is as follows: After baseline hemodynamics have stabilized, prostacyclin, inhaled NO, or adenosine is administered in incremental doses until either a beneficial effect, no change, or adverse effect is observed. It is imperative that, in addition to monitoring pulmonary artery and right atrial pressures, systemic blood pressure, arterial oxygen saturation, and cardiac output are also measured during the trial.

The criteria for a "response" to acute vasodilator testing that is sufficient to justify embarking on a course of chronic oral vasodilator therapy remains only partially defined (15,58,59). Most investigators agree that a reduction in pulmonary artery pressure accompanied by an increase in cardiac output and little change in systemic pressure constitutes a potentially beneficial response, and patients with this pattern of vasoreactivity tend to experience sustained hemodynamic and symptomatic improvement as well as prolonged survival (14,23). Similarly, patients who experience a symptomatic fall in systemic pressure or arterial oxygen saturation, an increase in pulmonary artery or right atrial pressure, or a reduction in cardiac output are more likely to derive harm than benefit from oral therapy. Patients who experience an increase in cardiac output accompanied by little change in pulmonary or systemic blood pressures may experience symptomatic improvement with chronic therapy; however, they are less likely to manifest hemodynamic regression or improved survival. Thus, long-term benefit from vasodilator therapy in these patients remains in question. An outline of the hemodynamic assessment of acute vasodilator testing is shown in Table 1.

G. Chronic Vasodilator Therapy

Approximately 25–30% of patients will meet the criteria for responsiveness as described above, and long-term improvement with therapy in such individuals has been documented (14,23). Chronic treatment should be reserved for those patients who responded acutely in a manner that is considered potentially efficacious. In general, the doses of calcium channel-blocking agents required to produce sustained hemodynamic improvement are higher than those conventionally used to treat other cardiovascular disorders (23), although variability exists. The optimal dose should be identified for each patient based on both acute testing and tolerance, as well as serial noninvasive and invasive assessments. The two most widely used agents are nifedipine and diltiazem, and there does not appear to be a uniform advantage of one over the other. Both drugs can lower systemic blood pressure and produce salt and water retention; more serious adverse effects include worsening right heart dysfunction owing to the negative inotropic effects of these drugs, and worsening hypoxemia due either to a reduced cardiac output, increased right-to-left shunting through a foramen ovale, and decreasing V/Q relationships by increasing blood flow to poorly ventilated lung units. Acute discontinuation of chronic therapy should be assiduously avoided, since this has been reported to be fatal, presumably due to rebound pulmonary vasoconstriction in highly vasoreactive individuals (23). There is insufficient experience with the newer calcium-channel blockers to determine their utility in the management of PPH.

Until recently, there were no alternatives to transplantation for patients who were unresponsive or refractory to therapy with calcium channel antagonists, and up to 30% of those awaiting transplantation died prior to receiving a graft. Continuous intravenous infusion prostacyclin therapy has now been shown to improve hemodynamics and exercise tolerance and prolong life in severe [New York Heart Association (NYHA) functional classes III and IV] PPH (60–62);

recently, prostacyclin became the first drug ever approved by the Food and Drug Administration for the treatment of pulmonary hypertension.

While the rationale for administering prostacyclin continuously was based initially on its pulmonary vasodilator properties, it appears that other effects of the drug may be equally important, since even patients who do not manifest acute vasodilator responses to the drug have shown symptomatic and hemodynamic improvement with chronic therapy (61,62). Prostacyclin inhibits platelet aggregation and may have inhibitory effects on vascular growth and remodeling, and these properties may facilitate the restoration of endothelial-dependent functions that normally serve to maintain the low-resistance state of the pulmonary vascular bed. Accordingly, in contrast to calcium-channel-blocker therapy, which should be reserved for patients who experience potentially beneficial acute hemodynamic responses, treatment with continuous prostacyclin should be considered even in the absence of acute hemodynamic effects. The single exception to this statement may be patients with pulmonary veno-occlusive disease (PVOD), who have been reported to develop acute, reversible pulmonary edema with prostacyclin (60). This effect, which is probably the result of increasing pulmonary blood flow in the setting of downstream fixed vascular obstruction, is virtually diagnostic of PVOD and constitutes a contraindication to chronic therapy.

Prostacyclin can only be administered by continuous intravenous infusion since its half-life in circulation is brief (3–5 min) and it is inactivated at low pH. Minor adverse effects with chronic therapy are common and include rash, joint and jaw pain, and diarrhea. The serious complications of chronic therapy are usually attributable to the delivery system and include catheter-related infections and thrombosis and pump malfunctions resulting in overdosing or underdosing of the drug. Patients must be extensively trained in drug preparation and in troubleshooting the delivery system so that the potential risks of this complex treatment are minimized. In addition to these clinical criteria, however, patients should undergo rigorous emotional and psychological screening to ensure that they are sufficiently informed about the potential benefits and drawbacks of this unconventional treatment and are sufficiently motivated to safely manage the delivery system.

Patients who remain in NYHA functional classes III and IV despite maximal "conventional" therapy—typically consisting of anticoagulants, diuretics, oral vasodilators, cardiac glycosides, and supplemental oxygen, when appropriate—are deemed potential candidates for continuous prostacyclin therapy. There is little experience with less seriously ill patients treated with prostacyclin. An assessment of the risks and benefit of continuous-infusion therapy in patients in NYHA class II has not been performed; accordingly, we do not currently advocate prostacyclin therapy, in its present form, in these patients.

Therapy with prostacyclin is initiated once intravenous access with a permanent central venous line has been established. Dose increments (1–2 ng/kg/min) are made based on an assessment of both symptoms and drug tolerance. Although the dose requirements are variable, they tend to increase over time. This effect is more likely due to enhanced metabolic degradation with chronic therapy rather than tachyphylaxis. Some experienced physicians have followed a protocol of routinely increasing the infusion by 2 ng/kg/min every 2–3 weeks to preempt symptomatic recurrences. As with other approaches to therapy, noninvasive and invasive monitoring of therapy is crucial, and abrupt discontinuation of the infusion should be avoided since recrudescence of symptoms is likely to occur.

Prostacyclin has been used in two ways: as a bridge to transplantation and as a primary mode of therapy. Since the average wait for a lung transplant in the United States exceeds 1 year and there are no baseline demographic or hemodynamic variables that predict responsiveness to prostacyclin, some clinicians list patients for transplantation at the same time as continuous prostacyclin therapy is initiated. When improvement is seen with prostacyclin, it is usually sustained, although frequent dose adjustments may be necessary. Nevertheless, deciding whether to proceed with or defer transplantation in a patient being treated with

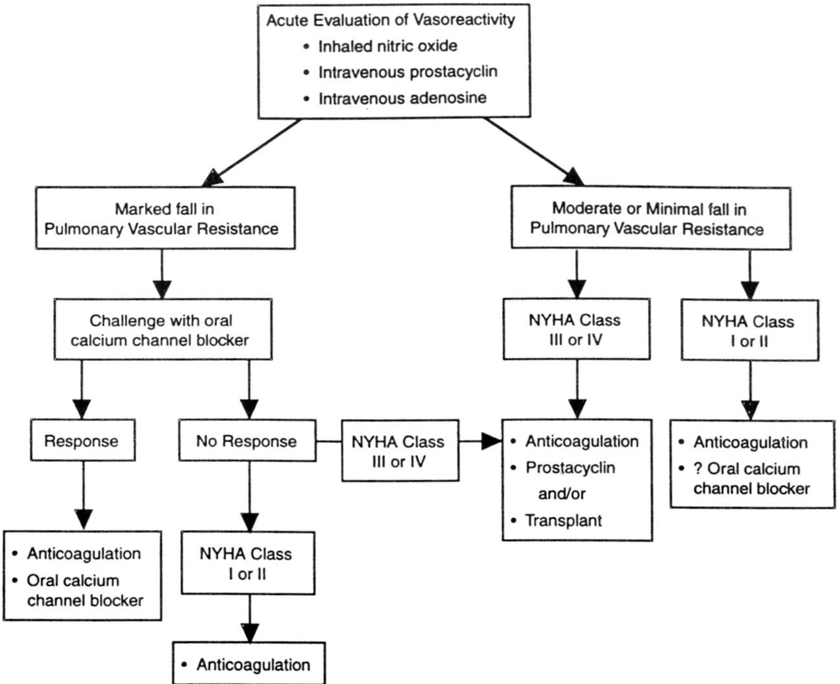

Figure 2 Algorithm for the management of PPH.

prostacyclin is often difficult, since sudden deterioration while on prostacyclin has occurred, even in patients who appeared to be doing well. Our algorithm for the management of PPH is shown in Figure 2.

As our understanding of the pathogenesis of PPH continues to evolve, more effective therapeutic approaches are likely to result. Oral or transdermal delivery of prostacyclin or an analog should be possible, eliminating the cumbersome and dangerous delivery mode currently in use. Recent studies have suggested that pulmonary endothelial production of endothelin may be increased and that synthesis of nitric oxide may be impaired in PPH (29,30). These observations could serve as a rationale for pharmacological manipulation using newly developed endothelin receptor antagonists or long-term inhaled nitric oxide (63). Alternatively, chronic diet supplementation with arginine, the precursor of nitric oxide, or administration of other compounds that stimulate endogenous nitric oxide synthesis may be useful therapeutic modalities, either alone or in combination with prostacyclin.

References

1. Dresdale DT, Schultz M, Michtom RJ. Primary pulmonary hypertension. I. Clinical and hemodynamic study. Am J Med 1951; 11:686–705.
2. Janiki JS, Weber KT, Likoff MJ, et al. The pressure-flow response of the pulmonary circulation in patients with heart failure and pulmonary vascular disease. Circulation 1985; 72:1270–1275.
3. Levin DL, Fixler DE, Morriss FC, Tyson J. Morphologic analysis of the pulmonary vascular bed in infants exposed in utero to prostaglandin synthase inhibitors. J Pediatr 1978; 92:478–483.
4. Manchester D, Margolis HS, Sheldon R. Possible association between maternal indomethacin therapy and primary pulmonary hypertension of the newborn. Am J Obstet Gynecol 1975; 126:467–473.
5. McCaffrey RM, Dunn LJ. Primary pulmonary hypertension in pregnancy. Obstet Gynecol Surg 1964; 19:567–591.
6. Demas NW. Maternal death due to primary pulmonary hypertension. Trans Pacif Coast Obstet Gynecol Soc 1972; 40:64–65.
7. Nelson DM, Main E, Crafford W, et al. Peripartum heart failure due to primary pulmonary hypertension. Obstet Gynecol 1983; 62:58S–63S.
8. Kleiger RE, Boxer M, Ingham RE, Harrison DE. Pulmonary hypertension in patients using oral contraceptives. Chest 1976; 69:143–147.
9. Oakley C, Somerville J. Oral contraceptives and progressive pulmonary vascular disease. Lancet 1968; 1:890–891.
10. Nootens M, Rich S. Successful management of labor and delivery in a patient with primary pulmonary hypertension. Am J Cardiol 1993; 71:1124–1125.
11. Fishman AP. Hypoxia on the pulmonary circulation: how and where it acts. Circ Res 1976; 38:221–231.

12. Macnee W. Pathophysiology of cor pulmonale in chronic obstructive pulmonary disease. Am J Respir Crit Care Med 1994; 150:833–852.
13. Fuster V, Steele PM, Edwards WD, Gersh BJ, McGoon MD, Frye RL. Primary pulmonary hypertension: natural history and the importance of thrombosis. Circulation 1984; 70:580–587.
14. Rich S, Kaufmann E, Levy PS. The effect of high doses of calcium-channel blockers on survival in primary pulmonary hypertension. N Engl J Med 1992; 327:76–81.
15. Rubin LJ, Barst RJ, Kaiser LR, et al. ACCP consensus statement: Primary pulmonary hypertension. Chest 1993; 104:236–250.
16. Yuceoglu YZ, Dresdale DT, Valensi QJ, et al. Primary pulmonary hypertension with hoarseness and massive (fatal) hemoptysis. Vasc Dis 1967; 4:290–292.
17. Nocturnal Oxygen Therapy Trial Group. Continuous or nocturnal oxygen therapy in hypoxemic chronic obstructive lung disease. Ann Intern Med 1980; 93:391–398.
18. Timms RM, Khaja FU, Williams, GW, and the Nocturnal Oxygen Therapy Trial Group. Hemodynamic responses to oxygen therapy in chronic obstructive pulmonary disease. Ann Intern Med 1985; 102:29–36.
19. Salvaterra CG, Rubin LJ. Investigation and management of pulmonary hypertension in chronic obstructive pulmonary disease. Am Rev Respir Dis 1993; 148:1414–1417.
20. Morgan JM, Griffiths M, du Bois RM. Hypoxic pulmonary vasoconstriction in systemic sclerosis and primary pulmonary hypertension. Chest 1991; 99:551–556.
21. Mathur PN, Powles RCP, Pugsley SO, et al. Effect of digoxin on right ventricular function in severe chronic airflow obstruction. Ann Intern Med 1981; 95:283–288.
22. Salvaterra CG, Rubin LJ, Schaeffer J, Blaustein MP. The role of Na/Ca exchange in the responses of pulmonary arteries to decreases in PO_2. Am Rev Respir Dis 1989; 139:933–939.
23. Rich S, Brundage BH. High dose calcium channel blocking therapy for primary pulmonary hypertension: evidence for long-term reduction in pulmonary arterial pressure and regression of right ventricular hypertrophy. Circulation 1987; 76:135–141.
24. Nootens M, Kaufmann E, Rector T, et al. Neurohormonal activation in patients with right ventricular failure from pulmonary hypertension: relation to hemodynamics and endothelin levels. J Am Coll Cardiol 1995; 26:1581–1585.
25. Ferguson DW. Digitalis and neurohormonal abnormalities in heart failure and implications for therapy. Am J Cardiol 1992; 69:24G–33G.
26. Wood P. Pulmonary hypertension with special reference to the vasoconstrictive factor. Br Heart J 1958; 20:557–570.
27. Wagenvoort CA, Wagenvoort N. Primary pulmonary hypertension: a pathologic study of the lung vessels in 156 clinically diagnosed cases. Circulation 1970; 42:1163–1184.
28. Christman BW, McPherson CD, Newman JH, et al. An imbalance between the excretion of thromboxane and prostacyclin metabolites in pulmonary hypertension. N Engl J Med 1992; 327:70–75.
29. Giaid A, Yanagisawa M, Langleben D, et al. Expression of endothelin-1 in the lungs of patients with pulmonary hypertension. N Engl J Med 1993; 328:1732–1739.
30. Giaid A, Saleh D. Reduced expression of endothelial nitric oxide synthase in the lungs of patients with pulmonary hypertension. N Engl J Med 1995; 333:214–221.

31. Shettigar UR, Hultgren HN, Specter M, et al. Primary pulmonary hypertension: favorable effect of isoproterenol. N Engl J Med 1976; 295:1414–1415.
32. Ruskin JN, Hutter AM. Primary pulmonary hypertension treated with oral phentolamine. Ann Intern Med 1979; 90:772–774.
33. Klinke WP, Gilbert JAL. Diazoxide in primary pulmonary hypertension. N Engl J Med 1980; 302:91–92.
34. Rubin LJ, Peter RH. Oral hydralazine therapy for primary pulmonary hypertension. N Engl J Med 1980; 302:69–73.
35. Cohen ML, Kronzon I. Adverse hemodynamic effects of phentolamine in primary pulmonary hypertension. Ann Intern Med 1981; 95:591–592.
36. Buch J, Wennevold A. Hazards of diazoxide in pulmonary hypertension. Br Heart J 1981; 46:401–403.
37. Packer MB, Greenberg B, Massie B, et al. Deleterious effects of hydralazine in patients with primary pulmonary hypertension. N Engl J Med 1982; 306:1326–1331.
38. Tolins M, Weir EK, Chesler E, et al. Pulmonary vascular tone is increased by a voltage-dependent calcium channel potentiator. J Appl Physiol 1986; 60:942–948.
39. McMurtry IF, Davidson AB, Reeves JT, Grover RF. Inhibition of hypoxic pulmonary vasoconstriction by calcium antagonists in isolated rat lungs. Circ Res 1976; 38:99–104.
40. Rubin LJ, Nicod P, Hillis LD, Firth BG. Treatment of primary pulmonary hypertension with nifedipine. Ann Intern Med 1983; 99:433–438.
41. Douglas JS. Hemodynamic effects of nifedipine in primary pulmonary hypertension. J Am Coll Cardiol 1983; 2:174–179.
42. Olivari MT, Levine TB, Weir EK, Cohn JN. Hemodynamic effects of nifedipine at rest and during exercise in primary pulmonary hypertension. Chest 1984; 86:14–19.
43. Brown G. Pharmacologic treatment of primary and secondary pulmonary hypertension. Pharmacotherapy 1991; 11:137–156.
44. Packer M, Medina N, Yushak M. Adverse hemodynamic and clinical effects of calcium channel blockade in pulmonary hypertension secondary to obliterative pulmonary vascular disease. J Am Coll Cardiol 1984; 4:890–901.
45. Berkenboom G. Failure of nifedipine treatment in primary pulmonary hypertension. Br Heart J 1982; 47:511.
46. Wood BA, Tortoledo F, Luck JC, Fennell WH. Rapid attenuation of response to nifedipine in primary pulmonary hypertension. Chest 1982; 82:793–794.
47. Weir EK, Rubin LJ, Ayres SM, et al. The acute administration of vasodilators in primary pulmonary hypertension: experience from the National Institutes of Health Registry on Primary Pulmonary Hypertension. Am Rev Respir Dis 1989; 140:1623–1630.
48. Rubin LJ, Groves BM, Reeves JT, et al. Prostacyclin-induced acute pulmonary vasodilation in primary pulmonary hypertension. Circulation 1982; 66:334–338.
49. Uren NG, Ludman PF, Crake T, Oakley CM. Response of the pulmonary circulation to acetylcholine, calcitonin gene-related peptide, substance P and oral nicardipine in patients with primary pulmonary hypertension. J Am Coll Cardiol 1992; 19:835–841.
50. Pepke-Zaba J, Higenbottam TW, Dinh-Xuan AT, Stone D, Wallwork J. Inhaled nitric oxide as a cause of selective pulmonary vasodilatation in pulmonary hypertension. Lancet 1991; 338:1173–1174.

51. Morgan JM, McCormack DG, Griffiths MJD, et al. Adenosine as a vasodilator in primary pulmonary hypertension. Circulation 1991; 84:1145–1149.
52. Groves BM, Badesch DB, Donnellan K, et al. Acute hemodynamic effects of iloprost in primary (unexplained) pulmonary hypertension. Semin Respir Crit Care Med 1994; 15:237.
53. Groves BM, Rubin LJ, Frosolono MF, Reeves JT. A comparison of the hemodynamic effects of prostacyclin and hydralazine in primary pulmonary hypertension. Am Heart J 1985; 110:1200–1204.
54. Barst RJ. Pharmacologically induced pulmonary vasodilatation in children and young adults with primary pulmonary hypertension. Chest 1986; 98:497–503.
55. Schrader BJ, Inbar S, Kaufmann E, et al. Comparison of the effects of adenosine and nifedipine in pulmonary hypertension. J Am Coll Cardiol 1992; 19:1060–1064.
56. Nootens M, Schrader B, Kaufmann E, Vestal R, Long W, Rich S. Comparative acute effects of adenosine and prostacyclin in primary pulmonary hypertension. Chest 1995; 107:54–57.
57. Sitbon O, Brenot F, Denjean A, et al. Inhaled nitric oxide as a screening vasodilator agent in primary pulmonary hypertension. Am J Respir Crit Care Med 1995; 151: 384–389.
58. Reeves JT, Groves BM, Turkevitch D. The case for treatment of selected patients with primary pulmonary hypertension. Am Rev Respir Dis 1986; 134:342–346.
59. Rich S. Primary pulmonary hypertension. Prog Cardiovasc Dis 1988; 31:205–238.
60. Rubin LJ, Mendoza J, Hood M, et al. Treatment of primary pulmonary hypertension with continuous intravenous prostacyclin (epoprostenol). Ann Intern Med 1990; 112: 485–491.
61. Barst RJ, Rubin LJ, McGoon MD, et al. Survival in primary pulmonary hypertension with long-term continuous intravenous prostacyclin. Ann Intern Med 1994; 121: 409–415.
62. Barst RJ, Rubin LJ, Long WA, et al. A comparison of continuous intravenous prostacyclin versus conventional therapy in primary pulmonary hypertension. N Engl J Med 1996; 334: 296–301.
63. Snell GI, Salamonsen RF, Bergin P, et al. Inhaled nitric oxide used as a bridge to heart-lung transplantation in a patient with end-stage pulmonary hypertension. Am J Respir Crit Care Med 1995; 151:1263–1266.

12

Transplantation for Primary Pulmonary Hypertension

YOSHIHIKO KATAYAMA, GEORGE CREMONA, JOHN WALLWORK, and TIM HIGENBOTTAM

Papworth Hospital NHS Trust
Cambridge, England

I. History of Thoracic Transplantation

Although successful human lung transplantation is a recently developed clinical procedure, lobe homograft transplantation was successfully performed in dogs as far back as 1947 by Demikhov (1). In 1950 canine pulmonary lobe allografts were successfully transplanted, but underwent rejection after 6–8 days (2). Demikhov also performed heart–lung transplantation (HLT) in dogs, which required a sequence of anastomoses timed to avoid prolonged cerebral ischemia. As a result of denervation of the heart and lungs, the dogs failed to sustain adequate ventilation, and irregular breathing patterns resulted from a loss of proprioceptive afferents from the lung. The concern about disruption of the normal-breathing pattern was allayed in later experiments, in which normal breathing was maintained with complete denervation of both lungs (3,4).

The first human lung allograft transplantation (LT) was performed in 1963 by Hardy in a patient with squamous cell carcinoma and chronic obstructive lung disease (5). In spite of successful reperfusion of the lung and the use of azathioprine and hydrocortisone, the patient died of renal failure and malnutrition after 18 days. Subsequent attempts at LT met with a similar fate, with only one patient who survived for 10 months. Human HLT was first performed by Cooley in

1968 (6) in an infant with an atrioventricular canal who died of respiratory failure 14 hr postoperatively.

The disappointing early clinical experience of both HLT and LT stimulated further laboratory developmental work. The discovery of the antilymphocytic effects of cyclosporine in animals (7) and its successful use in renal transplantation (8), was the first real advance in immunosuppressive therapy for 20 years. Meanwhile, improvements occurred in ventilatory support of the critically ill, and hemodynamic monitoring after cardiopulmonary bypass allowed the reintroduction of heart transplantation in the late 1970s. Reitz et al. (9) redeveloped the en bloc HLT in primates and achieved satisfactory tracheal anastomotic healing. The preservation of mediastinal collateral blood supply from the coronary arteries to the lower trachea and carina contributed to this result. This led, in turn, to the first successful long-term heart–lung transplant at Stanford, in a patient with primary pulmonary hypertension (PPH; 10).

Problems with bronchial anastomotic healing in the immediate postoperative period beleaguered single-lung transplantation (SLT). This was thought to be due to the effects of poor organ preservation, graft ischemia, immunosuppressive therapy with high-dose steroids, and rejection. The experimental use of omental pedicles to revascularize bronchial autografts in dogs (11), and the elimination of steroids in the immediate postoperative period (12), led to successful SLT for interstitial lung disease in 1983 (13). Subsequently, double-lung transplantation (DLT) was developed, initially involving median sternotomy, cardiopulmonary bypass, and tracheal anastomosis (14). This approach is no longer preferred, having been replaced with sequential bilateral lung transplantation (BLT) with two bronchial anastomoses, with considerable success (15).

Since the 1980s, both HLT and LT (16) have become established treatments for a wide range of end-stage cardiopulmonary diseases. Because of its poor prognosis PPH has been one of the principal indications for transplantation from the outset. With Eisenmenger's syndrome, PPH patients constituted much of the early heart–lung transplant population (17).

II. Preoperative Management

A. Assessment of Patients for Transplantation

Lung transplantation has been limited to relatively few patients, owing to a paucity of suitable donors. It must be remembered that, in most centers, the 5-year survival rates after SLT and HLT do not exceed 55% (18). The patients who are selected, therefore, have a poorer chance of survival with untreated PPH. The assessment programs are designed to allow a decision not only from the medical point of view, but also from the patient's perspective.

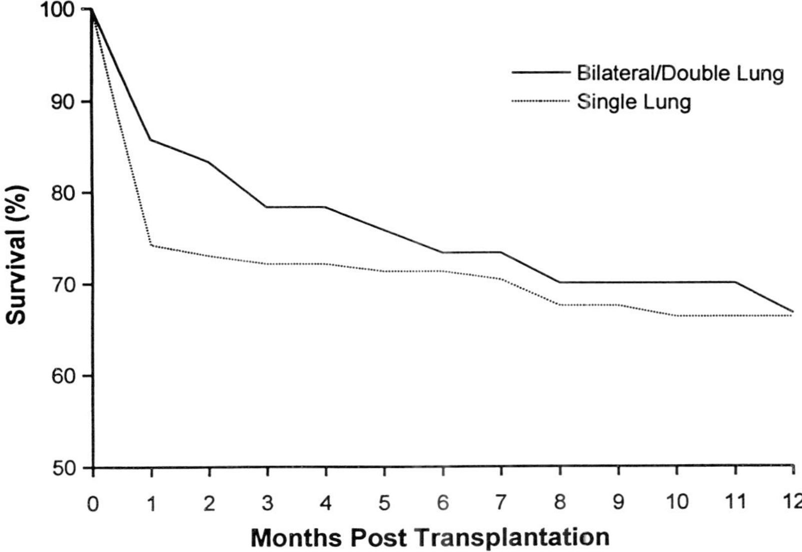

Figure 1 Survival curve with single- and double-lung transplantation. (From Ref. 18.)

The recipient and family are assessed by the transplant team and are allowed to assess the transplant team as well. During this period, they are encouraged to meet other transplant patients and to become familiar with all aspects of the transplant program. A formal interview between the surgeon and patient is then conducted. A number of different medical specialists are also involved in the selection process.

B. Diagnosis of Primary Pulmonary Hypertension

The first step in the assessment of patients for transplant surgery is to confirm the diagnosis of PPH (see Chapter 9 for a complete description of the approach to the diagnosis of PPH).

A ventilation–perfusion lung scan is undertaken to exclude chronic thromboembolic pulmonary hypertension (19,20), since changes suggestive of this disease should be pursued with pulmonary arteriography. Evidence of proximal large artery thromboembolism is an indication for consideration for thromboendarterectomy (21).

Right heart catheterization is undertaken to confirm the diagnosis of pulmonary hypertension. Additionally, hemodynamic measurements provide an accurate assessment of prognosis (22,23) and may also provide an indication of potential success with medical treatment.

C. Criteria for Recipient Selection

The natural history of PPH is now well described (23–25; see Chapter 13). In the absence of medical treatment, survival can be predicted from the hemodynamic results from right-sided heart catheterization.

Data from the National Institutes of Health (NIH) registry provide a simple equation to predict survival (26):

$$A(x,y,z) = e^{(0.007325x) + (0.0526y) - (.3275z)}$$

where x is the mean PAP, y is the mean right atrial pressure, and z is the cardiac index. The probability of surviving 1, 2, and 3 years would be then given by

$$p(1) = 0.75^{A}$$
$$P(2) = 0.65^{A}$$
$$P(3) = 0.55^{A}$$

Similar results have been reported by our group. Fuster et al. (23) have also reported a poorer prognosis in patients with a mixed venous oxygen saturation (Svo_2) below 60%.

Exclusion criteria for transplantation in PPH are in general the same as those for other pulmonary diseases (Table 1).

D. Opportunities for Alternative Medical Treatment

Approximately 20% of PPH patients have either a hemodynamic profile that indicates a favorable prognosis, including a CI $>$ 2.5 L min^{-1} m^{-2}, PAP $<$ 80 mmHg, and RAP $<$ 15 mmHg or Svo_2 greater than 60%, or show the ability to vasodilate with agents such as intravenous prostacyclin (PGI_2). These patients often respond to prolonged therapy with oral vasodilators, particularly the calcium channel blockers nifedipine and diltiazem (27,28). Up to 95% survival at 5 years has been reported for such patients, particularly when they also receive anticoagulants (27–31). In those patients with no capacity to immediately vasodilate, oral anticoagulants may also improve survival (28).

In patients with poor indices for survival, with or without the capacity to briefly vasodilate, long-term intravenous infusion of prostacyclin (PGI_2) can not only improve survival, but can also improve quality of life (30–32). Of, interest, excellent results may be seen in patients with Svo_2 of less than 60% and poor vasodilation capacity (31).

We now consider patients for transplant surgery only if they have failed to respond to prostacyclin or are deteriorating despite increased doses.

Table 1 Recipient Criteria for Lung Transplantation in Patients with PPH at Papworth Hospital

Absolute contraindications
Nonreversible organ dysfunction
Significant systemic or cerebrovascular disease
Malignancy
Ventilator dependence
Steroid dependence (> 10 mg/day of prednisolone)
Drug or alcohol abuse
Active systemic infection or aspergilloma
Relative contraindications
Age > 55 years (HLT, DLT)
Age > 60 years (single-lung transplantation)
Previous pleurectomy or pleurodesis
Insulin-dependent diabetes mellitus
Steroid dependence (< 10 mg/day of prednisolone)
Presence of *Aspergillus* in the sputum

E. The Choice of Transplantation Operation for Patients with Primary Pulmonary Hypertension

The earliest form of transplantation for PPH was HLT, which eliminates the failing right ventricle and removes the high pulmonary vascular resistance (10). As an alternative, both SLT and BLT have been used for the treatment of patients with PPH (33–36). We have used HLT principally because of the early excellent results. Additionally, in the United Kingdom, we can often undertake a "domino" operation that allows the recipient's heart to be used in another cardiac recipient. This is not as feasible in other countries, where cardiac and lung transplant surgery are run as separate programs. The use of SLT offers some advantage, as it does not use the heart, and potentially two or three recipients can benefit.

The HLT offers immediate correction of the hemodynamic problems. The Stanford group reported no recurrence of PPH in these patients. Long-term survival in PPH patients who have received HLT is the same as in other disease groups, with 1-year survival at 82% and 5-year survival at 44%. In our total population of 167 HLT patients, only 4 have developed coronary artery disease, a complication that is common in heart transplant patients.

Single-lung transplantation has achieved similar excellent results in patients with PPH (16). Patients experience restoration of near-normal pulmonary hemodynamics and resolution of right ventricular failure. The native lung receives only limited perfusion and most blood flow is diverted through the transplanted lung.

However, this can pose a major long-term problem (37,38): If the transplant lung develops obliterative bronchiolitis and underventilation, substantial hypoxemia develops with return of the patient's dyspnea. This has led to the use of sequential bilateral lung transplantation for PPH patients. Although experience is still too early for a comparison to be made, BLT may offer improvement comparable with HLT.

F. Criteria for Donor Selection and Organ Procurement

Donor Organ Selection

The intrinsic perversity of lung transplantation as a treatment lies in the necessity of someone's death to save the life of another. The improvements in automobile safety and treatment of head injury and stroke have appropriately impeded lung transplant programs. This scarcity was initially compounded by the strict exclusion criteria, so that only 10–15% of suitable cardiac donors were accepted as pulmonary donors. Since 1990, we have adopted a policy of sending a donor team, consisting of a surgeon, anaesthetist, and perfusionist experienced in organ harvesting, to support the intensive care personnel at the referring hospital. The team is equipped with facilities for invasive cardiopulmonary monitoring and bronchoscopy to ensure proper management of the donor. This approach has improved donor management and allowed harvesting of lungs from approximately 40% of heart donors. Our selection criteria are listed in Table 2. When a potential donor becomes available, information is requested on gas exchange and chest radio-

Table 2 Donor Selection Criteria for Lung Transplantation

Age < 55 years
No history of cardiopulmonary disease including asthma and neoplasm
No major thoracic trauma
No pulmonary or systemic infection
Normal chest radiograph
Minimal secretions on endotracheal suction (microorganisms may be present)
Satisfactory gas exchange ($PaO_2 > 100$ mmHg with FIO_2[a] = 30%)
Short period of mechanical ventilation (within 4 days)
Normal lung compliance (peak inspiratory airway pressure < 30 mmH_2O when tidal volume < 15 ml kg^{-1} and respiratory rate 10–14 min^{-1}
Additional conditions for HLT
Normal electrocardiogram
Minimal inotropic requirement with adequate left and right atrial pressures (dopamine or dobutamine < 10 μ kg^{-1} min^{-1})

[a]Fractional inspired oxygen.

graphic appearance. If these are satisfactory, the donor team is sent to evaluate the organs on site and decide on harvesting.

Organ Procurement

The donor lung is usually harvested, together with the heart, as a part of multiple organ retrieval. Active resuscitation is undertaken, with replacement of intravascular volume and hormone replacement with antidiuretic hormone and thyroxin. Fluid management is optimized by the routine use of a Swan–Ganz catheter, which permits adequate replacement without incurring edema. Ventilation is adjusted to maintain high volumes and low positive end-expiratory pressure (PEEP). Regular suctioning of the airways is carried out and fiberoptic bronchoscopy is performed, as clinically indicated. Blood and endotracheal secretions are then taken for Gram stain, culture, and sensitivity testing. A standard median sternotomy is performed, the pleurae are opened and the lungs inspected. After thymectomy and division of the innominate vein, the pericardium is opened and the innominate artery is divided. The superior vena cava (SVC) is then mobilized, and the azygous vein is divided. A pulmonary artery catheter is inserted and the heart–lung block is heparinized (250–300 U/kg).

Different methods of organ preservation are currently in use. Preservation systems provide for about 4–6 hr of ischemia (Table 3). The cold, single pulmonary artery flush with prior infusion of prostacyclin into the pulmonary artery (40 ng $kg^{-1}min^{-1}$ for 10 min) is both simple and effective (39). After prostacyclin infusion, the SVC is ligated and the inferior vena cava (IVC) is clamped. The heart is arrested with a cardioplegic solution (St. Thomas's solution, 10 ml/kg at 4°C), and the left atrial appendage is excised to prevent overload. The pulmonary vasculature is then perfused with Papworth solution (500 ml donor blood, 700 ml Ringer's solution, 200 ml of 20% salt-poor albumin, 100 ml 20% mannitol, 63 ml citrate-phosphate-dextrose, and 10,000 U heparin) at 4°C under gravity. Before removal, the lungs are hand-ventilated with air to approximately 80% of maximum, and special containers are used to avoid injury to the lungs by excessive cooling (40). If the heart–lung block is split, dissection is carried out after excision. The recipient is matched for ABO compatibility and predicted total lung capacity for the donor and recipient. We use the same approach to preserve the single lung for transplantation.

Recipient Procedures

On arrival at the hospital the recipient is prepared for the operation and a complete microbiology screen is carried out. Antimicrobial and immunosuppressive treatment begin on induction of anesthesia (Table 4). To avoid prolonged ischemic time for the donor lungs and long anesthetic and bypass time for the recipient, close coordination between the donor and the recipient teams is maintained.

Table 3 Preservation Methods for Heart–Lung Transplantation

Center	Pretreatment	Perfusion solution	Inflation	Storage
Papworth Hospital Cambridge, England	Prostacyclin flush solution 5–40 ng/kg/min into pulmonary artery for 10 min before cardiac arrest	Ringer's solution 700 mg 20% albumin 200 ml 20% mannitol 100 ml CPD 63 ml Donor blood 400 ml Heparin (100 IU/ml) 10 ml	80% with room air	Saline solution 4°C: maintained by eutectoid techniques
Harefield Hospital London, England	None	Core cooling by CPB less than 10°C	50% with room air	Collins solution 4°C ice chest
Toronto Lung Transplant Group Canada	None	None	Collapsed	Collins solution 4°C ice chest
Johns Hopkins Hospital Baltimore, MD	Isoproterenol 0.02 μ/kg/min 10–20 min prebypass	Core cooling by CPB	50% with room air	Collins solution 4°C ice chest
Univ. of Pittsburgh Pittsburgh, PA	None	Magnesium sulfate 12 mEq/L		Univ. of Wisconsin solution 100 ml/kg
Stanford University Stanford, CA	Prostaglandin E_1 10–80 μ/kg/min 15 min before removal	Collins solution with added 50% dextrose (65 ml/L) 60 ml/kg	50% with room air	Physiol solution (Abbott Labs) 4°C ice chest

Table 4 Immunosuppression Regimen for Heart–Lung, Double-Lung and Single-Lung Transplantation at Papworth Hospital

On arrival:	Azathioprine	100–150 mg iv/po (2 mg/kg)
On induction:	Methylprednisolone	500 mg iv
On CPB:	RATG[a] 0.5–1.5 mg/kg	250 ml N saline over 10 hr preceded by 1 g acetaminophen (paracetamol) orally and 10 mg chlorpheniramine iv
Reperfusion:	Methylprednisolone	500 mg IV
Immediate after surgery:	Methylprednisolone	125 mg × 3 doses (at 8, 16, 24 hr) after surgery for 2 days (as above).
	RATG	T cell count < 20% or 100 cells/ml
Maintenance therapy:	Predisolone	1 mg/kg per day in two doses reducing to 0.2 mg/kg/day
	Azathioprine	2 mg/kg per day (maximum daily dose) po Maintain WBC > 4500
	Cyclosporine[b]	Start at 50 mg, increasing to 10 mg/kg per day in two doses, po
Rejection:	Methylprednisolone	0.5–1.0 g iv for 3 days, followed by prednisolone 1 mg/kg per day to 15 mg/day po, tapering for 2 weeks

[a]RATG, rabbit antilymphocyte globulin.
[b]Cyclosporine is adjusted to renal function. Aim for cyclosporine trough levels of 300–500 ng/ml in the first 3 months (whole blood, SYVA emit assay).

G. Surgical Procedure

Heart–Lung Transplantation

The technique for en bloc HLT was described by Reitz et al. (10) and has remained virtually unchanged, except for some modification for a domino procedure. Aprotinin (Trasylol) is administered as a bolus of 2×10^6 kIU into the cardiopulmonary bypass circuit at the beginning of the procedure and then continuously infused at 5×10^5 kIU/hr during cardiopulmonary bypass to decrease postoperative bleeding. Peripheral arterial and central venous lines and urinary catheters are placed for perioperative monitoring. The incision is a median sternotomy. The patient is fully heparinized and placed on cardiopulmonary bypass by a single aortic cannula to the superior aspect of the ascending aorta and two venous cannulae in the junction between the IVC and the right atrium and in the SVC, or in the innominate vein in a domino procedure. After cardiopulmonary bypass is established, the aorta is cross-clamped, and the heart is excised, taking care not to

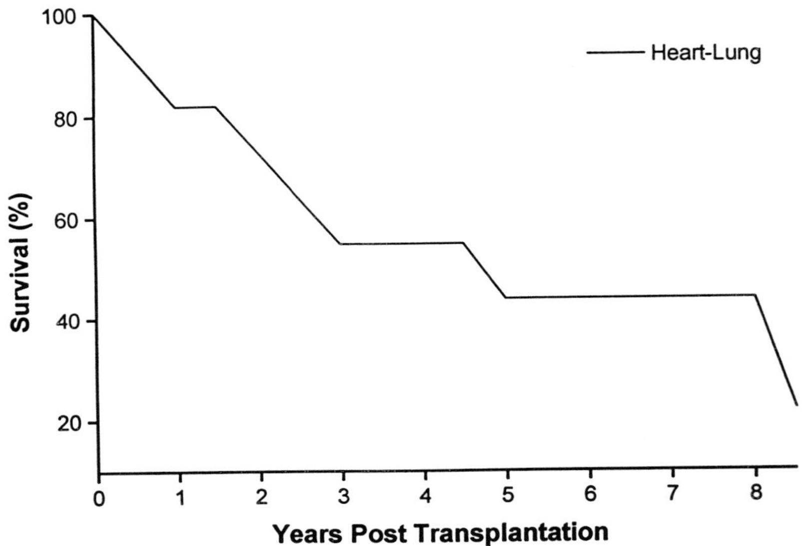

Figure 2 Survival curve from PPH with heart–lung transplantation (Papworth experience).

injure the phrenic, vagus, or recurrent laryngeal nerves. Cardioplegia is used for domino hearts, and the sinoatrial node and the coronary sinus are left in the excised heart. The right pulmonary artery is then dissected free from the SVC. This allows the hila of both lungs to be incised, with attention to preservation of the phrenic nerve anteriorly and the vagi posteriorly. The left and right bronchi are occluded with staples, and the lungs are removed. The thoracic cavity and trachea are irrigated with poviodine solution.

The trachea of the heart–lung block is trimmed to within two rings of the carina, and the bronchial tree is irrigated with normal saline. The heart–lung block is then maneuvered into position, passing the lungs through the windows in the pericardium into the respective pleural cavities. The trachea is anastomosed with a 3-0 monofilament suture just above the carina and is reinforced anteriorly and posteriorly with donor and recipient peritracheal tissue. The atrial anastomosis is accomplished with a continuous 3-0 monofiiament suture. In the case of a domino operation, the donor's SVC and IVC are individually anastomosed to the recipient's SVC and IVC with continuous 4-0 monofilament suture. The patients are rewarmed, and the aortic anastomosis is completed. Pacing wires are applied in right and left ventricles and drains are inserted into the apices and the posterior costophrenic angles of both sides of the thoracic cavity. The heart is de-aired the standard way, normothermic ventilation is commenced, and the patient is weaned from cardiopulmonary bypass. Despite the technical modifications that are required for the domino operation, no disadvantage has been imposed on live donors in our experience.

Single-Lung Transplantation

The SLT has undergone a number of developments since its introduction in 1983. Initially, bronchial anastomotic omentopexy was employed in an attempt to revascularize the bronchial circulation; however, this practice generally has been discontinued. The lung transplant procedure is performed with the adoption of one-lung ventilation. One of the advantages of SLT is that cardiopulmonary bypass is usually unnecessary, except for patients who do not tolerate pulmonary artery clamping or single-lung ventilation, such as those with a pulmonary artery pressure greater than 50 mmHg. However, cardiovascular bypass should be available. Indeed, in many centers, bypass is always used for SLT in patients with PPH.

The patient is placed in the lateral decubitus position, and a standard posterolateral thoracotomy is performed through the bed of the excised fifth rib. The main pulmonary artery is isolated and temporarily clamped to determine whether the operation can be performed without bypass. The pulmonary clamp is removed after this trial, the pulmonary veins are isolated, and the mainstem bronchus is mobilized just proximal to the upper lobe bronchus. Once hilar mobilization has been completed, cardiopulmonary bypass is instituted, if necessary. The recipient's bronchus is stapled and cut. Then the pulmonary clamp is replaced and the lung is extracted.

Following the removal of the recipient's lung, the donor lung is placed in the posterior thorax. After a cuff of atrium is trimmed to meet the orifice of the donor atrium, atrial anastomosis is performed, first with 4-0 monofilament; then the pulmonary artery anastomosis is performed with continuous 4-0 monofilament. Before removal of the vascular clamp, the bronchial anastomosis is performed with continuous 3-0 monofilament and wrapped with hilar lymphatic tissue. The graft lung vasculature is de-aired, by either the antegrade or retrograde method. After the completion of the anastomosis, ventilation is started, and hemostasis is secured. Chest closure is performed in standard fashion leaving two chest tubes.

Sequential Bilateral Lung Transplantation

A modified approach is to perform bilateral proximal bronchial anastomoses, instead of a tracheal anastomosis. A further innovation was the induction of bilateral fifth intercostal space, anterolateral thoracotomy, with a transfer sternotomy or bilateral thoracotomy. With this access, it was possible to control bleeding in the apices of the thoracic cavities. This enabled sequential SLT, with two distal main bronchial, two left atrial, and two pulmonary artery anastomoses.

This particular operation has been quite successful, but does require cardiopulmonary bypass for PPH patients. The main disadvantage of this procedure is that the first transplanted lung receives the entire cardiac output during second lung grafting and may develop high-flow pulmonary edema. An additional problem is longer ischemic time, particularly for the second graft lung.

H. Postoperative Management

Early extubation and mobilization of the patients, negative fluid balance and an induction of immunosuppressant regimen must be established immediately after lung transplantation.

Early extubation and subsequent mobilization of the patients are essential to avoid airway complications, because the denervated lung is not responsive to secretions below the tracheal anastomosis. There is often a transient period of deterioration of gas exchange within 24 hr after surgery, associated with bilateral roentgenographic pulmonary infiltrates (41,42). The etiology of this disorder may relate to graft ischemia during preservation, excessive intravascular fluid, surgical trauma, or lymphatic interruption. Fluids are initially restricted, and diuretics are administered to achieve a negative fluid balance by the second postoperative day.

In SLT for patients with PPH, despite early hemodynamic improvement, early postoperative complications are critical and dependent on the transplanted lung function (43). In some cases, transplanted lungs have severe pulmonary edema, which is believed to be accentuated by massive blood flow diversion to the grafted lung (44). To avoid these problems, fluid administration should be carefully restricted. A sudden rise in pulmonary artery pressure with concurrent arterial desaturation during the immediate postoperative period can be life-threatening (36). Prostaglandins (PGE_1 or PGI_2; 36) may be used as a pulmonary vasodilator in this setting. The problem with either of these agents is systemic hypotension, and potent inotropic drugs are often needed. Nitric oxide, which has been recently introduced as a selective pulmonary artery vasodilator (45), offers considerable assistance after SLT for PPH.

Immunosuppressive Therapy

Immunosuppressive therapy in lung and heart lung transplantation consists of azathioprine, cyclosporine, prednisolone, and rabbit antithymocyte globulin (Table 4). All patients begin oral azathioprine on arrival at the hospital. Methylprednisolone is administered at the induction of anesthesia and at the reperfusion of donor organs. Rabbit antithymocyte globulin is administered when cardiopulmonary bypass is initiated and is continued for 3 days. Since low-dose prednisolone does not increase the risk of postoperative airway complications (33,46), we use 0.2 mg/kg per day of prednisolone for maintenance therapy.

Rejection, Transbronchial Lung Biopsy, Pulmonary Function Monitoring

Patients are given pocket battery-operated spirometers that measure FEV_1 and vital capacity. Pulmonary function is monitored on the basis that many episodes of rejection and infection are associated with a fall in FEV_1 and vital capacity. Changes in function as little as 5% are sufficient for patients to be admitted to the hospital for further investigation (47). Histological confirmation of suspected rejection episodes is achieved using specimens of lung obtained by transbronchial lung biopsy through a fiberoptic bronchoscope. The procedure requires five biopsies from one lung, usually taken from different sites (16).

The treatment for acute rejection is a standard regimen of 3 days of 0.5–1.0 g of methylprednisolone each day, followed by oral administration of prednisolone at decreasing doses over the next 3 weeks.

Obliterative Bronchiolitis

Obliterative bronchiolitis (OB) is the major cause of long-term death from lung transplantation. This disorder consists of submucosal scarring of membranous and respiratory bronchioles that may be eccentric, concentric, or associated with total obliteration of the bronchiolar lumens (48) (Fig. 3). Once OB develops, deterioration of lung function may be stabilized by high-dose methylprednisolone, followed by oral prednisolone, but it is not reversible. Studies in HLT patients have shown that there are significant correlations between the frequency of episodes of acute rejection in the first 3 months after surgery and both the risks of dying of OB (49) and the severity of airflow obstruction in those who survive (50). In addition, more frequent or persistent rejection is also correlated with the development of OB (51,52).

To monitor graft function after HLT and S/BLT, a bronchiolitis obliterans syndrome-grading system has been introduced (53; Table 5). Once the diagnosis of OB grade 2 or 3 is achieved, we do not enhance immunosuppressive treatment, since there is little evidence that any salvage treatment is effective. However,

Table 5 Bronchiolitis Obliterans Syndrome (BOS) Grading

Grade		FEV_1
0	No significant abnormality	80% or more of baseline value
1	Mild obliterative bronchiolitis syndrome	66–80% of baseline
2	Moderate obliterative bronchiolitis syndrome	51–65% of baseline value
3	Severe obliterative bronchiolitis syndrome	50% or less of baseline value

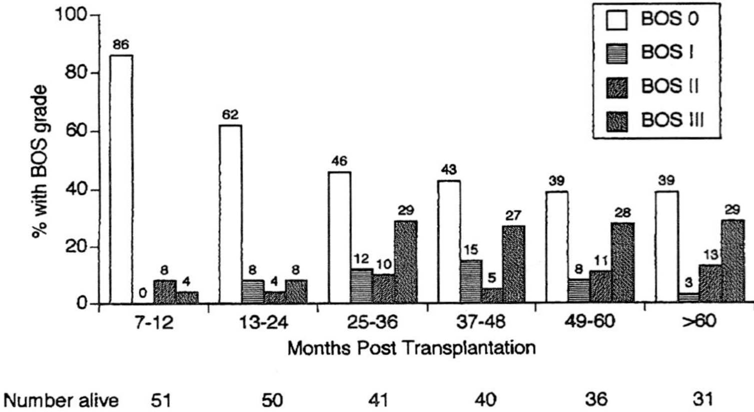

Figure 3 Degrees of severity of bronchiolitis obliterans syndrome (Papworth experience), indicating the worst grade of BOS observed in each period.

nebulized high-dose budesonide (a steroid for asthma care), when given for 1 year to high-risk patients, reduces the incidence of OB and stabilizes airflow obstruction (54).

Infection in the Transplanted Lung

Transbronchial lung biopsy is also essential to diagnose pulmonary infection, since it is often impossible to distinguish between infection and rejection using other clinical or physiological data (55). In the early postoperative phase, gram-negative bacteria and *Staphylococcus aureus* are the most frequent causes of pneumonia and are usually diagnosed easily and respond to antibiotic therapy. More serious infections occur later and are usually due to viruses, fungi, and protozoa, and these cause not only pulmonary complications, but also systemic infections. Therefore, we monitor the patient's serological status for cytomegalovirus (CMV), herpes simplex virus (HSV) and *Toxoplasma*.

Infections with CMV and HSV are the two major viral infections after lung transplantation. Infection with CMV is most common 4–8 weeks after transplantation, particularly if the patient has been treated recently for rejection. To minimize the risk of developing CMV infection posttransplantation, we currently avoid using organs from serologically positive donors for serologically negative recipients. The difficulties in diagnosing CMV and herpes simplex infections are that neither symptomatic nor histological features of these infections are easy to distinguish from rejection. Furthermore, both coexist with some frequency. A CMV infection is treated with intravenous ganciclovir, which is also prophylactically administered for a period of at least 14 days when CMV seronegative recipients receive a graft from CMV seropositive donors. An HSV pneumonia tends to occur in patients who have a positive HSV serology before surgery and is an infection that is associated with augmented immunosuppression. The diagnosis of HSV infection is made by lung biopsy, which shows the characteristic inclusions and evidence of bronchiolitis. Acyclovir is prophylactically given to those patients who are HSV-positive perioperatively and during a period of augmented immunosuppression.

Protozoal infection with *Toxoplasma* can cause significant deterioration of graft function. Prophylactic administration of pyrimethamine has eliminated toxoplasmal infection in most centers when recipients who are seronegative for toxoplasma receive grafts from seropositive donors.

I. Long-Term Prospects for Lung Transplantation for Primary Pulmonary Hypertension

With the advances in medical care, transplantation should be reserved for PPH patients who have failed medical treatment. New immunosuppressive treatments should lessen the prevalence of OB and improve survival. A constant review of outcomes should result in adjustments in the selection criteria in the future.

The continued shortage of organs may be overcome by the introduction of xenograft transplantation. For example, transgenic pig organs, expressing the DAF of human complement on their endothelium, do not experience acute rejection in primates. This approach could offer and alternative to human organs and, thereby, increase the availability of transplantation to patients in need in the future.

References

1. Demikhov VP. Some essential points of the technique of transplantation of the heart, lung and other organs. In: Anonymous Experimental Transplant Vital Organs. Moscow: Medgiz State Press for Medical Literature, 1960:29–48.
2. Staudacher V, Bellinazzo P, Pulin A. Primi rilievi su tentativi di reimpianti autoplastici e di trapianti omoplastici lobi polmonari. Chirugia (Milan) 1950; 5:223–227.
3. Nakae S, Webb WR, Theodorides T, Sugg WL. Respiratory function following cardiopulmonary denervation in dog, cat and monkey. Surg Gynecol Obstet 1967; 125:1285–1292.
4. Castaneda AR, Arnar O, Schmidt-Habelman P, Moller J, Zamora R. Cardiopulmonary autotransplantation in primates. J Cardiovasc Surg 1972; 37:523–531.
5. Hardy JD, Webb WR, Dalton ML, Walker GR. Lung homotransplantation in man. JAMA 1963; 186:1065–1074.

6. Cooley DA, Bloodwell RD, Hallman GL, Nora JJ, Harrison GM, Leachman RD. Organ transplantation for advanced cardiopulmonary disease. Ann Thorac Surg 1969; 8:30–42.
7. Borel JF, Feuer C, Magnee C, Stahelin H. Effects of the new antilymphocytic peptide cyclosporin A in animals. Immunology 1977; 32:1017–1025.
8. Calne RY, White DJG, Rolles K. Prolonged survival of pig orthotopic heart grafts treated with cyclosporin A. Lancet 1978; 1:1183–1185.
9. Reitz BA, Burton NA, Jamieson SW. Heart and lung transplantation, autotransplantation, and allotransplantation in primates with extended survival. J Thorac Cardiovasc Surg 1980; 80:360–372.
10. Reitz BA, Wallwork J, Hunt SA, et al. Heart–lung transplantation: successful therapy for patients with pulmonary vascular disease. N Engl J Med 1982; 306:557–564.
11. Lima O, Goldberg M, Peters WJ, Ayabe H, Townsend E, Cooper JD. Bronchial omentopexy in canine lung transplantation. J Thorac Cardiovasc Surg 1982; 83:418–421.
12. Saunders NR, Egan TM, Chamberlain D, Cooper JD. Cyclosporin and bronchial healing in canine lung transplantation. J Thorac Cardiovasc Surg 1984; 88:993–999.
13. Toronto Lung Transplant Group. Unilateral lung transplantation for pulmonary fibrosis. N Engl J Med 1986; 314:1140–1145.
14. Patterson GA, Cooper JD, Goldman B, et al. Technique of successful clinical double-lung transplantation. Ann Thorac Surg 1988; 45:626–633.
15. Pasque MK, Cooper JD, Kaiser LR, Haydock DA, Triantafillou A, Trulock EP. Improved technique for bilateral lung transplantation: rationale and initial clinical experience. Ann Thorac Surg 1990; 49:785–791.
16. Cooper JD, Patterson GA, Trulock EP. Results of single and bilateral lung transplantation in 131 consecutive recipients. Washington University Lung Transplant Group. J Thorac Cardiovasc Surg 1994; 107:460–470 (discussion).
17. Fragomeni LS, Kaye MP. The Registry of the International Society for Heart Transplantation: fifth official report—1988. J Heart Transplant 1988; 7:249–253.
18. Hosenpud JD, Novick RJ, Brun TJ, Daily PO. The Registry of the International Society for Heart and Lung Transplantation. The 11th official report 1994. J Heart Lung Transplant 1994; 13:561–570.
19. Hull RD, Raskob GE, Hersh J. The diagnosis of clinically suspected pulmonary embolism. Practical approaches. Chest 1986; 89(suppl):417–425.
20. Fishman AJ, Moser KM, Fedullo PF. Perfusion lung scans vs pulmonary angiography in evaluation of suspected primary pulmonary hypertension. Chest 1983; 84:679–683.
21. Moser KM, Spragg RG, Utley J, Daily PO. Chronic thrombotic obstruction of major pulmonary arteries. Results of thromboendarterectomy in 15 patients. Ann Intern Med 1983; 99:299–305.
22. Rich S, Dantzker DR, Ayres SM, et al. Primary pulmonary hypertension. A national prospective study. Ann Intern Med 1987; 107:216–223.
23. Fuster V, Steele PM, Edwards WD, Gersh BJ, McGoon MD, Frye RL. Primary pulmonary hypertension: natural history and the importance of thrombosis. Circulation 1984; 70:580–587.

24. Rich S, Levy PS. Characteristics of surviving and nonsurviving patients with primary pulmonary hypertension. Am J Med 1984; 76:573–578.
25. Rozkovec A, Montanes P, Oakley CM. Factors that influence the outcome of primary pulmonary hypertension. Br Heart J 1986; 55:449–458.
26. D'Alonzo GE, Barst RJ, Ayres SM, et al. Survival in patients with primary pulmonary hypertension. Results from a national prospective registry. Ann Intern Med 1991; 115:343–349.
27. Rich S, Brundage BH. High-dose calcium channel-blocking therapy for primary pulmonary hypertension: evidence for long-term reduction in pulmonary arterial pressure and regression of right ventricular hypertrophy. Circulation 1987; 76: 135–141.
28. Rich S, Kaufmann E, Levy PS. The effect of high doses of calcium channel blockers on survival in primary pulmonary hypertension. N Engl J Med 1992; 327:76–81.
29. Rich S, Kaufmann E. High dose titration of calcium channel blocking agents for primary pulmonary hypertension: guidelines for short-term drug testing. J Am Coll Cardiol 1991; 18:1323–1327.
30. Rubin LJ, Mendoza J, Hood M, et al. Treatment of primary pulmonary hypertension with continuous intravenous prostacyclin (epoprostenol). Results of a randomized trial. Ann Intern Med 1990; 112:485–491.
31. Jones DK, Higenbottam TW, Wallwork J. Treatment of primary pulmonary hypertension intravenous epoprostenol (prostacyclin). Br Heart J 1987; 57:270–278.
32. Higenbottam TW, Wells F, Wheeldon D, Wallwork J. Long-term treatment of primary pulmonary hypertension with continuous intravenous epoprostenol (prostacyclin). Lancet 1984; 1:1046–1047.
33. Pasque MK, Trulock EP, Kaiser LR, Cooper JD. Single-lung transplantation for pulmonary hypertension. Three-month hemodynamic follow-up. Circulation 1991; 84:2275–2279.
34. Levine SM, Gibbons WJ, Bryan CL, et al. Single lung transplantation for primary pulmonary hypertension. Chest 1990; 98:1107–1115.
35. Starnes VA, Stinson EB, Oyer PE, Theodore J, Kramer MR, Marshall SS. Single lung transplantation: a new therapeutic option for patients with pulmonary hypertension. Transplant Proc 1991; 23:1209–1210.
36. Maurer JR, Winton TL, Patterson GA, Williams TR. Single-lung transplantation for pulmonary vascular disease. Transplant Proc 1991; 23:1211–1212.
37. Hutter JA, Scott J, Wreghitt T, Higenbottam TW, Wallwork J. The importance of cytomegalovirus in heart-lung transplant recipients. Chest 1989; 95:627–631.
38. Levine SM, Jenkinson SG, Bryan CL, et al. Ventilation–perfusion inequalities during graft rejection in patients undergoing single lung transplantation for primary pulmonary hypertension [see comments]. Chest 1992; 101:401–405.
39. Hakim M, Higenbottam TW, Bethune D, et al. Selection and procurement of combined heart and lung grafts for transplantation. J Thorac Cardiovasc Surg 1988; 95:474–479.
40. Wheeldon DR, Wallwork J, Bethune DW, English TA. Storage and transport of heart and heart–lung donor organs with inflatable cushions and eutectoid cooling. J Heart Transplant 1988; 7:265–268.

41. Jamieson SW, Baldwin J, Stinson EB, et al. Clinical heart–lung transplantation. Transplantation 1984; 37:81–84.
42. Montefusco CM, Veith FJ. Lung transplantation. Surg Clin North Am 1986; 66:503–515.
43. Low DE, Trulock EP, Kaiser LR, Pasque MK, Dresler C, Ettinger NC. Morbidity, mortality, and early results of single versus bilateral lung transplantation for emphysema. J Thorac Cardiovasc Surg 1992; 103:1119–1126.
44. Chapelier A, Vouhe P, Macchiarini P, et al. Comparative outcome of heart–lung and lung transplantation for pulmonary hypertension. J Thorac Cardiovasc Surg 1993; 106:299–307.
45. Pepke-Zaba J, Higenbottam TW, Dinh-Xuan AT, Stone D, Wallwork J. Inhaled nitric oxide as a cause of selective pulmonary vasodilator in pulmonary hypertension. Lancet 1991; 338:1173–1174.
46. Calhoon JH, Grover FL, Gibbons WJ, et al. Single lung transplantation. Alternative indications and technique. J Thorac Cardiovasc Surg 1991; 101:816–824.
47. Otulana BA, Higenbottam T, Ferrari L, Scott J, Igboaka G, Wallwork J. The use of home spirometry in detecting acute lung rejection and infection following heart-lung transplantation [see comments]. Chest 1990; 97:353–357.
48. Yousem SA, Burke CM, Billingham ME. Pathologic pulmonary alterations in long-term human heart lung transplantation. Hum Pathol 1985; 16:911–923.
49. Sharples L, Scott J, Dennis C, et al. Risk factors for survival following combined heart–lung transplantation. Transplantation 1994; 57:218–223.
50. Sharples LD, Tamm M, McNeil K, Higenbottam T, Wallwork J. Risk factors for the development of bronchiolitis obliterans syndrome (BOS) in heart–lung transplant patients (abstr). J Heart Lung Transplant 1995; 14:S66.
51. Higenbottam TW, Stewart S, Penketh A, Wallwork J. Transbronchial lung biopsy for the diagnosis of rejection in heart–lung transplant patients. Transplantation 1988; 46:532–539.
52. Scott JP, Sharples L, Mullins P, et al. Further studies following heart–lung transplantation. Transplant Proc 1991; 23:1201–1202.
53. Cooper JD, Billingham M, Egan T, et al. A working formulation for the standardization of nomenclature and for clinical staging of chronic dysfunction in lung allografts. J Heart Lung Transplant 1993; 12:713–716.
54. Takao M, Higenbottam TW, Audley T, Otulana BA, Wallwork J. Effects of inhaled nebulized steroids (budesonide) on acute and chronic lung function in heart–lung transplant patients. Transplant Proc 1995; 27:1284–1285.
55. Penketh AR, Higenbottam TW, Hutter J, Coutts C, Stewart S, Wallwork J. Clinical experience in the management of pulmonary opportunist infection and rejection in recipients of heart–lung transplants. Thorax 1988; 43:762–769.

13

Prognosis and Natural History

MICHAEL D. McGOON

Mayo Clinic
Rochester, Minnesota

I. Introduction

Primary pulmonary hypertension (PPH) historically has exhibited a course of relentless deterioration and early death. With increasing clinical experience and the systematic accrual of data, the natural history of primary pulmonary hypertension among subgroups of patients is becoming more clearly defined. Newer modalities of both pharmacological and surgical treatments have demonstrably altered not only the symptomatic status of patients, but have had an effect on the progression of the disease and duration of survival. Thus, any discussion of the natural history and longevity of patients with primary pulmonary hypertension in the 1990s must take into account the clinical and hemodynamic characteristics of the population under discussion and the therapeutic modalities employed.

Although various vasodilator agents have been employed in the treatment of primary pulmonary hypertension, until recently, none had been convincingly demonstrated to alter life expectancy. Several large survival studies of general populations of heterogeneously treated patients conducted in the 1980s, therefore, provide a basis of comparison for patients treated with subsequently evolving modalities. These retrospective and prospective studies yield quite uniform results: among the general population of patients with primary pulmonary hypertension who do not undergo heart–lung transplantation, actuarial survival at 1 year is 68–77%, 2 years 52–58%, 3 years 40–56%, 4 years 30–43%, and 5 years 22–38% (Fig. 1) (1–3).

The usual causes of death in these patients are right ventricular failure (63%), pneumonia (7%), and sudden death (7%) (1). Less common causes of mortality in the past include iatrogenic complications from cardiac catheterization (although this appears to be less frequent in more recent reports; 4). Despite the overall dismal prognosis, duration of survival ranges up to 10 years or more. Instances of survival up to several decades have been reported (5–7), as have rare cases of apparent regression of the disease (8,9).

II. Hemodynamic Predictors of Survival

Predicted survival based on hemodynamics at the time of evaluation has been investigated in 194 patients followed prospectively after enrollment between July 1981 and December 1985 in the Patient Registry for the Characterization of Primary Pulmonary Hypertension (PRCPPH) (3). Given the data from this registry, the probability of survival can be described as a function of right atrial pressure, mean pulmonary arterial pressure, and cardiac index, using the following equations:

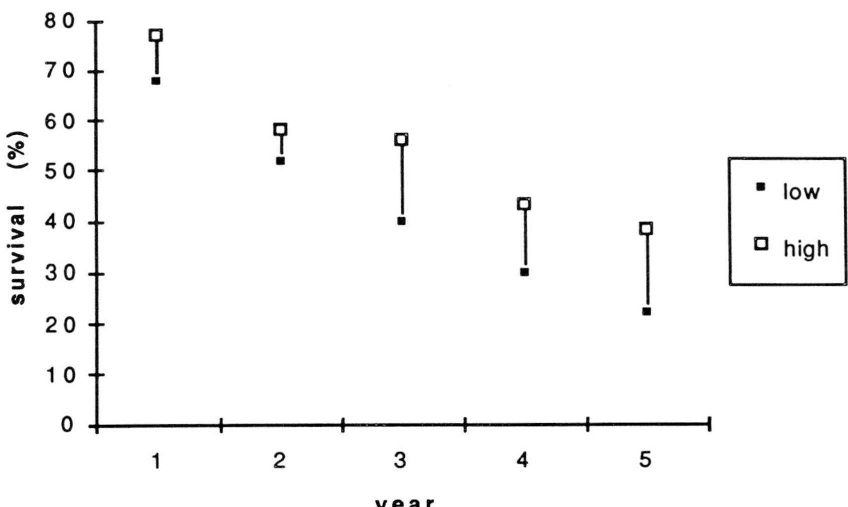

Figure 1 Range of reported actuarial survival in three large studies of patients with primary pulmonary hypertension. (From Refs. 1–3.)

$$P(t) = [H(t)]^{A(x,y,z)}$$
$$H(t) = [0.88 - 0.14t + 0.01t^2]$$
$$A(y,y,z) = e^{(0.007325x + 0.0526y - 0.3275z)}$$

Where:

P(t) = a patient's chances of survival at t years
t = 1, 2, 3, 4, or 5 years
x = mean pulmonary arterial pressure
y = mean right atrial pressure
z = cardiac index

Application of these equations can offer predicted survival of individual patients, although it must be clearly acknowledged that these predictions represent *probability* of survival duration only (Fig. 2). As these curves have been derived from a general population of patients with primary pulmonary hypertension, they also may provide the basis for comparison of other groups of hemodynamically equivalent patients subjected to specific treatment regimens.

A variety of individual hemodynamic indicators have been identified that have predictive value for duration of survival. These include the following:

A. Pulmonary Vascular Resistance and Pressure

Most studies have found an inverse correlation between the degree of pulmonary hemodynamic abnormality and survival (2,3). Among the 194 patients in the PRCPPH, median survival for those with a mean pulmonary arterial pressure of less than 55 mmHg was 48 months, compared with 12 months for those with mean pulmonary arterial pressure of 85 mmHg or more (3).

Mean pulmonary arterial pressure is one of the predictive indices contributing to the estimated probability of survival. The observation that elevated pulmonary arterial pressure is associated with reduced survival suggests that, in these patients, the disease is more advanced or has progressed to a more severe level relatively rapidly. The higher pressure exposes the right ventricle to a greater workload, ultimately progressing to death from right ventricular failure.

B. Right Atrial Pressure Elevation

Among measurable hemodynamic indices of right ventricular failure, right atrial pressure elevation is highly predictive of survival. Right atrial pressure higher than 20 mmHg corresponds to a median survival of 1 month, compared with 46 months survival for patients with right atrial pressures less than 10 mmHg (3). Other less specific markers of right ventricular involvement, such as radiographic cardiomegaly and right ventricular strain pattern on electrocardiography, also qualitatively suggest shorter survival.

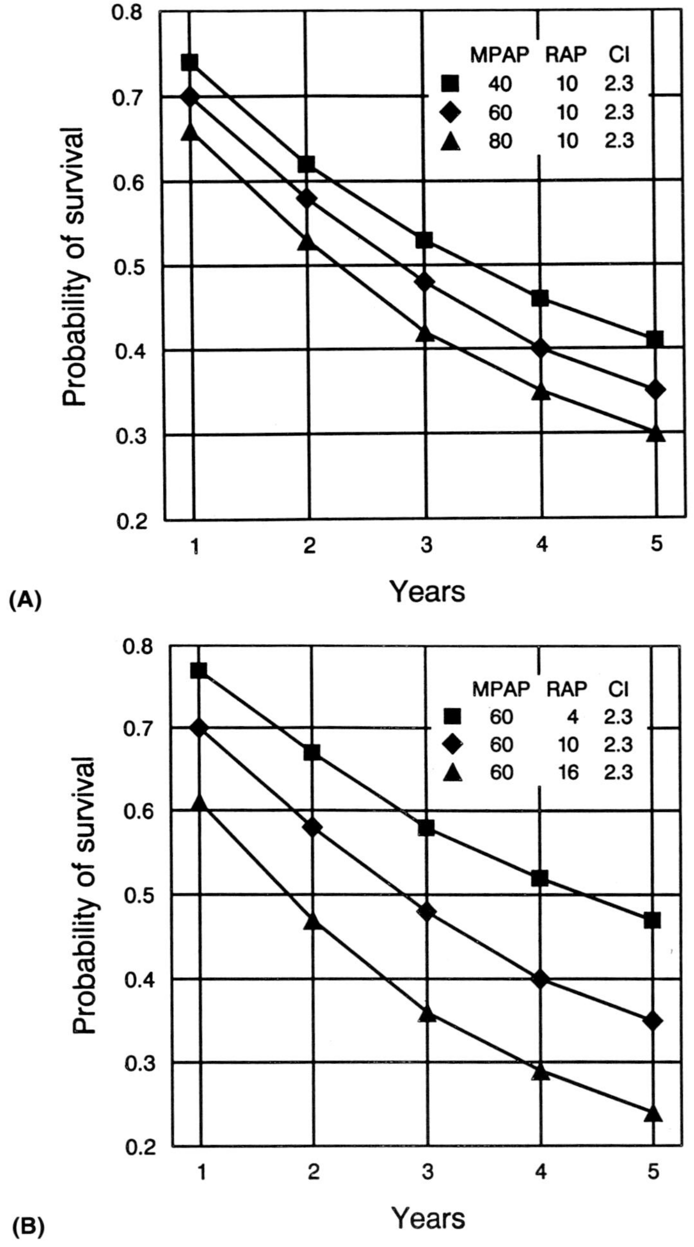

Figure 2 Probability of survival for medically treated patients with primary pulmonary hypertension. Differences in survival probability are depicted based on variation of baseline mean pulmonary artery pressure (MPAP, mmHg) (A); right atrial pressure (RAP; mmHg) (B); and cardiac index (CI, L min^{-1} m^{-2}) (C). (From Ref. 12.)

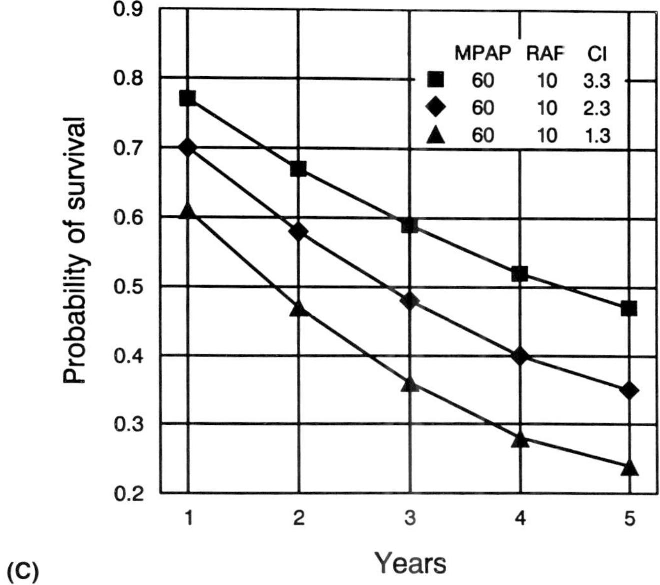

(C)

C. Depressed Cardiac Output

Decreased cardiac output is associated with severity of primary pulmonary hypertension. It is caused by high, fixed resistance to blood flow through the pulmonary vasculature and by right ventricular failure. Reduced cardiac output also correlates with reduced survival (1,3,10). A cardiac index less than 2.0 L·m^2/min is associated with a median survival of 17 months; a cardiac index of 4.0 L·m^2/min or more increases median survival to 43 months (3).

D. Low Pulmonary Arterial (Mixed Venous) Oxygen Desaturation

Low (less than 63%) Svo_2 predicted a mean 3-year survival of 17%, whereas a higher Svo_2 predicted a mean survival of 55% at 3 years (1). The predictive power of this factor probably derives from its combined reflection of poor oxygenation owing to low diffusing capacity, arterial hypoxemia, and low cardiac output.

III. Clinical Predictors of Survival

Several clinical parameters are indicative of future outcomes in primary pulmonary hypertension:

A. Functional Classification

Although most patients with primary pulmonary hypertension are symptomatic at the time of diagnosis, symptoms are considered to be a late development in the course of disease. The extent of symptomatic deterioration is essentially a global clinical index of hemodynamic dysfunction and of end-organ (right ventricular) status. Thus, patients exhibiting more advanced symptoms have shorter subsequent survival (11). In the PRCPPH, the median survival for patients in New York Heart Association class I or II was 58.6 months; class III, 31.5 months; and in class IV, 6 months (3).

B. Presence of Raynaud's Phenomenon

Raynaud's phenomenon, noted almost exclusively in females with primary pulmonary hypertension, correlates with reduced median survival (11.8 months, compared with 43.9 months without Raynaud's). When subjected to multivariate analysis this association is not significant (3).

C. Associated Conditions

Clinical primary pulmonary hypertension is occasionally associated with other conditions of unclear etiologic relations (12). Although survival data are imprecise because of limited numbers and variable reporting, there appears to be an effect on survival that is contributed to by these additional features.

Patients with primary pulmonary hypertension and coexisting portal hypertension have a reduced mean survival of 15 months (13). The 49 patients who died among the 78 reported in the literature had a very short survival (Fig. 3). Although insufficient data are available to make reliable comparisons with the PRCPPH population, survival in patients with associated portal hypertension appears substantially worse.

Syndromes of primary pulmonary hypertension-type features associated with human immunodeficiency virus (HIV) infection (14) or crack cocaine inhalation have been reported. Survival in HIV-related pulmonary hypertension is comparable to that in primary pulmonary hypertension (14a).

Pulmonary hypertension associated with exogenous substances, such as the anorexic agent aminorex, toxic rapeseed oil (15), or L-tryptophan (16) has occurred in epidemic patterns after temporary exposure of broad populations. Survival data are not reliably available, and the frequently regressing or phasic course of these illnesses prohibits meaningful correlation of survival with pulmonary hemodynamics.

D. Age

Patients with primary pulmonary hypertension at either end of the age spectrum appear to have worse prognoses. Among 111 patients reviewed at the Mayo

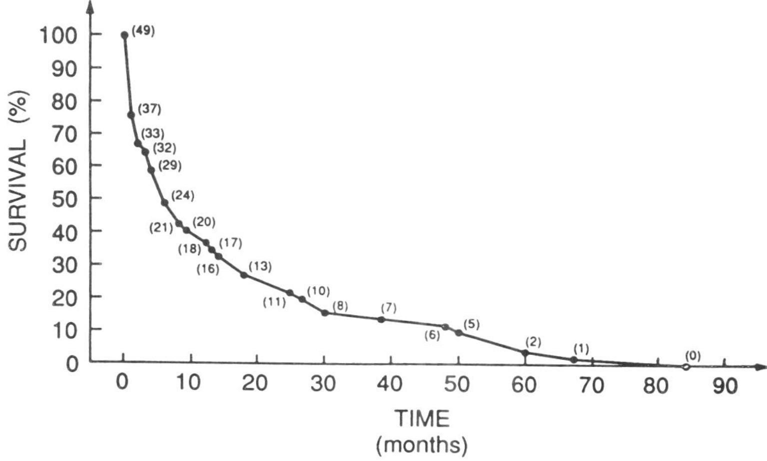

Figure 3 Survival duration among 49 patients who died with primary pulmonary hypertension associated with portal hypertension. Numbers in parentheses indicate surviving patients at each point. (From Ref. 13.)

Clinic, the 11 patients 14 years old or younger had a higher mortality within 1 year of follow-up, than did the older patients (Fig. 4), though the difference was not statistically significant because of the small population (1).

Elderly patients (mean age 73, range 65–85 years) also have substantially reduced survival (mean 29.9 months, range 3–80 months), which is exacerbated by the presence of other coexisting diseases or short prior symptom duration (17).

IV. Treatment-Related Predictors of Survival

Medical therapy has an increasingly recognized influence on survival of patients with primary pulmonary hypertension.

A. Response to Vasodilator Therapy

The immediate response to administration of a vasodilator is predictive of survival. The capacity of the pulmonary vasculature to vasodilate in response to pharmacological stimuli identifies patients at a relatively vasoreactive stage of the disease. An unproved hypothesis presumes that such patients are at an earlier phase of the disease than are those with fixed, high pulmonary vascular resistance, because of advanced or diffuse endothelial cell dysfunction, medial hypertrophy, and thrombosis in situ. Patients who demonstrate improved pulmonary arteriolar resistance with brief administration of vasodilators tend to survive longer (since

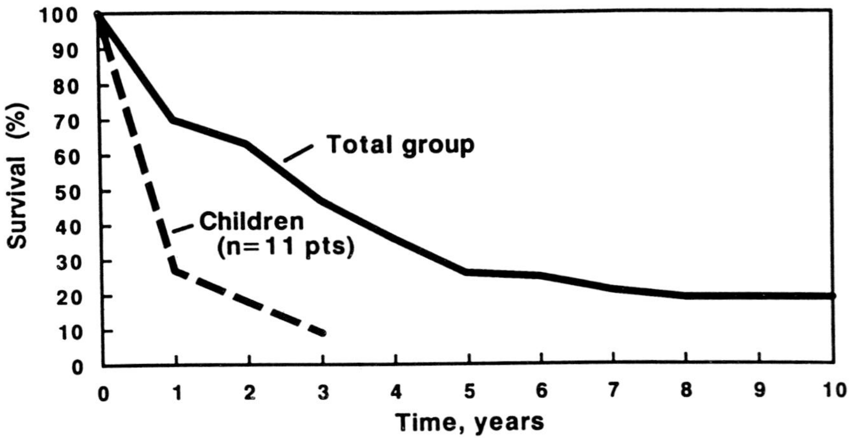

Figure 4 Probability of survival among 100 patients older than 14 years and 11 patients 14 years old or younger. (Data from Ref. 1.)

they have been identified earlier in the course of their illness) and, to some extent, this is independent of subsequent treatment status (18).

B. Treatment with Certain Vasodilators

In addition to the predictive role of acute vasodilator response, long-term treatment with vasodilators may enhance survival. This observation represents a major advance in the role of pharmacological management of primary pulmonary hypertension. Among 64 patients evaluated for response to high-dose calcium channel blockers (18), 26% exhibited reductions in pulmonary artery pressure and resistance of 39 and 53%, respectively. These responders, who were treated long-term with high doses of calcium channel blockers, had a 5-year survival of 94%. Nonresponders had a survival of 55% at 5 years (Fig. 5), although these patients also received lower doses of calcium blockers. The fact that treatment with high doses of calcium blockers substantially improved long-term survival over expectations, based on initial hemodynamic studies, or when compared with the PRCPPH registry population, suggests that survival is at least partially attributable to ongoing treatment (18,19).

Additional evidence is derived from patients treated continuously with intravenously administered prostacyclin (20). The use of this agent appeared to improve survival, compared with the predicted survival curve of patients with similar baseline hemodynamic indices, as determined by PRCPPH data. When compared with the entire PRCPPH cohort, the difference in survival imparted by

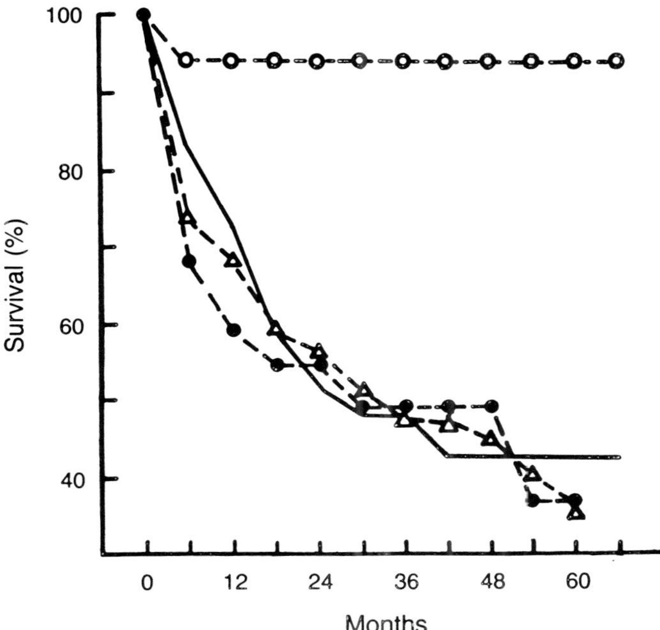

Figure 5 Probability of survival of primary pulmonary hypertension patients who responded to treatment with high doses of calcium blockers (open circles), compared with nonresponders (solid line), PRCPPH patients at the same institution (solid circles), and the entire PRCPPH cohort (triangles). The difference between the responders and the other groups was highly significant ($p = 0.003$). (From Ref. 18.)

prostacyclin was even more apparent (Fig. 6). Interestingly, this survival advantage was observed, despite the absence of an immediate improvement in the pulmonary pressure of the group as a whole (21) and with only a slight decrease in pulmonary arterial and right atrial pressures after 6 months of treatment (20). This suggests that the survival benefit is due to more than the predictive value of the agent's immediate effect. Moreover, it may confer its benefit by unclear mechanisms other than vasodilatation alone. A more recent, larger study confirmed a significant survival benefit among patients randomized to treatment with prostacyclin (21a).

C. Anticoagulation

Uncontrolled observations have suggested that survival is higher among patients who are anticoagulated during the course of their illness. Survival after 1 and 2

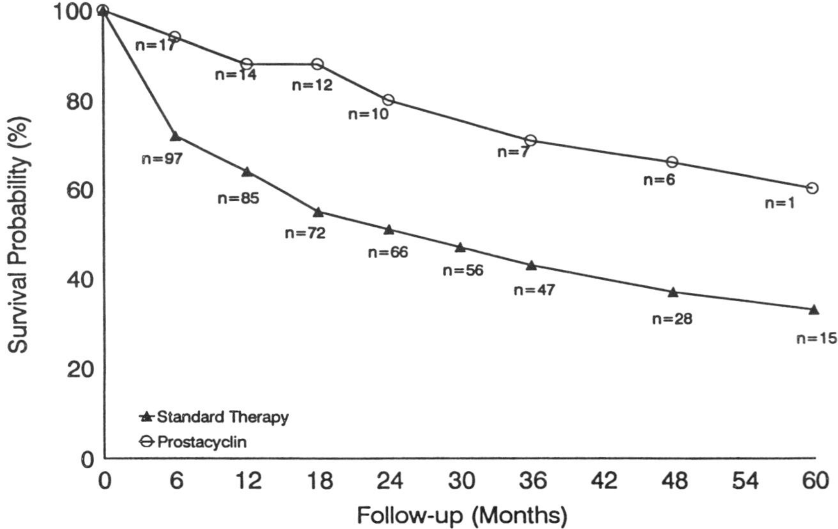

Figure 6 Probability of survival for symptomatic primary pulmonary hypertension patients treated with prostacyclin (n = 18) compared with PRCPPH patients treated with standard therapy (n = 138). Survival was significantly better in the prostacyclin-treated group (p <0.05). (From Ref. 20.)

years among patients who receive anticoagulants is 80 and 60%, respectively, compared with 60 and 35% among those who do not (Fig. 7; 1). The survival benefit conferred by anticoagulation is seen both in patients who have responded to treatment with high-dose calcium blocker vasodilators and in those who have failed to respond (Fig. 8). Whether anticoagulation impinges on the pathogenesis of the disease, or whether it reduces thrombotic sequelae, is uncertain.

V. Histopathological Predictors of Survival

A. Plexogenic Versus Thromboembolic Subtype

Although lung biopsy cannot be recommended to establish a prognosis, biopsy and postmortem evidence suggests that the predominant histopathological lesion in an individual patient may correlate with survival duration and mode of death. Patients with primary plexogenic pulmonary hypertension reportedly survive longer, on the average, (63 months, range 2–180, from onset of symptoms to death) than those who have thrombotic lesions and eccentric intimal proliferation and fibrosis in the absence of plexiform lesions (48 months, range 1–204; 22). Sudden death, however, may be 2.5 times more likely in association with plexogenic pulmonary hypertension (22).

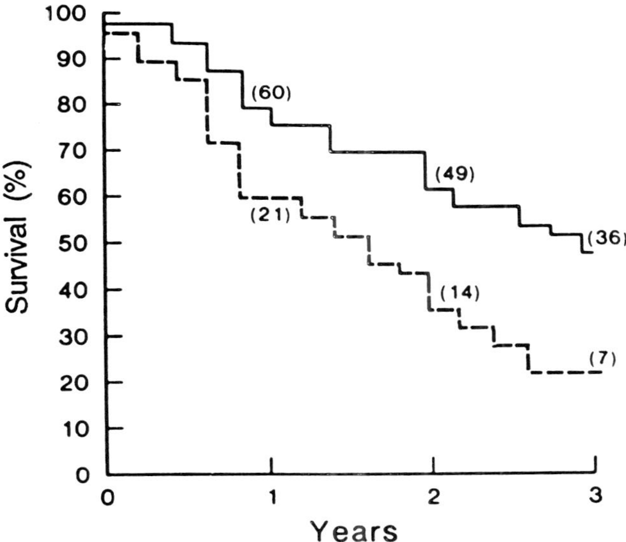

Figure 7 Probability of survival with and without anticoagulant treatment in patients with primary pulmonary hypertension. The difference between the two groups is significant ($p = 0.02$, log-rank test). Numbers in parentheses indicate number of patients surviving at any point. (From Ref. 1.)

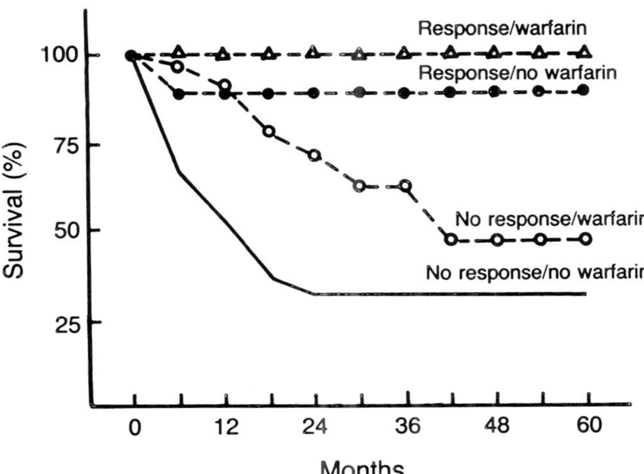

Figure 8 Probability of survival according to the presence or absence of a response to calcium blocker vasodilator administration, and to the use of concurrent anticoagulation with warfarin. Overall survival was significantly improved by treatment with warfarin. (From Ref. 18.)

References

1. Fuster V, Steele PM, Edwards WD, et al. Primary pulmonary hypertension: natural history and the importance of thrombosis. Circulation 1984; 70:580–587.
2. Glanville AR, Burke CM, Theodore J, et al. Primary pulmonary hypertension: length of survival in patients referred for heart–lung transplantation. Chest 1987; 91: 675–681.
3. D'Alonzo GE, Barst RJ, Ayres SM, et al. Survival in patients with primary pulmonary hypertension: results from a national prospective registry. Ann Intern Med 1991; 115:343–349.
4. Rich S, Dantzker DR, Ayres SM, et al. Primary pulmonary hypertension: a national prospective study. Ann Intern Med 1987; 107:216–223.
5. Anderson TJ, Larsen ET, Wyse G, Lester WM. Primary pulmonary hypertension for 30 years. Am J Cardiol 1991; 68:284–285.
6. Suarez LD, Sciandro EE, Llera JJ, Perosio AM. Long term follow-up in primary pulmonary hypertension. Br Heart J 1979; 41:702–708.
7. Trell E. Benign idiopathic pulmonary hypertension. Acta Med Scand 1973; 193:137–143.
8. Cohen M, Edwards WD, Fuster V. Regression in thromboembolic type of primary pulmonary hypertension during 2½ years of antithrombotic therapy. J Am Coll Cardiol 1986; 7:172–175.
9. Bourdillon PD, Oakley CM. Regression of primary pulmonary hypertension. Br Heart J 1976; 38:264–270.
10. Kanemoto N, Sasamoto H. Pulmonary hemodynamics in primary pulmonary hypertension. Jpn Heart J 1979; 20:395–405.
11. Rich S, Brundage BH, Levy PS. The effect of vasodilator therapy on the clinical outcome of patients with primary pulmonary hypertension. Circulation 1985; 71: 1191–1196.
12. American College of Chest Physicians Consensus Statement. Primary pulmonary hypertension. Chest 1993; 104:236–250.
13. Robalino BD, Moodie DS. Association between primary pulmonary hypertension and portal hypertension: analysis of its pathophysiology and clinical, laboratory and hemodynamic manifestations. J Am Coll Cardiol 1991; 17:492–498.
14. Speich R, Jenni R, Opravil M, et al. Primary pulmonary hypertension in HIV infection. Chest 1991; 100:1268–1271.
14a. Petitpretz P, Brenot F, Azarian R, et al. Pulmonary hypertension in patients with human immunodeficiency virus infection: comparison with primary pulmonary hypertension. Circulation 1994; 89:2722–2727.
15. Gomez-Sanchez MA, De la Calzeda CS, Gomez-Pajuelo C, et al. Clinical and pathologic manifestations of pulmonary vascular disease in the toxic oil syndrome. J Am Coll Cardiol 1991; 18:1539–1545.
16. Tazelaar HD, Myers JL, Drage CW, et al. Pulmonary disease associated with L-tryptophan-induced eosinophilic myalgia syndrome: clinical and pathologic features. Chest 1990; 97:1032–1036.
17. Braman SS, Eby E, Kuhn C, Rounds S. Primary pulmonary hypertension in the elderly. Arch Intern Med 1991; 151:2433– 2438.

18. Rich S, Kaufmann E, Levy PS, et al. The effect of high doses of calcium-channel blockers on survival in primary pulmonary hypertension. N Engl J Med 1992; 327: 76–81.
19. Uren NG, Oakley CE. Primary pulmonary hypertension: the role of endothelial dysfunction and treatment implications. Clin Cardiol 1993; 19:59–66.
20. Barst RJ, Rubin LJ, McGoon MD, et al. Long-term continuous prostacyclin therapy improves survival in primary pulmonary hypertension. Ann Intern Med 1994; 121: 409–415.
21. Rubin LJ, Mendoza J, Hood M, et al. Treatment of primary pulmonary hypertension with continuous intravenous prostacyclin (epoprostenol): results of a randomized trial. Ann Intern Med 1990; 112:485–491.
21a. Barst RJ, Rubin LJ, Long WA, et al. A comparison of continuous intravenous epoprostend (prostacyclin) with conventional therapy for primary pulmonary hypertension. N Engl J Med 1996; 334:296–301.
22. Bjornsson J, Edwards WD. Primary pulmonary hypertension: a histopathologic study of 80 cases. Mayo Clin Proc 1985; 60:16–25.

14

Living with Primary Pulmonary Hypertension

CHARLES L. SELBY†

Germantown Hospital and Medical Center
Philadelphia, Pennsylvania

I did not enter middle-age gracefully.

By all indications as I went through my mid- and late-30s, I was very healthy. I had exercised regularly since childhood, even during the rigorous time-consuming years of medical school and residency. Basketball, bicycling, running, calisthenics, all were a part of my regimen—not in any all-consuming way (I didn't do triathlons or become a male anorectic), but in a three to four times a week program appropriate for maintaining cardiovascular fitness. I exercised because I liked it and felt invigorated after a workout. I always felt my baseline bradycardia was evidence of my level of fitness. I remember having a pulse of 55 in medical school, and in later years, as running became a mainstay of my exercise, it was between 45 and 50. I occasionally had pulses as low as 40, and wondered if there might be a pathological cause.

I had no medical problems, except labile systolic hypertension, which developed during my chief residency, and which appeared to be, at least initially, white-coat hypertension. For some reason, perhaps the flawed concept that I wound not really develop any medical illness until after I reached Medicare age, I

†Dr. Selby died October 28, 1995, following surgery for metastatic small bowel cancer.

simply got anxious when my blood pressure was checked, and I still do. After several years of intermittently checking, my blood pressure with initial readings 150–170 systolic (diastolics were generally running 70–80), and gradually decreasing over a few minutes to a more reasonable 130–140, the pattern began to change. By late 1988, the systolic would go up to 180–190, and only drop into the 150–160 range. The diastolic also began to run close to 90. It was obvious I was developing sustained systemic hypertension.

I placed myself under the care of a very capable nephrologist, and my blood pressure did well on monotherapy for a year or two, although the dose was increased on one or two occasions. However, over the course of several months, my diastolic pressures gradually began to skyrocket, up to 120 at times, with only mild stress. Combination therapy, up to three drugs, ultimately including minoxidil, did not seem to have any consistent effect. My pressures may have been normal one day, and then the next day very elevated. A workup for secondary causes of hypertension was negative. A 24-hour ambulatory blood pressure monitor was done during the summer of 1991 to see if my pressures were any different. But I knew the time at which my blood pressure would be checked (every 30 min) and would become anxious before each reading. Even during the night of the study, I slept poorly and was keyed up. Needless to say, my pressures averaged around 170/110, despite two drugs plus a diuretic.

It was at about this time that I began to develop my initial cardiac symptoms, albeit somewhat subtle. I noted while running up the steepest hill during my routine run that I was becoming somewhat more winded than usual. I didn't initially think that this was a cause for major concern. I had cut back somewhat on the frequency of running because of the birth of our first child several months earlier. I had attributed my symptoms to a drop off in conditioning plus the fact that I was turning 40. So this is what getting old is all about, I thought. I even felt older one day when a younger woman breezed past me running up the hill. I continued to run for several more months, with a gradual further decline in exercise tolerance. There was nothing precipitous. I had also noted a mild change in my resting pulse. For the first time in many years, it was consistently staying above 55, although still in the bradycardic range. Not a major change, but in retrospect, a significant harbinger. I also seemed to be fatiguing somewhat during my weekly 2-hour full-court basketball game. Again, the symptoms were subtle, but gradually progressive. I decided to get a chest x-ray to make sure I did not have cardiomegaly. The radiologist read it as normal.

By late 1991, however, rather precipitously, I could run only about one-third of a mile and then became so dyspneic that I had to stop. Previously, despite noticing a gradual decrease in my pace, I had been able to complete my 3.8-mile run. Finally, I realized something was wrong. This was not deconditioning and aging. My wife (an anesthesiologist) suggested that maybe I had exercise-induced asthma. I saw a pulmonologist. My blood pressure the night before that appointment was 110/80, yet the next day with some anxiety it was 160/120. He reviewed my recent chest x-ray films, thought the pulmonary arteries looked "plump," and felt maybe that was secondary to my systemic hypertension. I underwent pulmonary function studies with bronchodilators as well as a methacholine challenge test, both of which were unremarkable. I had a bicycle exercise test, and my heart rate increased significantly for the level of exercise, suggesting either significant deconditioning, or "cardiac disease." I didn't desaturate with exercise. I was told to see a cardiologist for further evaluation.

I next went to see the cardiologist. My ECG, which had been normal about a year earlier, was now read as consistent with left ventricular hypertrophy. My echocardiogram demonstrated septal hypertrophy consistent with left ventricular hypertrophy, and mildly elevated pulmonary pressures. A diagnosis of hypertensive hypertrophic cardiomyopathy was made. I was crushed. How could this have happened? I had had sustained hypertension for only about 3 years, had been compliant with my medications, and only in the last few months had I developed transient severe blood pressure elevation. The cardiologist felt my blood pressure had probably been poorly controlled for years, and the development of cardiac disease was not surprising. I didn't think my blood pressure had been bad enough for that long to cause symptomatic cardiac disease, but I wanted to be the "good patient," so I accepted the explanation. Besides, my knowledge of cardiac physiology was rusty after years of practicing clinical rheumatology.

The cardiologist reassured me that the process was potentially reversible with good blood pressure control. He readjusted my medications, and now I was taking four drugs (a β-blocker, an ACE-inhibitor, a calcium channel blocker, and a diuretic). I was instructed not to exercise until I had a standard treadmill stress test. Subsequently, I completed 13 minutes on the treadmill (somehow I was able to push myself to go that long) without any ECG changes or arrhythmias. The cardiologist reassured me that I had "done well" and that, although he was my contemporary, he probably could not last that long on the treadmill.

I was "cleared" for activity, as tolerated, but over the next few months whenever I tried to jog, I couldn't go more than two blocks. I could no longer play basketball because I became very short of breath after a couple of times up and down the court. Yet my blood pressure finally did improve on all the medication I was taking. It was 140/90 when checked by my physician, and was even lower at home. But, I was not improving clinically. In fact, I was getting worse, although at first I refused to admit it. I was starting to become symptomatic with normal activity—a flight of stairs or two, walking quickly on level ground, and so on. Again, the decline was gradual. Finally, an echocardiogram 4 months later documented further changes now consistent with clearcut right ventricular hypertrophy, moderate pulmonary pressures by Doppler, and a questionable "jet," suggesting a possible left-to-right shunt. The possibility of atrial septal defect was suggested. At this juncture, my condition clearly indicated the need for a cardiac catheterization.

My story became somewhat more complicated and frustrating because about this time, in May 1992, I suddenly developed blurred vision in my left eye. An ophthalmologist friend examined me and noted retinal hemorrhages. Although my blood pressure had appeared to be well-controlled over the prior few months, he informed me that the most common cause was hypertension. Perhaps I had had a transient surge in my blood pressure, causing the retinal hemorrhages. I became more depressed. I felt like I was a hypertensive time bomb. Hypertensive cardiomyopathy and now hypertensive retinopathy, all developing while on therapy with total compliance with medication. I sought a second opinion from a retinal specialist. Incomplete central retinal venous occlusion was his diagnosis. This was not secondary to hypertension, but he was not sure of the etiology. A workup, including a multitude of coagulation studies (some esoteric), was negative. What was going on, I thought? Am I falling apart? Why am I developing all of these problems?

I had always been a "lumper," rather than a splitter when it came to trying to make a diagnosis with multiple problems. Perhaps this is because in rheumatology there are often systemic problems with multisystem involvement. In any event, the blurred vision became more of a nuisance, and a side issue as my cardiovascular symptoms intensified.

As I readied for my cardiac catheterization, I felt somewhat helpless, but at least reassured that the definitive study would be done. But I am not sure I was prepared for the results. The catheterization demonstrated severe pulmonary hypertension, without evidence for any shunting. It had taken almost 1 year from the onset of symptoms until a diagnosis had been made. In the interim I had been seen by one nephrologist, one cardiologist, one pulmonologist, and two ophthalmologists.

I was crushed by the diagnosis, as was my wife. The depth of my immediate despair was unlike anything I had experienced before. I felt my days were numbered; my life was to be abruptly cut short. I felt cheated. I wouldn't see my young daughter grow up, I wouldn't grow old together with my wife, but mostly, it was despair. I cried more that first week than I had cried my entire adult life. I realized that a lifetime of subscribing to the societal custom of the male suppressing his emotions would not carry me through this crisis. As a physician, one must also bury one's emotional side to be able to effectively function amidst all the illness and death one is confronted with every day. This "coat of armor" begins being applied while in medical school, and with each succeeding year, additional coats are added, to the point that one is rarely shaken by a patient's illness or death. With the diagnosis of primary pulmonary hypertension, my emotional coat of armor dissolved immediately. The raw emotion that followed was painful.

As a practicing rheumatologist, I was familiar with pulmonary hypertension as a dreaded complication of connective tissue disease, particularly scleroderma and mixed connective tissue disease. I don't think I had ever had a patient with documented pulmonary hypertension, but could recall that 2-year survival in scleroderma was only 50% in patients with such complications. This was a condition not much better than cancer. I didn't recall any effective therapy, although I had read reports of the lack of effectiveness of nitrates, hydralazine, and other older vasodilatory agents in the early 1980s. I vaguely recollected that heart–lung transplant was a possible option.

My being a physician probably made it more difficult to be a patient. I understood immediately the gravity of the diagnosis, even if initially I was not aware of some of the newer treatment options. I had no false illusions about the power of medical science, no blind faith that somehow I would be saved. Advances would be made, but occurred slowly. I was very scared, and justifiably so. Support from family and friends was some consolation. But this would not make me better. I needed to find a center with a strong interest in my diagnosis to maximize my chances for survival. Through a network of professional friends, I ultimately found a physician with such an interest.

My new physician initially reassured me that perhaps all my problems were interrelated; that my labile systemic hypertension was probably a part of a generalized endothelial disorder of some sort that also caused my primary pulmonary hypertension. Also, central retinal venous occlusion had occasionally been seen in primary pulmonary hypertension, perhaps secondary to sludging induced by high right-sided pressures.

I underwent another cardiac catheterization. A pulmonary angiogram excluded the possibility of embolic disease as a cause. Then, a drug trial with the pulmonary vasodilating agent prostacyclin infused in gradually increasing doses documented some vasoreactivity of my pulmonary vessels. Although my pulmonary pressures didn't drop, my pulmonary vascular resistance did decrease, and my cardiac output increased. At least this was some positive news.

I was to be tried on an oral nifedipine regimen, one of the best oral pulmonary vasodilatory agents. Unfortunately, a trial with high-dose nifedipine (up to 210 mg/day) over 3 months proved to be a major therapeutic failure. I developed severe pedal edema, requiring large doses of diuretics just to put my shoes on in the morning. I seemed to be urinating all the time, I was continually thirsty, and developed a craving for salt-laden foods. I recall going through a jar of pickles in 1 day, and another time drinking a large can of tomato juice in one sitting.

Despite being intravascularly depleted of both salt and water (my BUN was running close to 40), I continued with significant pedal edema. To make matters worse, my dyspnea progressed. Minimal activity tired me out. It became an effort to climb stairs, a real problem in my older three-level Tudor home with long staircases.

Another right-sided heart catheterization confirmed what I had known clinically. I was getting worse. I was now in right ventricular failure, my pulmonary vascular resistance was higher, and my cardiac output was not good.

In the fall of 1992, 3 weeks after that cardiac catheterization, I had a Hickman catheter placed and began a prostacyclin infusion through an ambulatory infusion pump. Fortunately, there was gradual improvement in my dyspnea after starting the prostacyclin. After about 2 weeks, it became somewhat easier to climb steps and perform the usual activities of daily living. The chest heaviness that I had had became less pronounced. I diuresed most of the pedal edema as my nifedipine (Procardia) was tapered off. I began to feel halfway decent. My blurred vision also gradually improved over several months. I continued on the anticoagulant therapy that was begun about the time of my diagnosis.

I have now been receiving prostacyclin for about 1 year. I probably plateaued after 3–4 months. I'm better, but have nowhere near the exercise capacity I had at baseline. I still can't run, although I have started a walking regimen. I am able to walk about 3 miles at about a 13-minute mile pace with only mild dyspnea. I can no longer play basketball because of my lack of physical stamina, being on anticoagulant therapy, and my central line and ambulatory infusion pump. I have bicycled a little, and this may be one enjoyable activity I can further cultivate in the future. However, my area is somewhat hilly, and this could potentially make cycling less pleasurable.

Follow-up cardiac catheterization data at 3 and 9 months have confirmed some improvement. I am no longer in right-sided failure. Although there has been only minor reduction in my pulmonary pressures, my pulmonary vascular resistance has decreased by more than 50%, and my cardiac output is up significantly.

I have good and bad days in my symptoms. Sometimes I feel fine with light activity, other times I become fatigued and winded. I've learned to ignore the prostacyclin adverse reactions, which are more of a nuisance than anything else. I have hyperdefecation with frequent diarrhea, episodic flushing particularly of my trunk, and hypersensitivity of the tongue when I first start to eat.

I have tried to be philosophic about my condition, but at times I become depressed. It boils down to that glass of half-filled water. It's half-filled, I say, on my better days. I'm alive, still working full time, and am capable of doing the usual activities of daily living along with mild exercise. It's half-empty on my bad days. I can't run, bicycle long distances, or play basketball. I never truly feel great, but simply okay. And many times I become fatigued, or simply just feel "unwell."

Being attached 24-hours a day to an infusion pump (albeit ambulatory) is also an inconvenience. The medication must be changed every 8 hours and kept refrigerated until use. I need to plan my day in advance so I know where I'll be when I have to make a drug change. I need to know whether or not to carry my medication in a little bag with some ice. Life becomes less spontaneous on such a regimen.

The prostacyclin must be reconstituted nightly, and there is also daily catheter maintenance. These activities require 30–45 minutes daily. It doesn't seem like a lot of time, but at the end of a busy day, it can become burdensome, especially when it's done day-in/day-out. Fortunately, my wife shares in the drug preparation, and that makes it somewhat easier. But its still an imposition on our precious free time; so little do we seem to have now with a young child.

A chronic illness makes one aware of one's mortality very quickly. My future is uncertain. Perhaps I'll develop tolerance to the prostacyclin. My next option is a lung transplant, which I find to be a very scary proposition. I look upon the prostacyclin as a bridge to other therapy, perhaps prostacyclin by another route (transdermal), or perhaps another vasoreactive substance or antagonist that will more effectively lower my pulmonary pressure and vascular resistance. I've got to have faith in the medical system of which I am a part. What I have learned is that illness makes patients of us all.

AUTHOR INDEX

Italic numbers give the page on which the complete reference is listed.

A

D

G

M

N

O

P

Q

R

S

U

V

W

X

Y

Z

SUBJECT INDEX

A

B

R

S

T

V

W